MW00332377

Obesity

Obesity

Evaluation and Treatment Essentials

Edited by

G. Michael Steelman, MD, FASBP
American Society of Bariatric Physicians
The Steelman Clinic
Oklahoma City, Oklahoma, U.S.A

Eric C. Westman, MD, MHS
Lifestyle Medicine Clinic
Duke University Medical Center
Durham, North Carolina, U.S.A

informa
healthcare

New York London

First published in 2010 by Informa Healthcare, Telephone House, 69-77 Paul Street, London EC2A 4LQ, UK.

Simultaneously published in the USA by Informa Healthcare, 52 Vanderbilt Avenue, 7th floor, New York, NY 10017, USA.

Informa Healthcare is a trading division of Informa UK Ltd. Registered Office: 37–41 Mortimer Street, London W1T 3JH, UK. Registered in England and Wales number 1072954.

A CIP record for this book is available from the British Library.

Library of Congress Cataloging-in-Publication Data available on application.

ISBN-13: 9781420090024

Orders may be sent to: Informa Healthcare, Sheepen Place, Colchester, Essex CO3 3LP, UK
Telephone: +44 (0)20 7017 5540
Email: CSDhealthcarebooks@informa.com
Website: http://informahealthcarebooks.com/

For corporate sales please contact: CorporateBooksIHC@informa.com
For foreign rights please contact: RightsIHC@informa.com
For reprint permissions please contact: PermissionsIHC@informa.com

Typeset by Aptara, Delhi, India.

Foreword

Obesity: The word itself doesn't conjure up many positive emotions from people at- large or busy doctors. Perhaps, being fat was a good thing in the year AD 1000 when our ancestors were running around, and there were no supermarkets on the corners. Who survived when there was a famine and passed their gene pools down to us? Generally, it wasn't the skinny ones.

Significant corpulence was out of vogue by the 1860s, at the time of our Civil War. William Banting, a 5′ 5″, 202 lb, undertaker in merry old England tried nearly everything to lose weight without success. A hearing problem led him to see Dr. William Harvey, an ear, nose, and throat doctor of some renown. Dr. Harvey thought Banting's hearing problem might be related to his obesity and suggested a reduced carbohydrate diet (with still a few spirits allowed). Low-carbohydrate diets were used to treat diabetes in the pre-insulin era. Following this eating plan, Banting lost weight nicely and kept it off. He was so happy that he wrote and distributed a pamphlet about his success. This stirred up considerable discussion at the time, and, by the early 1900s, some people, instead of saying, "its time to diet" were saying, "its time to Bant."

No, I wasn't there then, but I do remember the "Great Depression" (what was so *great* about the depression of the 1930s?). Anyway, in the 1950s and 1970s curbing the intake of carbs was more in vogue than keeping the dietary fat down. Yudkin, in England, was a low-carbohydrate advocate and was published several times in this regard in the 1970s.

Then the "experts" came along, telling us to keep the fat down and load up on nonrefined carbohydrates, etc. Low and behold, we've continued getting fatter. They've been fattening Iowa hogs with a nonrefined carbohydrate, namely corn, for decades. The last I checked, they weren't using the fibrous veggies, like cabbage or zucchini.

So, it's nice to have a book like ***Obesity: Evaluation and Treatment Essentials*** that covers it all. It's written primarily by practicing Bariatricians, who make their living treating patients with obesity problems. There are also chapters written by academicians who have been doing research involving human obesity for quite some time, plus chapters by experts on exercise, behavior modification, and nutrition. All in all, you have an outstanding group of experts who bring it all together. This book is an excellent read for those of us who have been treating the obese for years and need to be brought up to date. It's especially beneficial for doctors who are getting into, or thinking about getting into, the field of Bariatric Medicine. In essence, this book is a must have for practicing Bariatricians.

Let me give you a short history regarding the appetite suppressants. Starting in 1969 I lead the American Society of Bariatric Physicians (ASBP) from 35 obesity-treating, dues paying physician members to approximately 450 by 1974. Currently, the ASBP has over 1000 members. In the late 1960s and early 1970s, the mothers of America were crying for the Feds to take the amphetamine appetite suppressants off the market, so their kids wouldn't be abusing them. I flew back to Washington, D.C., and spent time at the FDA presenting the ASBP's position that at least some of the appetite suppressants should remain available for the treatment of obesity.

Barrett Scoville, MD, a career FDA bureaucrat involved with the issue, said he had reviewed the studies submitted in the 1960s to get approval for the non-amphetamine appetite suppressants and that, over the 12-week study periods, those getting the appetite suppressants lost about a pound a week and those taking the placebos lost about one-half pound a week. To him that wasn't a significant difference. Therefore, he opined that all appetite suppressants should be taken off the market. I made the ASBP's position clear that we strongly opposed such action. Charles Edwards, MD, was another physician working at the FDA at the time. He had a little cooler head. After much discussion, the upshot was that the amphetamines moved up to schedule II (no appetite suppressant usage) and the other three, phentermine, diethypropion, and phendimetrazine, went into Schedule III or IV, with the "few week" limitation being put in the package insert material. So, we do have them and most of us Bariatricians use them "off label." I do, and I've had patients on them more or less continuously for 30 years. I saw a patient a few weeks ago who is still fighting the weight battle at age 69, and she was 27 years old when I first saw her. Certainly, this doesn't make me feel any younger. Obviously, she wouldn't be coming back to see me if she wasn't needing and getting ongoing help.

So, let's get back to the FDA and the BNDD (now DEA). I asked Barrett at the time to define what a "few weeks" meant. He said they weren't going to do that. I had my appetite suppressants, so, "be gone." Over the next several years, "few weeks" came to be interpreted as 12 weeks, which was the length of time most studies were done to get these drugs approved by the FDA in the 1960s.

I've had patients come in and say "I didn't think the medication was helping but, boy, when I didn't have it...." If the appetite suppressants continued working like they do the first few weeks, we wouldn't have much of an obesity problem—they don't, but even with long-term usage, they do help to keep the hunger levels down enough so that patients can make intelligent food choices. If they do, they won't be so hungry.

I've always said "You won't keep very many patients, if they're very hungry, very long." So, I welcome the way this book covers the appetite suppressants plus much, much more. Thank you, Michael Steelman, MD, FASBP, and Eric Westman, MD, MHS, as the editors for ***Obesity: Evaluation and Treatment Essentials***, and thanks to all chapter contributors for doing a fine job covering the other aspects of the obese state, its treatment, and what may be in store for Bariatricians and our patients in the not too distant future.

In short, I highly recommend ***Obesity: Evaluation and Treatment Essentials***. On winding down my history lesson, I'm reminded of the story of a seven-year-old boy in church who kept looking around and generally appeared bored. On the way out the pastor, who had noted the boy's behavior, shook his hand and asked if there was anything he could help him with. The seven-year-old asked "What are those plaques on the wall with the name and dates on them?" To which the pastor replied, "Son, those are our members who have died in the service." To this, the young lad asked, "In the 8 o'clock service or the 10 o'clock service?"

Thus, I wind down my commentary before the readers start asking, "... the 8 o'clock or the 10 o'clock?"

W. L. Asher
Littleton, Colorado, U.S.A.

Preface

It is clear that obesity is one of our nation's biggest health care challenges. It is associated with our most common causes of mortality and morbidity as well as with producing considerable psychosocial discomfort. The incidence of this killer disease has been steadily increasing and has reached epidemic proportions.

Most physicians receive little or no training in nutritional matters or the treatment of obesity. Perhaps because the treatment of obesity is less glamorous and more frustrating than the treatment of other conditions, too many physicians are unable or unwilling to deliver effective medical assistance to overweight patients struggling to manage their weight. Too often, this void is filled by commercial interests more focused on "the bottom line" rather than on the health of the consumer.

The treatment of obesity has been hindered by myths, misconceptions, and prejudices about its causes and consequences. The obese individual is not simply a lazy, metabolically normal adult with too much adipose tissue; rather, he or she is a metabolically complex individual who may respond differently to nutritional intake and exercise/activity.

The causes of obesity are complex and multifactorial. Its treatment, therefore, must be multimodal and tailored to meet the individual needs of the particular patient. This book will discuss the essential, clinical guidelines, and standards of each treatment option from dietary interventions to bariatric surgery, as well as the bariatrician's role in this treatment option.

Dietary intervention is the mainstay of bariatric treatment. In order to individualize treatment, the physician needs to be familiar with various approaches, including low calorie diets, low-carbohydrate diets, and very low-carbohydrate diets (VLCD). It is our hope that nutritionists and dieticians will benefit from the detail and level of discussion of these dietary interventions in addition to the bariatric physician.

Exercise is an important part of weight loss efforts and is probably essential for long-term weight maintenance. It provides numerous benefits in addition to its effect on weight. While patients are willing to follow almost any diet plan, it is often difficult to get them to initiate and sustain a meaningful exercise regimen.

Weight loss and maintenance require that individuals make changes in the way they interact with their environment. In this effort, they battle with a culture that, on one hand, values being fit and trim and, on the other, promotes obesogenic food patterns and sedentary lifestyles. To succeed, the overweight individual must be armed with effective strategies to deal with internal and external forces that favor the overweight state.

Various pharmaceutical agents have been used to help facilitate weight loss. Anorectic agents have been in use for over four decades and have been shown to be both safe and effective. Newer agents that inhibit the absorption of fat or carbohydrate are also available. Various other pharmaceuticals and some natural substances may also play a role in helping with the process of weight management. On the other hand, there are many common medications that promote weight gain, and replacing these with ones that are similarly effective but less likely to impact weight negatively can often bring rewarding results.

We must also consider, when treating the bariatric patient, that children represent a special population with special needs. The increasing incidence of obesity (and attendant type II diabetes) in this population is alarming. Clearly, something must be done to stem this tide or, as has been suggested, today's generation of children will be the first generation of Americans with a life expectancy less than that of their parents. The chapter on Childhood Obesity clearly identifies the special needs of children and outlines approaches for managing the obese child.

For some individuals, obesity and its comorbidities advance to such a degree that their life is at considerable risk. For them, bariatric surgery may be warranted. It is essential that they be properly evaluated before surgery, skillfully treated during surgery, and followed appropriately afterwards. The bariatric physician plays an important role in treating the patient perioperatively if bariatric surgery is a determined method of treatment for a particular patient.

Those of us who have developed a special interest and specialize in the field of bariatric medicine find great satisfaction in the work we do and the role we play in helping our patients live healthier, happier, and longer lives. We are excited about the potential for better understanding of this complex and fascinating disease and for the development of better weapons to use in its treatment.

To our colleagues engaged in academic and clinical research, we offer our sincere appreciation for your efforts and eagerly await the fruits of your labor.

To our colleagues engaged in clinical practice who are awakening to this field and want to improve their skills and expertise in the medical management of obese patients, we extend our heartfelt encouragement and support.

G. Michael Steelman, MD, FASBP
Eric C. Westman, MD, MHS

Contents

Contributors

James L. Bland Family Health Care, Aiken, South Carolina, U.S.A

Erin Chamberlin-Snyder American Weight Loss Center, Indianapolis, Indiana, U.S.A.

John B. Cleek Carolinas Weight Management & Wellness Center, Charlotte, North Carolina, U.S.A.

James T. Cooper Private Practice, Marietta, Georgia, U.S.A.

Howard J. Eisenson Duke University Diet & Fitness Center, Duke University Health System, Durham, North Carolina, U.S.A.

Frank L. Greenway Pennington Biomedical Research Center, Louisiana State University System, Baton Rouge, Louisiana, U.S.A.

Ed J. Hendricks Center for Weight Management, Roseville, California, U.S.A.

Deborah Bade Horn Private Practice, Houston, Texas, U.S.A.

Jeffrey D. Lawrence Lake Otis Medical Clinic, Anchorage, Alaska, U.S.A.

Larry A. Richardson Doctor's Weight Control Center, Spring, Texas, U.S.A.

Scott Rigden Private Practice, Chandler, Arizona, U.S.A.

Harold C. Seim Weight Management, Stillwater, and University of Minnesota, Minneapolis, Minnesota, U.S.A.

Steven R. Smith Molecular Endocrinology Laboratory, Pennington Biomedical Research Center, Louisiana State University System, Baton Rouge, Louisiana, U.S.A.

G. Michael Steelman American Society of Bariatric Physicians, The Steelman Clinic, Oklahoma City, Oklahoma, U.S.A.

Mary C. Vernon Private Practice, Lawrence, Kansas, U.S.A.

Eric C. Westman Lifestyle Medicine Clinic, Duke University Medical Center, Durham, North Carolina, U.S.A.

James A. Wortman First Nations and Inuit Health Branch, Health Canada, Vancouver, British Columbia, Canada

1 Obesity: the scope of a growing problem

Harold C. Seim

It is common knowledge that obesity has reached epidemic proportions in the United States and in the rest of the world. We come across obese people in every walk of life and hear about them on the nightly news on TV as well as read about them in the newspaper.

Dr. C. Everett Koop, former Surgeon General of the United States (1982–1989), said "Except for smoking, obesity is now the number one preventable cause of death in this country." Casket makers are now making larger caskets. So what has caused this epidemic and what remedial action is taken to prevent it?

CAUSE

in 1965, a study was conducted with 12,000 Japanese men 45 to 69 years old, living in Japan, Hawaii, and California. The mean body mass index (BMI) for Japanese men living in Hawaii and California were similar, but it was substantially lower for those living in Japan. Although total calorie intake was not greatly different between Japan and Hawaii, the percentage intake of fat was two times greater in Hawaii compared with Japan. This put these immigrants at risk for increases in body weight and subsequent cardiovascular risk. Because of this and other studies like it, there has been a concerted public health effort to curtail fat in the diet. Unfortunately, the low fat diet has been a major contributor to the fattening of America. When fat is removed from a food product, sugar or another carbohydrate is added in its place. Many people, especially those who are insulin resistant, are unable to process sugar and other easily digested carbohydrates for energy. Insulin is released when sugar is eaten and it helps convert sugar into triglyceride that is stored in the fat cells. Also, when insulin is present, we become hungry and eat more carbohydrates and put more fat on our bodies. Insulin is also a very atherogenic hormone that causes inflammation in the cells of the body, which may lead to cardiovascular disease, diabetes, and kidney disease (1).

As our society has become more urban and more affluent, diets high in complex carbohydrates have decreased, and now we eat a higher proportion of saturated fats and sugars. Also, there has been a shift to less physical work and less activity in our leisure time. Americans eat large amounts of food at meals. Plates are larger than they were 50 years ago and Americans tend to fill them. We see this especially when eating out.

Fast foods have been a large contributor to this epidemic, and supersizing makes the situation worse. Fast foods are high in carbohydrate calories and high in saturated fats. Calories do count, and for persons who are insulin resistant, carbohydrate calories are a worse choice. For example, drinking one soda a day for a year (150 cal) will add 15 extra pounds.

RESULTS

Children in America

Our children have become obese as they have been immersed in high calorie, high carbohydrate eating patterns, and are now developing type 2 diabetes—a disease that was formerly seen only in obese adults (2).

World Health Organization (WHO) statistics on children estimate that approximately 22 million children younger than 5 years old are overweight. In the United States, the percentage of overweight children (5–14 yr) has gone from 15% to 32% over the last 30 years (3).

National Health and Nutrition Examination Surveys (NHANES) are conducted periodically by the National Center for Health Statistics using measured heights and weights. Tables 1 and 2 below show the progress of obesity over the years of children and adolescents and of adults (4,5).

Must et al. in JAMA, October 1999 noted serious health problems in children associated with excess weight: high blood pressure 3 times more prevalent, type 2 diabetes 13–18 times

Table 1 Prevalence of Overweight Among Children and Adolescents (Percentage)

Age	NHES I	NHANES I	NHANES II	NHANES III	NHANES		
	1963–1970	1971–1974	1976–1980	1988–1994	1999–2000	2001–2002	2003–2004
2–5		5	5	7.2	10.3	10.6	13.9
6–11	4.2	4	6.5	11.3	15.1	16.3	18.8
12–19	4.6	6.1	5	10.5	14.8	16.7	17.4

Source: Ref. 2 from Table 4 and Ref. 5 from Table 2.

more common among the heaviest individuals, gall bladder disease 21 times more common, heart disease 3 to 5 times more prevalent, and osteoarthritis 30 times more common (3).

Adults in America

A study conducted by the Centers for Disease Control (CDC) found that from 1971 to 2000 obesity in the United States increased from 14.5% to 30.9%. During that period, there was a calorie increase for women of 335 calories per day (1542–1877) and for men the increase was 168 calories per day (2450–2618). This increase was mainly due to an increase in carbohydrate consumption rather than fat consumption (6).

Worldwide

Obesity is a problem not just in the United States but also is increasing at an alarming rate throughout the world.

WHO estimates that there are 1.6 billion *overweight* people in the world, which ironically is about the same number of people who go to bed hungry each night.

It is estimated that there are more than 400 million *obese* people worldwide (www.who.int). It is becoming an increasing problem in many developing countries. Studies have found that the prevalence of obesity varies from less than 5% in rural China, Japan, and some African countries to as high as 75% in urban Samoa. In the United States, where 65% are overweight, there are also large differences in obesity between people of different ethnic origins.

PREVENTION: SO WHAT IS BEING DONE ABOUT THIS EPIDEMIC?

Several government agencies have weight loss campaigns designed for use in schools.

There is a move in schools to have less soda, and more water and milk in vending machines. Fast food concessions are disappearing from schools, and less high carbohydrate, government surplus foods are being served. Most magazines at the grocery store checkouts have articles about losing weight to raise awareness about the problem.

Exercise is being promoted in schools and by local gyms. Some parents have started to limit the time their children spend on computers, internet games, and TV. People are walking more often than in the past.

The following are the American Medical Association Expert Committee Recommendations for childhood obesity (paraphrased):

- Address the issue of weight once yearly at the child's clinical visit. Assess dietary habits, especially the consumption of sweetened beverages, physical activity habits, readiness to change lifestyle habits, and family history of obesity and related illnesses.

Table 2 Age-Adjusted Prevalence of Overweight and Obesity Among U.S. Adults Aged 20 to 74 (Percentage)

	NHANES I	NHANES II	NHANES III	NHANES		
	1971–1974	1976–1980	1988–1994	1999–2000	2001–2002	2003–04
Overweight or obese (BMI 25+)	55.9	64.5	65.7	64.5	65.7	66.3
Obese (BMI 30+)	14.5	15.0	23.3	30.5	30.6	32.2

Source: From Ref. 4, Table 1 and Ref. 5, Table 4.

- Limit sweet drinks and fast food, eat breakfast and have family meals most days of the week. Limit screen time and engage in physical activity for 60 minutes daily.
- For children in the 85th to 94th percentile with comorbidities, do a lipid profile, liver profile, and blood glucose. Add kidney function tests for those above the 95% percentile (7).

WHO has suggested the following actions to help prevent obesity:

- Creating supportive population-based environments through public policies that promote low-fat, high fiber foods, and provide opportunities for physical activity.
- Promoting weight loss by eating more fruit and vegetables, nuts, and whole grains.
- Cutting the amount of fatty, sugary foods in the diet; moving from animal-based fats to unsaturated vegetable oil-based fats; engaging in physical activity for 30 minutes daily.
- Establishing clinical programs to aid losing weight and avoiding further weight gain. (www.who.int)

SOCIAL IMPLICATIONS

Obesity is the only remaining issue in our society in which discrimination seems to be acceptable. Obese persons have been thought of as being gluttonous and slothful. People say, "Why don't they take care of themselves?" There is discrimination in the work place.

In Japan, a national law mandates that a waist circumference of 33.5 in. for men and 35.4 in. for women is where health risks begin. Those exceeding the limits will get dieting help if they do not lose weight by themselves after three months. Further education will be given after six months if they have not met the goal.

A survey in the United States found that the average waist size of men was 39 in., just under the 40 in. threshold of the International Diabetes Federation. Women were 36.5 in. approximately 2 in. above the threshold of 34.6 in.

COST OF OBESITY

Cost to Society

The annual U.S. obesity-attributable medical expenditures were estimated at $75 billion in 2003 dollars, and about one-half of these expenditures are financed by Medicare and Medicaid. If all obesity-attributable medical expenditures were financed by federal taxes, it would cost approximately $350 per adult to cover the cost. This figure would be reduced by one-half if limited to expenditures financed by Medicare and Medicaid (8).

Costs to Insurance Companies

The Milliman Research Report in 2004 by Fitch et al., presented findings from examination of a large 2001 database from a single plan employer/employee group coverage (9):

- Per-person claim costs for obese persons were triple those for the average member
- Hospital admission rate for obese was 350 per 1000 contrasted to 50 per 1000 for an average population
- Cesarean section rate was 50% of deliveries of obese mothers, more than double that of a typical insured population.

Employers bear most of the costs associated with treating obesity-related conditions, primarily in terms of lost productivity and paid sick leave and the increased cost of health, life, and disability insurance. Obese employees are twice as likely to have high-level absenteeism (seven or more absences in six months) and one and one-half times more likely to have moderate absenteeism (six absences in six months) (10).

Thus, there are many prevention programs in place but how do we help the 65% of Americans who are obese? That is the subject of this book that is written by experienced bariatricians, physicians who are devoted to, and specialize in, the treatment of individuals with obesity.

REFERENCES

1. Curb JD, Marcus EB. Body fat and obesity in Japanese Americans. Am J Clin Nutr 1991; 53:1552S–1555S.
2. Ogden CL, Flegal KM, Carroll MD, et al. Prevalence and trends in overweight among US children and adolescents, 1999–2000. JAMA 2002; 288:1728–1732.
3. Must A, Spadano J, Coakley E, et al. The disease burden associated with overweight and obesity. JAMA 1999; 282:1523–1529.
4. Flegal KM, Carroll MD, Ogden CL, et al. Prevalence and trends in obesity among US adults, 1999–2000. JAMA 2002; 288:1723–1727.
5. Ogden CL, Carroll MD, Curtin LR, et al. Prevalence of overweight and obesity in the United States, 1999–2004. JAMA 2006; 295:1549–1555.
6. Centers for Disease Control and Prevention (CDC). Trends in intake of energy and macronutrients, United States, 1971–2000. MMWR Morb Mortal Wkly Rep 2004; 53(4):80–82.
7. Rao G. Childhood obesity: highlights of AMA expert committee recommendations. Am Fam Physician 2008; 78(1):56–63.
8. Finkelstein EA, Fiebelkorn IC, Wang G. State-level estimates of annual medical expenditures attributable to obesity. Obes Res 2004; 12(1):18–24.
9. Fitch K, Pyenson B, Abbs S, et al. Obesity: A big problem getting bigger. Milliman Research Report, 2004; New York.
10. Tucker LA, Friedman GM. Obesity and absenteeism: An epidemiologic study of 10,825 employed adults. Am J Health Promot 1998; 12(3):202–207.

2 Etiologies of obesity

Larry A. Richardson

INTRODUCTION

As has been said many times in various fields and disciplines, "The more we know, the more we know that we don't know." This is quite true when exploring the etiologies of overweight and obesity. Just like a trip to the moon, the concept can seem outwardly simple—rocket, command capsule, astronauts, space suits, lunar landing module, and re-entry vehicle. Yet, each one of these concepts, and the thousands more that tie them all together, can take years of study, design, and training to understand the complexity of the various components. Such is our threshold in the field of obesity, wherein we once were instructed that the fat cell (adipocyte) was just a simple storage vessel for excess fat, nothing more and nothing less. We were also told that fat kept us warm and helped protect our organs. This was an infantile conceptualization of the greater truth.

By similar inference, many researchers and health personnel were taught that overweight and obesity were simply due to an energy imbalance: too much eating (excess calories in) and too little exercise (not enough calories burned) (1). It therefore seemed logical for physicians to view obesity as a lack of willpower (slothfulness) and all too often dispense the admonition, "Just push yourself away from the table and join a gym"—advice that persists until this day.

The etiologies of obesity described in this chapter can be considered, on a basal level, to serve as a foundation for additional knowledge and understanding, not as a simple or complete answer to the complexities. If lean body mass remains stable and energy output is less than energy intake, body fat will increase. It would be quite simple if the explanation stopped here, but it does not. What we will examine later in this chapter are the multifaceted keys to susceptibility to obesity that are strongly influenced by genetic, environmental, and other factors. Family and twin studies show that genetics determine a moderate portion of weight variation, but the almost exponential increase in U.S. obesity prevalence over the past several decades cannot be blamed on sudden genetic changes (2).

It is estimated that about 133.6 million U.S. adults are either overweight or obese, with approximately 72.3% of men and 64.1% of women ($\geq$20 years) meeting these criteria (3). Obesity prevalence in U.S. children has risen markedly between the National Health and Nutrition Examination Survey (NHANES) II and III. Currently, it is estimated that 20% to 25% of them are either overweight or obese, with the prevalence being even higher in some minority groups, including African-Americans, Mexican-Americans, and Pima Indians. Even as we thought childhood obesity in the U.S. was stabilizing (4), the latest data shows that the rate of childhood obesity continues to rise (5).

Conservative estimates imply that more than 250 million people worldwide are obese. Unfortunately, double or triple this amount are probably overweight (1). While these current numbers are staggering, the fact that they are continuing to rise mandates that we better understand the various factors influencing adiposity and devise new and innovative medical alternatives and social strategies to stem this true, worldwide pandemic.

Trying to detail the many aspects of the etiologies of obesity is much like trying to describe a major superhighway, with its many entrances and off-ramps, as well as all the things that are associated with it during its course—heat, cold, rain, snow, traffic conditions, and so on. Suffice it to say that the journey we will embark upon has at least three major thoroughfares: (*i*) Global & Community Influences, (*ii*) Personal Characteristics, and (*iii*) Behavioral factors. Each thoroughfare is comprised of many smaller segments, which will also be briefly described. Even though the routes vary, they can all lead to the final destination of *Adipose City* (adiposity).

Major Highway: Global & Community Influences

As we look at the first major highway heading toward corpulence, **Global & Community Influences**, we need to identify several of the "mile markers" (kilometer posts for the metric minded) that are seen along this part of the journey. These could be labeled: (a) food environment,

(b) socioeconomic status, (c) family structure variations, (d) community dynamics, (e) health care, and (f) nontraditional factors. A readily apparent fact is that food and societal environments have a large influence in promoting what is termed an "obesogenic environment"—one which promotes both overindulgence in caloric intake and diminished activity during daily living. They have a major impact on influencing food acquisition, eating, and lifestyle habits.

Food environment is not an isolated marker but just a flag to direct attention to some of its supportive and surrounding components. Globalization and urbanization around the world has led to marked economic and social changes, which, in turn, influence environmental and behavioral changes, which can lead to obesity. Technical advances in both food production and transportation, coupled with the global marketing of modern commerce, have led to the introduction of relatively cheap, energy-dense foods into the domestic food markets of many developing countries. One does not have to strain to see the expansion of fast food franchises on a global scale. Couple this availability with reduced expenditure of energy, and we witness worldwide weight gain that seems to be escalating.

One of the most controversial areas of obesity research deals with the role of diet composition upon body weight. There is evidence to suggest that obesity is more likely to occur and be maintained in the presence of a high-fat, rather than a low-fat, diet. From the late 1970s to the early 1990s, the percentage of dietary fat decreased in the United States, although the actual grams per day of fat did not decline. Rather, there was an actual increase in the total energy intake due to addition of more refined carbohydrates to the diet.

Even the amount of essential omega-3 fatty acids in the diet has been linked with weight status and abdominal obesity. Higher plasma levels of total n-3 PUFA (polyunsaturated fatty acids) are associated with a healthier BMI, waist circumference and hip circumference (6).

Besides fat intake, there seems to be a trend toward increased intake of processed and prepared foods. Such foods tend to have higher energy content, fats, and carbohydrates (including simple sugars), as well as being served in oversized portions that are highly appetizing. It is of note that highly palatable high-fat and sucrose diets blunt the signals of the satiety neuropeptides (supposed to decrease appetite), insulin, and cholecystokinin (CCK). As if this were not enough to promote overeating, such palatable food also activates a brain reward system that reinforces the eating behavior.

The average U.S. caloric intake has increased 200 kcal/day over the past 20 years. This includes the increased consumption of sweetened beverages by young adults to constitute almost 25% of their daily calories. A recent study found high fructose corn syrup (a common sweetener) to be the most adipogenic of all dietary carbohydrates (7). The consumption of energy-dense foods and beverages typically results in greater energy intake because many adults respond to the volume of food consumed rather than to the energy content of the food itself. Remember that high-fat foods can be low volume (e.g., salad dressings, sauces, cooking oils, gravy) but energy dense.

There are many factors leading to an increase in the consumption of energy-dense foods and dietary fats. The commercial food environment influences these through numerous small changes, including the following:

- Increased, inexpensive, energy-dense foods: soft drinks, cheese, fat/sugary foods
  - Processed food up-regulates hunger and blunts satiety signals
- Numerous convenient eating sites promoting non–home-cooked meals
  - Neighborhood fast food restaurants
  - Delivery options (pizza)
  - Convenience marts/gas stations
  - Sports venues (snack bars)
  - Movie theaters, playhouses, symphonic halls
  - Snack and soda machines (airports, hotels, schools, offices)
- High variety of foods at mealtime
  - Especially high-energy content but low-nutrient density
  - Increased fatness and food intake seen with more choices of entrees, sweets, snacks, and other refined carbohydrates
  - Increased variety of vegetables is NOT associated with increasing fatness or energy intake

- Unreasonably large portion sizes
    - Seen in affluent societies: Omnipresent food and larger portion sizes translate into greater intake of food and beverages
    - Overconsumption of palatable food leads to shift in set point (energy balance/body weight) similar to adaptation in drug addiction

Another major marker along this highway to adiposity is *socioeconomic status*. The prevalence of obesity in most developed countries, including the United States, seems to be negatively correlated with socioeconomic class. A postulate is that financial growth and industrialization lead to a shift in daily routine activity patterns. Many blue- and white-collar occupations no longer involve much physical activity. There are also differences in the mix of external and social networking resources available to those at various levels of socioeconomic status and educational experience. Those differences may influence the trend and shape parenting, also.

It should be noted that a positive correlation between status, education, and excess weight is seen in undeveloped areas, including parts of South America, Malaysia, China, and sub-Saharan Africa. It may be that wealthier, more educated people in these countries can afford more of the processed and refined items, as well as have larger portion sizes and variety of foods (see the previous text).

The next road flag we see is *family structure variations*. This heading includes the subsets of cultural influences and parenting behaviors. A discussion of environmental causes for obesity could not occur without the consideration of cultural factors, most of which impact through attitudes, beliefs, and behaviors. Some of the culturally defined contributors to body size and shape which are conveyed from parents to their children include the following:

- Types and amounts of food and beverages
- Textures, flavors, and food combinations
- Traditional uses and symbolic meanings of food
- Foods used to create social interactions as well as for pleasure and punishment
- Conceptualization of which foods are healthful, harmful, or protective
- Dietary celebration of various holidays
    - Behavioral holiday changes contribute to winter seasonal weight gain
    - Can contribute up to one-half of individual's annual weight gain
- Media influence
    - Influences all cultures to promote enhanced food intake
    - Enhances "addiction" to excessive fat and sugar intake

Even some governmental policies take on a cultural tone when dealing with certain ethnic groups. Subtle societal influences on energy intake and expenditure can foster the development of obesity. One such example involves the Pima Indians in Arizona. Because of U.S. imposed dietary modifications and altered manual labor and hunting activity resulting from reservation life, they have developed tremendous rates of diabetes and obesity.

Parenting is, indeed, a subset of family structure variations and includes feeding practices and monitoring activity. Behaviors associated with parenting are a culmination of the family's food and physical environments, family resources (structure, parental education, and income), and beliefs and norms reinforced through kin and nonkin groups. Even after correcting for genetic influence, parental beliefs, attitudes, and practices correlate with children's weight (8).

Before birth, eating patterns of the mother can impact one of the associated causes of obesity development—that of prenatal exposure to over- or undernutrition. This marker, taken along with rapid growth in early infancy, early adiposity rebound in childhood, and early pubertal development can alert one to increased risk of obesity development in later life [see road marker regarding *health care*].

Feeding practice during infancy, particularly breastfeeding and its longer duration (greater than three months), promotes a lower risk of being overweight during childhood and adolescence. Support for breastfeeding in the work environment and in kin/nonkin networks of new mothers is to be encouraged. As a side note, the initial taste preferences of infants are for sweet-tasting foods, with a tendency to reject foods that are bitter, such as vegetables.

During childhood and adolescence, dietary predictors of increased adiposity include increased energy intake and greater percentages of energy supplied by fat and refined carbohydrates. Preferences and selections of foods, along with regulation of energy intake, are affected by parental feeding practices, including the foods made available to them, portion sizes, frequency of eating occasions, and the social context in which eating occurs. When children self-select their own food portion size, their consumption is usually reduced.

The Feeding Infants and Toddlers study (FITS) further implicates feeding practices and patterns of food intake that seem to fuel the obesity epidemic in children. French fries are the most commonly consumed vegetable among toddlers. Current child-feeding practices seem to be creating diets that promote excessive weight gain during the first years of life.

Patterns of eating are an integral part of feeding practices within families. Some healthy models include regular, "sit down" meals by the family versus haphazard, "grab-on-the run" eating, snacking, or grazing. While some longitudinal studies are neutral on the topic, others show significant correlation between snacking and body weight increase. It seems to be important that healthy snacks be readily available to children.

Monitoring of activity is another integral subset of parenting. This includes computer usage, video gaming, television watching, and the encouragement of physical activity (biking, swimming, sports, etc.). The amount of television watched seems to have some correlation with overweight. Children and adolescents spend up to four hours per day watching television or related media. Some of this time displaces physical activity time and encourages increased snacking due to advertising of such items. Parents need to be role models for healthy eating and activity, as this decidedly has more impact upon their children than empty words or imposed rules. Even such things as insuring adequate sleep for their children and themselves impacts weight within the entire family. Sleep duration has been identified recently as a risk factor for adolescent and child overweight. The theorized pathway involves changes in ghrelin and leptin levels associated with shorter periods of sleep (9).

Looking forward, we see that another of our significant highway markers is *community dynamics*. The term "built environment" has been coined to try to summarize the living and working conditions which are key determinants of both restrictions and opportunities for food consumption and for physical activity that are collectively created by societies. In order to reverse currently unhealthy trends in these areas, major changes in urban planning, transportation, public safety, and food production and marketing need to occur. As an example of this phenomenon, it is estimated that between 1982 and 1992, energy expenditure in the workplace declined approximately 50 kcal/day. Considering the additional changes that have taken place in that milieu since 1992, most studies indicate that an even greater reduction of employment-related physical activity has occurred (2).

Other factors relating to the dynamics of the community and how it interplays with eating behavior and physical activity within that community include the following:

- Population density—urban living is associated with lower energy demands than rural life
- Street connectivity—impedes or facilitates access to travel and acquisition of food
  - Poor connectivity encourages more vehicle usage versus walking or biking
- Access to fast-food restaurants, supermarkets, or nutritious food sources
- Access to parks and recreational facilities—importance of walking paths and sidewalks
- Public transportation systems
  - Centers for Disease Control and Prevention data: Children walked/biked to school 42% in 1969; only 16% in 2001
  - Adults and children rarely need to be physically active for transportation
    - Subways, cars, buses—automatic transmissions reduce even driving activity
- Schools
  - As the child's experience moves beyond the family into school and peer environments, these new settings assume greater influence over diet and activity patterns.
  - Features of schools believed related to childhood and adolescent obesity risk include
    - nutritional content of foods made available in schools, including cafeterias and vending machines offering sodas and snacks;

- availability of (and requirements for) regular physical education classes and involvement in organized sports; and
- patterns of transportation to and from school.

Yet another major road marker along our highway to adiposity is *health care*. Studies show the importance of good nutritional counseling and monitoring during all trimesters of pregnancy in regard to risk factors (and outcomes) for both obesity and diabetes, among other concerns. The prenatal period is extremely important in setting the stage for later weight.

Reduced, increased, or imbalanced growth during gestation and early postnatal life due to abnormal perinatal environments (e.g., malnutrition, maternal diabetes) can result in the permanent programming of physiological systems that will predispose individuals to develop obesity and diabetes. Inadequate nutrition in the first two trimesters actually increases the risk of obesity. Undernutrition in the last trimester of pregnancy, and in the early postnatal period, results in a decreased risk of adult obesity but increases the risk of hypertension, abnormal glucose tolerance, and adult cardiovascular disease.

One possible mechanism whereby these prenatal nutritional environments affect undesirable changes in long-term energy balance involves changes in leptin secretion that, in turn, result in central defects in neural systems controlling behavior and autonomic regulation. Other postulated pathways include influence on insulin metabolism and formation of hypothalamic pathways regulating feeding and metabolism (10).

The effects of prenatal development on subsequent obesity risk are clearest with respect to accelerated fetal growth (macrosomia), which is associated with an increased risk for obesity. It is most often related to maternal hyperglycemia or diabetes (11). This intrauterine exposure to the diabetic environment results in an increased risk of both diabetes mellitus and obesity in the offspring.

A specific subset of prenatal markers which have had a great deal of study has been malnutrition during the first and second trimesters. Undernutrition limited to the first two trimesters of pregnancy is associated with an increased probability of adult obesity. Other early "environmental" effects that were previously mentioned were that infants of diabetic mothers tend to be fatter than those of nondiabetic mothers, and children of diabetic mothers have a greater prevalence of obesity when they are 5 to 19 years of age, independent of their mother's obesity status (2).

One major "on-ramp" at this causative road marker is how these prenatal nutritional factors affect development of the central nervous system (CNS). A number of epidemiologic studies have highlighted the role of fetal nutrition in the development of the CNS early in life. Developmental abnormalities rooted in abnormal in-utero conditions provide evidence that environmental factors related to inadequate nutrition affect brain development in ways that will predispose to obesity. The first clearly defined example of this abnormality came from studies of effects of long-term starvation on the development of fetuses in pregnant women during the Dutch famine in the winter of 1944 to 1945. Some of the findings from these studies were as follows:

- High prevalence of obesity and comorbidities (e.g., diabetes mellitus) later in life.
    - Hypothesized mechanism was that altered fetal brain development shifted fetal CNS regulation of energy homeostasis toward favoring enhanced energy storage to compensate for deficient nutrition.
    - Additional theories assigned changes in hypothalamic circuitry toward supporting positive energy balance through increased food consumption during times of improved nutrition, leading to obesity and its comorbidities.
- Malnourished first- and second-trimester infants with low birth weights compensated with enhanced growth in childhood and were predisposed to adult obesity and type 2 diabetes. It is of note that rapid growth in infancy and childhood in these individuals had a particularly strong association with adult obesity (12).

One of the principles of the Hippocratic Oath is "first, 'do no harm.'" However, in an attempt to treat other issues, health care providers often use treatments and pharmacological agents that can contribute to obesity—the so-called "iatrogenic" or secondary factors. Many of

Table 1 Drugs That May Promote Weight Gain

Psychiatric–neurologic medications
Antipsychotics: olanzapine, clozapine, risperidone, quetiapine, and aripiprazole
Antidepressants
Tricyclics: imipramine and amitriptyline
Triazolopyridines: trazodone
Serotonin reuptake inhibitors: paroxetine, fluoxetine, and citalopram
Tetracyclics: mirtazapine
Monoamine oxidase inhibitors
Antiepileptic drugs: gabapentin (higher does), valproic acid, carbamazepine, and divalproex
Mood stabilizers: lithium, carbamazepine, lamotrigine, and gabapentin (higher does)
Steroid hormones
Progestational steroids
Corticosteroids
Hormonal contraceptives
Antidiabetes agents
Insulin (most forms)
Sulfonylureas
Thiazolidinediones
Antihistamines—commonly reported with older agents; also oxatomide, loratadine, and azelastine
Antihypertensive agents
α- and β-Adrenergic receptor blockers
Calcium-channel blockers: nisoldipine
Highly active antiretroviral therapy

the neurological, mood stabilizing, hormonal, and steroidal drugs promote appreciable weight gain; for examples, see Table 1 (2).

The last road marker we will examine under this "environmental influence" stretch of our highway is what can be termed *nontraditional factors*. They include such things as

- Ambient temperature variability reduction
  - Thermoneutral zone is the range of ambient temperature in which energy expenditure is not required for homeothermy. More Americans are living in such a zone during the past several decades.
  - Exposure to temperatures above or below the thermoneutral zone increases energy expenditure, which all other things being equal, decreases energy stores (i.e., fat).
- Reduced sleep time (also see Hypothalamus section later in this chapter)
  - Decreases leptin, thyroid-stimulating hormone, and glucose tolerance
  - Increases ghrelin
- Endocrine disruptors
  - Lipophilic, environmentally stable, industrially produced substances that can affect endocrine function
    - Examples—dichlorodiphenyltrichloroethane, some polychlorinated biphenyls (PCBs), and some alkylphenols
  - Some endocrine disruptors are antiandrogens
- Decreased smoking
  - Nicotine has both thermogenic and appetite-suppressant effects
  - Centers for Disease Control and Prevention estimates that, for 1978 to 1990, smoking cessation is responsible for about one-quarter of the increase in prevalence of overweight in men and about one-sixth of the increase in women
- Increasing gravida age
  - Mean age at first birth increased 2.6 years among U.S. mothers since 1970
  - One study of girls aged 9 to 10 years found that odds of obesity increased 14.4% for every 5-year increment in maternal age (13).

Major Highway: Personal Characteristics

While we could continue along this first thoroughfare for more in-depth discovery, it is time to merge onto the second major highway leading to *Adipose City*. This multilane road is called **Personal Characteristics** and is laid down upon bedrock of DNA. Just as many factors (heat, cold, water, frequency and tonnage of traffic utilizing road) affect the integrity and structure of physical highways, so does the influence of genes and genetic variability and mutations affect the backbone of the metaphorical highways leading to obesity.

The impact of *genetic influences* on body mass index (BMI—an imperfect surrogate for excess adiposity) is estimated to be between 25% and 90%, with most researchers adopting a midrange of these estimates (40–60%) as the true influence. The size and shape of the human body is markedly influenced by heredity. Risk of obesity is about two to three times higher for an individual with a family history of obesity. This risk increases with the severity of the obesity (14). We also know that there is considerable interindividual difference in the response of plasma lipid concentrations to alterations in the amount of dietary fat and cholesterol, a fact that again points to genetic susceptibility (15).

Studies of twins suggest that genes account for more than 50% of the variation in body mass (8). These same twin studies have shown genetic influences on the following parameters which can, in turn, be associated with increased adiposity:

- Resting metabolic rate (RMR)
- Feeding behavior
- Energy expenditure changes in response to overfeeding
- Lipoprotein lipase activity
- Basal rate of lipolysis

There is firm evidence that genes influencing energy homeostasis and thermogenesis, adipogenesis, leptin–insulin signaling transduction, and hormonal signaling peptides play a role in the development of obesity (15). Newer evidence does seem to suggest that the genetic foundations of childhood and adult obesity share some common ground (16). This includes the three major factors influencing body weight: diet, metabolic factors, and physical activity; each is modulated by genetic traits.

Obesity can be classified into three primary categories on the basis of genetic etiology: monogenic, syndromic, and polygenic. In contrast to the monogenic animal models of obesity and rare genetic syndromes of human obesity, predilection toward the common types of obesity seen in current societies stems from the interplay of multiple susceptibility genes (polygenic) that can affect expenditure of energy, utilization of fuel, characteristics of muscle fibers, and, even, taste preferences. All of these factors, in turn, influence our behavioral responses to the environment.

The overall consensus of the scientific community is that excessive body fat is the end result of interactions among environmental, behavioral, and genetic factors (17). For example, it is estimated that approximately 40% of the variance in daily energy expenditure (excluding vigorous physical activity) is attributable to genotype (18). Genes have also been implicated in one-third of the variance in total caloric intake. Overall, more than 400 genes have been implicated in weight regulation (8). Genome-wide linkage studies have linked BMI to almost every chromosomal region except Y (15).

Monogenic obesity results from a single, yet dysfunctional, gene. It accounts for a small number of severe cases, first appearing in childhood and accompanied by various behavioral, developmental, and neuroendocrine disorders.

In 1992, the first obesity gene characterized at a molecular level was the agouti gene. Agouti is expressed in various tissues, including adipose, suggesting that it may be involved in the regulation of energy homeostasis. However, since then, a better-known gene mutation was discovered—that involving the satiety hormone leptin and its receptors, "ob" and "db" (19).

The 2005 Human Obesity Gene Map identified 11 different genes inducing obesity, including leptin, the leptin receptor, proopiomelanocortin (POMC), and melanocortin 4 receptor (MC4R). Mutations of these four have been associated with juvenile-onset morbid obesity. MC4R-related obesity is the most frequent type of monogenic obesity responsible for up to

4% of early-onset and severe childhood obesity (16). It is also the only locus contributing to a significant proportion of cases of severe adult obesity (20).

To date there are almost 200 different human obesity cases associated with single gene defects. Some examples include (15,21).

- Autosomal dominant—achondroplasia, Angelman syndrome, and IR syndromes
- Autosomal recessive—Alstrom-Hallgren syndrome, Cohen syndrome, Fanconi-Bickel syndrome

Syndromic obesity is that which occurs in association with distinct clinical phenotypes, such as organ specific developmental abnormalities, dysmorphic features, and mental retardation. There have been approximately 25 of these genetic obesity syndromes categorized to date (21). The most common syndromes in this group are Prader–Willi syndrome, Bardet–Biedl syndrome, and Alstrom syndrome (16).

- Prader–Willi syndrome—the most common (prevalence 1:25,000) and best-characterized human obesity syndrome. Includes obesity, reduced fetal activity, hypotonia at birth, short stature, hypogonadism, small hands and feet, and hyperphagia usually developing between 12 and 18 months (14).
- Bardet–Biedl syndrome—(also known as Laurence Moon syndrome) polydactyly, developmental delay, impaired vision, truncal obesity during infancy and hypogonadism
- Cohen syndrome—dysmorphic features, developmental delay, visual problems, and late childhood or adolescent truncal obesity
- Borjeson-Forssman-Lehmann syndrome—mental retardation, obesity, and hypogonadism
- Wilson-Turner syndrome—mental retardation, gynecomastia, and childhood onset obesity

Polygenic obesity results from the synergy of multiple altered genes acting in a permissive environment and is thought to constitute more than 90% of human obesity seen today (1,16). It seems that no single genotype will cause common obesity, with the exception of the monogenic mutations. The most recent obesity gene map includes a collection of more than 430 genes (16).

Research continues to look for "candidate genes" that can be identified on the basis of their putative roles in relevant metabolic pathways. Some of these candidate genes may pertain to body mass, body fat, or fat distribution, whereas others can be defined from their potential contributions to the regulation of energy intake, energy expenditure, or nutrient partitioning. Additional ones can also emerge from our present understanding of other metabolic, physiologic, or behavioral phenotypes involved in the predisposition to obesity (14).

Lest we need a reminder of the intricacies of human physiology, obesity and genetic interaction does not exist in a vacuum. For example, genetic variation at the FTO (fatso/fat mass and obesity associated gene) locus contributes to the etiology of obesity, insulin resistance, and increased plasma leptin levels (22). It is the first compelling example of a common variant impacting on variation in weight and fat mass and on the individual risk of obesity (20).

As we move on from our focus of the genetic foundation of this *Adipose City* highway, we should not lose sight of its interaction and interplay with the milieu around it, just like a real highway. Whatever the influence the genotype has on the etiology of obesity, it is generally attenuated or exacerbated by nongenetic factors, including an obesogenic environment (23). Since our genes have not changed appreciably during the last few decades, although the rates of obesity have, it has been suggested that "genes load the gun, but the environment pulls the trigger" (12).

Traveling down this major highway (personal characteristics), we now traverse the first portion of the road labeled *Biological factors,* remembering, all the while, the underlying genetic support layer for the entire trip. Obesity arises as a consequence of how the body regulates energy intake, energy expenditure, and energy storage (energy balance). Interestingly, the regulation of energy balance may be biased; negative energy balance may be defended more strongly than positive energy balance—our biology is geared to protect more strongly against weight loss than against weight gain (24).

At the outset of this journey we come across the first marker affecting this energy balance conundrum: "Age." Some specifics associated with varying stages of life are as follows:

Young

- Early maturation increases risk of subsequent obesity, since numerous biological mechanisms support significant increases in body fatness in the postpubertal period (9).
- Children and, particularly, adolescents who are obese have a high probability of growing to be adults who are obese (1).

Middle-aged

- Increasing age is associated with an increase in obesity. Changes in body weight and composition are attributable, in part, to the natural declines in growth hormone, dehydropeiandrosterone (DHEA), and testosterone with aging.
- The prevalence of obesity in adults tends to rise steadily from the ages of 20 to 60 years but does not increase and, in fact, begins to decrease in later years (2).

Elderly—

- There is evidence suggesting that the optimal BMI range for adults 65 years of age or older is higher than the range for younger adults.

Besides the hormonal alterations affecting weight that are associated with age in the perinatal, pubertal, midlife, and latter years of life, age also has a role in influencing human metabolism. RMR generally declines every decade of life. This reduction alters energy balance and can contribute to weight gain (18). Hill et al., noted metabolic susceptibility with fat-storing tendencies and differences in skeletal muscle composition (24).

In addition to age and hormonal effects on metabolism, other factors can influence its reduction also. This includes marked food restriction, weight-reduced state, activity diminution, and smoking cessation.

Our second mile marker on this highway is *gender*. Differences in patterns of weight gain, as well as the development of overweight and obesity, are apparent between the genders. These patterns are partially attributable to hormonal differences between men and women before menopause (testosterone and estrogen) and to hormonal changes in women during menopause. During the perimenopausal and postmenopausal periods, many women experience alterations in body weight, total body fat, and body fat distribution (18). Such alterations can also occur with pregnancy.

Following closely on the heels of the *gender* marker is our next milestone, *Race/Ethnicity*. It is known that the prevalence of being overweight and becoming overweight at any age during adolescence is approximately twice as high among African and Hispanic Americans as compared with European-American children. It is believed that inherent ethnic differences in metabolism and fat accumulation in combination with the obesogenic environment may put different population segments at greater risk for disease. Genetic background contributes to racial and ethnic differences in obesity and metabolic risk factors, independent of social and financial aspects (17).

Certain ethnic and racial groups appear to be particularly predisposed to obesity. The Pima Indians of Arizona and other ethnic groups native to North America have a particularly high prevalence of obesity. In addition, Polynesians, Micronesians, Anurans, Maoris of the West and East Indies, African-Americans in North America, and the Hispanic populations (both Mexican and Puerto Rican in origin) in North America also have particularly high predispositions to developing obesity (1).

Ethnicity is associated with differences in food-related beliefs, preferences, and behaviors. Cultural influences may contribute to the higher than average risk of obesity among children and youth in the U.S. ethnic minority populations (25).

Not only is our next mile marker a major one, there is a large service plaza associated with it. While at this *Well Known Hormonal Pathways* service center, we will visit many of the long-standing vendors known to be responsible for excess weight. If you do not see your favorite hormonal "vendor" at this stop, be patient; there are more of them just up the road. Of note is that all of these vendors seem to have the same parent company—Genetics Amalgamated!

The following is a listing of selected dealers at this roadside stop. Some have entire textbooks written about them, so we will only give a cursory overview of a few of their qualities here. While there are more than those listed, this will give a representative example of the variety and intricacies of these adiposity contributors. Visit them briefly and then we will return to our journey.

- Puberty
  - The extent to which pubertal timing is a cause and/or consequence of obesity remains a subject of debate.
  - There is evidence that early maturation increases the chance of subsequent obesity. Early maturing girls (menarche before age 11) were more than twice as likely to be overweight as young adults (9).
- Thyroid
  - The active component of thyroid is T3. There is a decline in active T3 activity with aging and weight reduction.
  - Hypothyroidism can lead to fluid retention, slower than normal metabolism, and weight gain.
- Growth hormone deficiency
  - Decreased lean body mass
  - Increased fat mass, especially visceral
- Testosterone
  - Male hypogonadism can predispose to central weight gain
  - Inverse relationship between testosterone levels and insulin resistance
  - Strong association with obesity, type 2 DM, and metabolic syndrome
- Estrogen
  - Inhibits the actions of peroxisome proliferator-activated receptors (PPAR)-alpha on obesity and lipid metabolism (26).
- Leptin
  - Fat-derived, anorexigenic hormone which acts at the arcuate nucleus of the hypothalamus to regulate energy homeostasis (27).
    - Reduces food intake by signaling satiety (1).
    - Increases activity of thermogenetic components of the sympathetic nervous system (8).
  - Of the six different isoforms of this receptor, the isoform OB-RB is expressed in hypothalamic nuclei, where leptin initiates inhibition of food intake and stimulation of energy expenditure (26).
  - The overwhelming majority of obese humans are not leptin deficient. Obesity results in high plasma leptin concentrations. Recent studies suggest that leptin is physiologically more important as an indicator of energy deficiency, rather than energy excess (28).
  - Animal data suggest that leptin's appetite suppressant effect may be overridden by access to highly palatable, energy-dense foods (29).
  - Cumulative new knowledge favors a unified central leptin insufficiency syndrome over the central resistance hypothesis to explain the global adverse impact of deficient leptin signaling in the brain. Both hypo- and hyperleptinemia are associated with reduced leptin entry into the brain. Excursions from the normal pattern can extinguish target response due to receptor downregulation.
  - Evidence suggests that extended periods of central leptin insufficiency orchestrate pathophysiological consequences that include
    - increased rate of fat accrual,
    - decreased energy expenditure and general activity level,
    - hyperinsulinemia,
    - hyperglycemia,
    - neuroendocrine disorders,
    - osteoporosis,
    - metabolic syndrome, and
    - impaired learning and memory (30).

- Ghrelin
  - Gut hormone which mediates sense of hunger
  - Levels increased in diet-induced weight loss
  - When administered intravenously (IV), found to decrease fat oxidation and increase food intake and adiposity (26).
  - May be regulator of long-term energy balance (8)
- Cushing's disease
  - Adenoma in the pituitary gland producing large amounts of adrenocorticotropic hormone, which in turn elevates cortisol, causing weight gain.
  - Cushing syndrome (also known as hyperadrenocorticism) is an endocrine disorder caused by high levels of cortisol in the blood.
- Polycystic ovarian syndrome (PCOS)
  - Usually associated with central obesity, insulin resistance, hyperinsulinemia, diabetes, and excess testosterone
  - Thought to be caused by insulin resistance, associated with obesity, triggering the development of PCOS in susceptible individuals (2)
  - Debate remains as to whether factors contributing to PCOS cause obesity or whether obesity and its predisposing factors can lead to the development of PCOS. (Classic "which came first question: Chicken or the egg?")
- Metabolic syndrome
  - Usually includes dyslipidemia and insulin resistance
  - May predispose to truncal obesity and diabetes, but not absolute

Once we restart our journey on this highway of personal characteristics, it is not long until we come to another mile marker also associated with a service center and multiple vendors, this time called the *Other Physiological Hormones and Contributors* service plaza. Multiple factors, including central and peripheral ones, are important for regulation of energy balance between fed and fasting states. These include uncoupling proteins, catecholamines, and heat production (27).

As before, this plaza is so voluminous that we will only have time to visit a sampling of the occupants. Here is a listing of just a few of these obesity-regulating vendors:

- Central melanocortin (MC) system
  - Involved in body weight regulation through its role in appetite and energy expenditure via leptin, ghrelin, and agouti-related protein (27; wikipedia)
  - Two receptors complement each other: MC4-R influences food intake and MC3-R regulates fat stores by an exclusive metabolic pathway (27).
- Peroxisome proliferator-activated receptors (PPAR)
  - Group of nuclear receptor proteins that function as transcription factors regulating the expression of genes.
  - Plays crucial role in the pathogenesis of obesity (see cannabinoids).
  - Consists of three isoforms (alpha, delta, and gamma):
    - PPAR-gamma is expressed highest in adipose tissue
      - Important therapeutic target in management of obesity and diabetes
    - PPAR-alpha is involved in energy balance
      - PPAR-alpha ligand fibrates increase hepatic fatty acid oxidation and thereby reduce levels of triglycerides causing adipose cell hypertrophy and hyperplasia
- Peripheral satiety signalers
  - Travel to the brain via vagus nerve or the systemic circulation (see Table 2). Peripheral signals indicating the size of adipose tissue stores as well as circulating factors indicating current nutritional status are received and integrated within the CNS (31).
  - Stomach stretch receptors (32).
- Lipoprotein lipase
  - Known as the fat-storage enzyme
  - Stimulated in the climacteric by testosterone and cortisol, unopposed by decreased progesterone and estradiol, causing increased visceral fat deposition (33)

Table 2 Suggested Biologic Modulators of Food Intake

Peripheral signal	Proposed effect on food intake
Vagal	–
Cholecystokinin	–
Apolipoprotein A-IV	–
Insulin	–
Glucagon-like peptide 1	–
Other glucagon-related peptides	–
Leptin	+ when leptin ↓↓
Ghrelin	+
Tumor necrosis factor-α	–
Obestatin	–

- Cannabinoids
  - Genetic variations at the endocannabinoid type-1 receptor (CB 1 R) gene are reported to be associated with obesity phenotypes.
  - PPAR and endocannabinoid-receptor polymorphisms alter the course of metabolic homeostasis.
  - The role of ghrelin, leptin, adiponectin, and PPAR-gamma activation on adipocyte production of the endocannabinoids is a significant and promising concept in the management of obesity (26).
  - Endocannabinoids are produced by human white adipose tissue. *N*-Palmitoylethanolamine is the most abundant cannabimimetic compound produced by the human adipocyte and its levels can be downregulated by leptin.
- Peptides that stimulate appetite
  - POMC is the polypeptide precursor of adrenocorticotropic hormone.
  - Regulation of body weight is linked to the action of Nhlh2 on prohormone convertase mRNA levels, supporting a direct role for transcriptional control of neuropeptide-processing enzymes in the etiology of adult onset obesity also seen in thyroid patients (27).
  - Factors known to regulate eating behavior include several brain-gut peptides, along with more than a dozen neuropeptides expressed in the CNS.
    - Neuropeptide Y (NPY)
      - NPY is the most potent central appetite stimulant known. It also reduces thermogenesis in brown adipose tissue, thus further promoting positive energy balance (8).
      - The first orexigenic factor from the hypothalamus to be identified. NPY may be a redundant signaling molecule in weight regulation (19).
    - Melanin-concentrating hormone (MCH)
      - Maintains feeding and mediates feeding-related functions via the hormone Orexin, which provokes hyperphagia (8).
    - Orexin A/B
      - Found in lateral hypothalamus
      - Increases food intake
      - Up-regulated by fasting
    - Galanin
      - Stimulates feeding (fat intake > carbohydrate)
      - Reduces energy expenditure by inhibiting sympathetic activity
- Hypothalamus
  - Obesity can be caused by structural damage—craniopharyngioma most common.
  - The arcuate nucleus is considered the primary site within the hypothalamus for reception of blood-borne signals of nutritional status (31).
  - A primary site of convergence and integration for redundant energy status signaling, which includes central and peripheral neural inputs as well as hormonal and nutritional factors (8,34).

- The key energy regulator resides in the CNS. This tightly regulated network resides within the hypothalamus. Two different neuron populations exist:
  - One synthesizes NPY and agouti-related peptide (AgRP)
  - The other synthesizes alpha-melanocyte stimulating hormone (alpha-MSH) from POMC neurons that impact MC4R receptors and thus affect energy intake and expenditure (32).
- Affected via emotions through depression
  - Factors that affect emotional behavior include psychologically induced stress that causes depression. Such depression stimulates the hypothalamic appetite centers to increase food intake, as well as parasympathetic input into the upper gut that enhances fat storage.
- Sleep time variance (e.g., night shift)
  - Changes in sleeping time from night shift work that affect the suprachiasmic center biologic clock also influence centers in the hypothalamus and forebrain that affect increased eating and depression, respectively (12).
  - Secular trends in reduced sleeping time have been implicated in weight gain via altered endocrine function, particularly increased cortisol and ghrelin levels and reduced appetite-dampening leptin.
  - Sleep deprivation contributes to weight gain by increased sympathetic activity and impaired carbohydrate handling (8).
- Hunger-increasing neuropeptides
  - Opioids
    - Released in response to intake of highly palatable foods that enhance appetite—maintain ingestion
    - Interact with cannabinoids to enhance food palatability
  - Dopamine
    - The availability of dopamine D2 receptors is decreased in morbidly obese individuals (BMI $\geq$ 40) in proportion to their BMI.
    - Deficit in dopamine D2 receptors may promote eating as a means to compensate for decreased activation of dopaminergic reward circuits.
  - Offset (−) by satiety neuropeptides insulin, serotonin, and CCK (12).

• Insulinoma
  - Rare: ≈4 cases per million/year.
  - This is usually seen with patients consciously eating to prevent spells of low blood sugar and eventually developing weight gain.

• Adipocyte
  - Obesity results from abnormal accumulation of fat deposits, which consists of an excessive storage of triacylglycerol within adipocytes located within subcutaneous tissue and intra-abdominal viscera (12).
  - Adiponectin is the most abundant adipokine and it causes increased insulin sensitivity and decreased tumor necrosis factor (TNF)-alpha–induced changes. In obesity, adiponectin levels are decreased (26).
  - In addition to their storage function adipocytes serve as endocrine cells by secreting hormones and growth factors that regulate fat metabolism through feedback mechanisms (18).
  - The adipokines, which affect metabolic functioning of fat cells and impact other tissues throughout the body, have been documented to mediate fat metabolism and obesity (17).
  - The adipocyte, which is the cellular unit of obesity, is increasingly found to be a complex and metabolically active cell. At present, the adipocyte is being perceived as an endocrine gland with several peptides and metabolites that may be relevant to the control of body weight, and these are being studied intensively. Among the products of the adipocyte that are involved in complex intermediary metabolism are cytokines, TNF-alpha, interleukin-6, lipotransin, adipocyte lipid-binding protein, acyl-stimulation protein, prostaglandins, adipsin, perilipins, lactate, adiponectin, monobutyrin, and phospholipid transfer protein.

- Among critical enzymes involved in adipocyte metabolism are endothelial-derived lipoprotein lipase (lipid storage), hormone-sensitive lipase (lipid elaboration and release from adipocyte depots), acylcoenzyme A (acyl-CoA) synthetases (fatty acid synthesis), and a cascade of enzymes (beta oxidation and fatty acid metabolism). The ongoing flurry of investigation into the intricacies of adipocyte metabolism in the last 5 years has not only improved our understanding of the pathogenesis of obesity but also offered several potential targets for therapy.
- Another area of active research is investigation of the cues for the differentiation of preadipocytes to adipocytes. With the fairly recent recognition that this process occurs in both white and brown adipose tissue, even in adults, its potential role in the development of obesity and the relapse to obesity after weight loss has become increasingly important. Among the identified factors in this process are transcription factors peroxisome proliferator-activated receptors-gamma (PPAR-gamma); retinoid-X receptor ligands; perilipin; adipocyte differentiation-related protein (ADRP); and CCAAT enhancer-binding proteins (C/EBP) alpha, beta, and delta (1).

After leaving the last service center, we soon see the next major marker on our road: *Psychological Considerations*. Less well-defined causes of obesity may be related to psychosocial factors, which may have cultural roots (mentioned earlier) and/or reflect behavioral expressions that cause excessive food intake, altered body image, and depression. Emotional stress appears to involve multiple brain centers that influence vagal input into the enteric neuromuscular system and its neurotransmitters that affect visceral hypersensitivity (12).

Several lines of evidence indicate that emotional modulation of food intake differs between lean and obese individuals (8). Since almost 30% of patients who are obese have eating disorders, it is important to screen for these in the history (1).

There are several subcomponents to this psychological stretch of highway. One is *vagus nerve mediation*. Like stoplights on a highway, there are a series of peripheral "satiety" signals that act to inhibit further food intake at some point during meal consumption. Some of the signals reach the brain through the vagus nerve and some through the systemic circulation (2).

Restraint disinhibition is like a broken traffic light and comprises another one of the psychological disorders. It involves the inability to refrain from overeating when there is an abundance of food (12).

Another important psychological aspect for obesity is *abuse*. This can take the form of emotional, physical, or sexual abuse, especially in women. Some of the long-term adverse consequences of abuse include obesity, both as a result of stress eating and sometimes to provide for protection against unwanted sexual attention (2).

Eating patterns and disorders complete our psychological subsets. Dietary patterns contribute substantially to the development of obesity. Modern society facilitates excessive consumption with an abundance of inexpensive, energy-dense foods, numerous conveniently located eating establishments that promote dining away from home, a high variety of food at mealtime, and unreasonably large portion sizes (18). Specific eating disorders, which include overeating syndromes, such as binge-eating disorder, bulimia nervosa, and night-eating disorder can contribute significantly to overweight and obesity (1,12).

Further down our traveled road a fairly new marker has arisen. Many of the previous markers have been known and considered for awhile but one newcomer to the scene is labeled: *Inflammatory State*.

A mild inflammatory response process plays a role in stimulation of weight gain. Studies show association of obesity with the presence of a chronic, mild state of inflammation (35). It is known that overweight individuals have elevated levels of C-reactive protein (8). There is also increasing evidence to suggest that the features of metabolic syndrome, including obesity and type II diabetes, have a common inflammatory basis (26).

Central visceral sites of white adipose tissue secrete inflammatory adipokines, such as tumor necrosis factor alpha (TNF-a), interleukin-1 (IL-1), and interleukin-6 (IL-6), that are the precipitating and/or aggravating factors that contribute to the comorbid conditions of obesity such as diabetes mellitus with insulin resistance (12).

- Inflammatory adipokines (white adipose tissue)
    - TNF-a—causes decreased adipose cell differentiation, increased lipolysis, and increased free fatty acids (26).
    - IL-1 and IL-6

Some adults recruit new adipocytes more readily than others do and thus gain weight more from adipocyte hyperplasia than from hypertrophy. Those who gain fat with large adipocytes are more likely to display inflammatory responses, both in adipose tissue (greater numbers of macrophages and increased expression of cytokines) and systemically (increased C-reactive protein) (2).

A fairly recent and quite intriguing field of study linking inflammatory inducers of obesity and other metabolic sequlae involves gut microbiota. Several mechanisms are proposed linking events occurring in the colon and the regulation of energy metabolism and the regulation of fat storage. High-fat diet feeding triggers the development of obesity, inflammation, insulin resistance, type 2 diabetes and atherosclerosis by mechanisms dependent on the bacterial lipopolysaccharide (LPS) and/or the fatty acids activation of the CD14/TLR4 receptor complex. These effects occur through various interactions with epithelial and endocrine cells. Large-scale alterations of the gut microbiota and its microbiome are associated with obesity and are responsive to weight loss (36,37).

Much as evidence showed an infectious agent (*Helicobacter pylori*) to be an etiological agent for peptic ulcer disease, evolving data suggest that a possibly infective etiology may exist for obesity. (1). Speaking of a possible infectious route taking us to Adipose City, this brings us to our next mile marker labeled: *Infectious.* A new term associated with this postulated theory is "infectobesity," meaning obesity of infectious origin. Clearly, not every case of obesity is of infectious origin, but infection attributable to certain organisms should be included in the long list of potential etiological factors for obesity (35).

It should be mentioned that production of obesity is not a characteristic of all animal or human pathogens. Many of the animal viruses that cause obesity do so by damaging the CNS (38).

In the last two decades, adipogenic (fat causing) pathogens have been reported: these include human and nonhuman viruses, prions, bacteria, and gut microflora (mentioned above). Two pathogens of note are the avian adenovirus SMAM-1 and the human virus Ad-36. SMAM-1 was the first virus to be implicated in human obesity. After its discovery, the human adenovirus AD-36 was found to be linked to obesity (35).

- SMAM-1
    - An avian adenovirus from India (38)
    - Acts directly on adipocytes. Causes fat deposition (adiposity) in chickens
    - The only animal virus to date to show a serological association with human obesity (35,38)
    - Dhurandhar et al. (39) screened 52 obese humans for antibodies to SMAM-1 virus. Approximately 20% of the subjects had antibodies to SMAM-1. The antibody (+) subjects had significantly greater body weight compared with the antibody (−) group.
- AD-36
    - First human adenovirus linked with obesity. Data show an association of AD-36 antibodies with human obesity but do not establish a causative relationship (35). Recent predicted molecular models of the AD-36 fiber protein seem to implicate a unique tissue tropism (40).
    - Has a direct effect on adipocytes to turn on the enzymes of fat accumulation and recruitment of new adipocytes
    - Present in 30% of obese humans and 11% of nonobese humans in one study (41). In the whole population, AD-36 antibody (+) individuals were nine BMI units heavier than antibody (−) individuals
    - Also causes obesity in chickens, mice, rats, and monkeys

    - Subsequent to discovery of the linkage of AD-36 with obesity, two additional human adenoviruses (out of 50 known serotypes) have been associated with obesity and shown to affect adipocytes directly, Ad-5 and Ad-37 (38)
- Chlamydia pneumoniae
    - The first bacterium reported to be associated with increased BMI in humans. At this time the link remains somewhat uncertain (35).

Major Highway: Behavioral Factors

Hopefully, our journey to this point, though long and sometimes encumbered with details and uncertainties, has been interesting and thought-provoking. Let us now look at the last and final superhighway leading to our ever-expanding metropolis—*Adipose City*. This is the mega highway called **Behavioral Factors** and may be the primary road upon which individuals and health care professionals can have their greatest impact for good. Our travel on this road, as compared with the previous two, can be much more easily modified, so that we can exit and head away from expanding waistlines and increasing health risk factors.

Take note that all of these highways, Global & Community Influences, Personal Characteristics, and Behavioral Factors are all interconnected, just like real highways, with side streets, crossroads, and alternate routes. Each has an influence upon the other ones and always will. It is up to us to decide which pathway we want to take and where we want to end up at the end of our journey.

Obesity is often considered a "problem of the belly rather than of the brain." However, neurobiology and neurology play a prominent role. Adiposity can be initiated by pathological conditions of the brain and various signaling mechanisms, as we have indicated earlier. Obesity is mediated by learned behavior and may, therefore, be better understood by disciplines concerned with cognition and behavior (8).

We cannot attribute the obesity epidemic solely to our biology. We must also examine the role of our behavior patterns regarding diet and physical activity (or inactivity) as key pathways for how our social environment influences energy balance, overweight, and obesity (11). These primary factors are the source of day-to-day variations in energy balance, superimposed on top of our genetic fabric (24).

Our last highway has three primary markers that will be addressed. The first and perhaps most critical milestone is *diet* or caloric intake. The reason it is ranked so highly is that it takes a lot of exercise to offset/undo just a little extra caloric intake. For example, just to burn the calories in a single, plain M&M candy®, one has to walk the entire length of a football field (100 yards). Another way of looking at the insidious effect of persistent, minute deviations from energy balance can be illustrated in another example. Consuming just 100 extra calories per day (e.g., 1 banana or 2/3 of a 12 oz. soda) in excess of your body's energy need can lead to an extra 10 lb of fat gained in a year.

Dietary recommendations are beyond the scope of this chapter and will be handled elsewhere in this book. There are definitely differences in body chemistry, hormonal response, and subsequent fat storage or utilization depending upon the quantity and mixture of the food substrate. Suffice it to say that we will touch on a few of the known dietary and caloric causes contributing to overweight and obesity. Some of these have already been addressed in the beginning of this chapter.

Over the short term, humans eat a constant volume of food at meals, so that total energy intake increases with the energy density of the diet. Excess energy is efficiently stored in the body regardless of its source; however, excess energy from dietary fat is stored with a greater efficiency than excess energy from carbohydrates and proteins (24). Fat is energy dense (1 g = 9 cal; technically kilocalories) compared with carbohydrate and protein (1 g = 4 cal). However, debate remains that these values were determined in a bomb calorimeter and whether the same values hold true 'in vivo' is still being sought.

Decisions, like what food to consume and at what quantities, may be explained by interplay of competing processes. Choices of food intake are not only based on homeostatic criteria but also on hedonic criteria. Ingestion of a high fat/sucrose diet increases gene expression of the opioid peptide dynorphin, which can have reinforcing properties on future intake (8).

One also cannot forget the cultural and societal effects on our behavior of eating. Studies examining peers have found a greater correlation of overweight BMI among peers than among siblings or spouses. We are just now realizing that peers have a larger impact on BMI than previously thought, as this influences physical activity/inactivity and diet (42).

The next major marker we note is that of *daily energy expenditure* and its subcomponents: physical activity, basal metabolic rate (BMR), thermic effect of food (TEF), and nonexercise activity thermogenesis (NEAT) (2). Genetic influences appear to affect resting energy expenditure, TEF, and adaptive body fat changes to short-term overfeeding. Resting energy expenditure, which generally represents about 60% of daily energy expenditures, depends largely on body mass, especially fat-free mass, which is more metabolically active than fat tissue.

Since we are dealing in this chapter with etiologies of obesity, we will not focus on the positive weight reducing and maintenance benefits of exercise but just mention a few physiologic facts regarding them. It is known that a higher body weight is associated with greater physiologic stress of exercise, which may add to the reasons some people avoid exercise and its benefits (29).

There may be a threshold of physical activity below which energy balance regulation is least sensitive. Disruption of energy balance toward a positive surplus is conducive to obesity. This causes an increase in energy flux. The two ways to deal with this increase in energy flux are to become more physically active or to become obese. Both serve to increase total energy expenditure, allowing energy balance to be regulated at a higher level. If it is easier to maintain energy balance at a high energy flux, this is an important consideration in the treatment of obesity (24).

In the average overweight person, the amount of energy expended in physical activity and exercise often is insufficient to counter the generally sedentary nature of the remainder of their lifestyle and the influence of excessive caloric consumption (18). For example, being seated rather than upright for an hour per day can result in approximately 6 kg weight gain over the course of one year (≈1 lb/mo). If this extra hour of sitting is coupled with television viewing, then there is the addition of exposure to food marketing, increased opportunity for snacking on high energy foods and drinks, decreased opportunity for physical activity, and reinforcement of sedentary behavior (8).

As we consider the various subcomponents of daily energy expenditure, one of the biggest contributors is the BMR and its quasi-surrogate the RMR. The BMR is the energy expenditure of laying still at rest, awake, in the overnight postabsorptive state. A true BMR is measured after awakening but before arising from bed. The RMR is similarly defined but is not necessarily measured before arising from bed. For most sedentary adult Americans, the RMR represents the major portion of energy expended during the day and may range from less than 1200 kcal to more than 3000 kcal/day.

Most of the BMR (≈80%) is directly proportional to the amount of lean tissue mass, although age, sex (women have slightly lower BMRs, even corrected for fat-free mass), and fat mass also affect it. Small changes in BMR occur during the menstrual cycle (luteal phase > follicular phase). There is also evidence that heritable or family factors do influence BMR, accounting for as much as 10% of the interindividual differences.

Not all components of lean tissue consume oxygen at the same rate. Visceral or splanchnic bed tissues account for approximately 25% of RMR but a much smaller proportion of body weight. The brain, which is only a small percentage of body weight, accounts for almost 15% of RMR. Likewise, the heart (≈7%) and kidneys (≈5–10%) account for greater portions of resting energy needs relative to their contribution to body mass. In contrast, resting muscle makes up 40% to 50% of lean tissue mass but accounts for only 25% of RMR. This contribution changes dramatically with exercise, at which time muscle can account for 80% to 90% of energy expenditure, especially during high-intensity exercise.

With an energy-restricted diet, significant reductions in BMR relative to the amount of fat-free mass occur. Reductions in the production of triiodothyronine from thyroxine are thought to contribute to this phenomenon. Likewise, during brief periods of overfeeding, it has been shown that RMR increases more than would be expected for the amount of lean tissue present.

The TEF is a component of energy expenditure that will be included for completeness. Approximately 10% of the energy content of food is expended in the process of digestion, absorption, and metabolism of nutrients. There is a significant interindividual variability in this value, however, ranging from a low of approximately 5% to a high of 15% of meal calories that are "wasted" in the postprandial interval. The thermic effect of a meal is related to the carbohydrate and protein calorie content of the meal (the fat content has little stimulatory effect).

Both obligatory and facultative components of the TEF have been identified. The obligatory components reflect the energy costs of digestion, absorption, and storage of nutrients. Approximately 60% to 70% of the thermic effect of meals is obligatory and the remaining 30% to 40% is facultative thermogenesis. The two factors thought to play a role in the facultative component of the TEF are the postprandial insulin response and activation of the sympathetic nervous system. The TEF is somewhat lower in insulin-resistant obese humans.

A fairly significant subcomponent of daily energy expenditure is NEAT. This is the calorie expense of performing all activities other than exercise. The range of observed NEAT under controlled (metabolic chamber) conditions has been from less than 100 to about 800 kcal/day. There is probably a much wider range in free-living individuals (2). Spontaneous activity-related energy expenditure represents about 30% of total energy expenditure and is the most variable component. The available evidence suggests that reduced activity-related energy expenditure is a potentially important contributor to the predisposition to obesity (29).

It has been shown that NEAT can increase in response to increased food intake in an unconscious manner. In fact, modulation of NEAT can be a significant factor that acts to stabilize weight despite variations in food intake. Low levels of NEAT have been reported to predict future weight gain in some populations, and there may be differences between lean and obese persons in the daily amount of NEAT, which could relate to differential tendencies to regulate weight (2).

At the beginning of the 20th century, 90% of the population of the world was rural. However, over the last century, more than 2 billion agriculturalists have become city dwellers. In the latter transition, physical activity has declined. In particular, chair use has replaced ambulation such that obese individuals tend to sit for approximately 2.5 hours/day more than lean counterparts. Walking is the principal component of NEAT. Even at slow velocities, walking doubles energy expenditure.

In one study by Levine et al. (43), it was found that on average, free living people walked about 7 miles/day. In sedentary people, walking represented the cumulative effort of many short duration, low intensity walks. The subjects with obesity walked one-third less distance per day than lean individuals. This difference represented approximately 3.5 miles or about 2 hours of walking per day. These differences occurred because the distance of each walking bout was one-third shorter in the obese subjects compared with the lean, whereas the number of walking bouts per day was similar between the groups. This suggests that walking distance progressively declines with increases in body fat. It was also noted that with overfeeding and experimental weight gain, free living walking distance decreased.

Other components of NEAT, the activities of daily living, are somewhat difficult to measure. A plethora of labor-saving conveniences (drive-through food and banking, escalators, remote controls, e-mail, and online shopping) have been introduced into the modern environment. Each of these further reduces the energy humans must expend to get through the day. Little hard data exist to document how much change has actually occurred, although future studies may help shed light on this topic.

There are certainly exercise strategies that can help prevent weight regain after loss, but one of the quickest ways to get back on the road to adiposity after weight loss is NOT to increase activity or change habits in favor of more energy use throughout the day. Many Americans get as few as 4000 to 5000 steps per day, whereas it may take as many as 15,000 to 17,000 steps per day to help those who have lost significant amounts of weight to maintain that lower weight (2).

The last subcomponent of our metaphorical highway is every bit as important as most of the other milestones we have covered to this point. The last marker we will mention which is almost guaranteed to steer us toward Adipose City in this highly energy dense, calorically laden, refined and processed dietary environment with continued trends toward sedentary behaviors is, of course, *physical inactivity*. It has been well known that a strong link exists between physical inactivity and overweight and obesity (23,44). Epidemiologically, the relationship of physical inactivity to weight gain appears to be more consistent than the relationship of excess energy intake to weight gain (29).

Information as to how differences in sedentary activity (television watching, video games, and computer use) relate to obesity is readily available. There is compelling evidence that more time spent in sedentary pursuits is associated with an increased risk of overweight and obesity. The striking aspect to these studies is that the adverse effect of sedentary activities is independent of participation in traditional exercise activities (2).

Obesity seems to track the sales of domestic labor-saving devices and vehicles more than trends in energy and fat intake (45). Domestic mechanization, in just four areas, decreased energy expenditure by 111 kcal/day. These areas were (*i*) clothes washing, (*ii*) dish washing, (*iii*) stair climbing, and (*iv*) walking to work. If not compensated by food/energy reduction, as a result of these changes, body weight could increase 10 lb (4.5 kg) per year—an amount exceeding progressive weight gain associated with the U.S. obesity epidemic.

More than half of the U.S. adult population maintains an almost totally sedentary lifestyle. Is it any wonder there is such a large population in *Adipose City*?

In the venue of today's rap music, listen carefully and one might hear this plea, "Hey people... we need motivation for a new location that will be the salvation for our expanding nation." The solution may be to take William Purkey's advice, and "Dance like there's nobody watching...." Or, perhaps, we can revise it for today's Americans to say "At the very least, just get up and move ... whether anyone's watching or not!"

REFERENCES

1. Uwaifo GI, Arioglu E. eMedicine—Obesity. 2009. http://emedicine.medscape.com/article/123702-overview. Accessed May 11, 2010.
2. Jensen MD. Obesity. In: Goldman L, Ausiello D, eds. Cecil Textbook of Medicine. 23rd ed. Philadelphia, PA: Saunders Elsevier, 2008:1643–1652.
3. U.S. Department of Health and Human Services, National Institutes of Health, National Institute of Diabetes and Digestive and Kidney Diseases. Statistics related to overweight and obesity. NIH Publication Number 04-4158. http://www.win.niddk.nih.gov/publications/PDFs/stat904z.pdf. Accessed May 12, 2010.
4. Ogden CL, Carroll MD, Flegal KM. High body mass index for age among US children and adolescents. 2003–2006. JAMA 2008; 299(20):2401–2405.
5. Bethell C, Simpson L, Stumbo S, et al. National, state and local disparities in childhood obesity. Health Aff(Millwood) 2010; 29(3):347–356.
6. Micallef M, Munro I, Phang M, et al. Plasma n-3 polyunsaturated fatty acids are negatively associated with obesity. Br J Nutr 2009; 102(9):1370–1374.
7. Parks EJ, Skokan LE, Timlin MT, et al. Dietary sugars stimulate fatty acid synthesis in adults. J Nutr 2008; 138(6):1039–1046.
8. Knecht S, Ellger T, Levine JA. Obesity in neurobiology. Prog Neurobiol 2008; 84(1):85–103.
9. Adair LS. Child and adolescent obesity: epidemiology and developmental perspectives. Physiol Behav 2008; 94(1):8–16.
10. Fox EA. Purdue ingestive behavior research center symposium 2007: influences on eating and body weight over the lifespan—childhood and adolescence. Physiol Behav 2008; 94(1):1–7.
11. The National Children's Study. Social environmental influences on child and adolescent obesity. 2002. http://www.nationalchildrensstudy.gov/about/organization/advisorycommittee/2003Sep/Pages/social-environment-document-11.pdf. Accessed May 11, 2010.
12. Redinger RN. The prevalence and etiology of nongenetic obesity and associated disorders. South Med J 2008; 101(4):395–399.
13. Keith SW, Redden DT, Katzmarzk PT, et al. Putative contributors to the secular increase in obesity: exploring the roads less traveled. Int J Obesity (London) 2006; 30:1585–1594.
14. Perusse L, Chagnon YC, Bouchard C. Etiology of massive obesity: role of genetic factors. World J Surg 1998; 22(9):907–912.
15. Yang W, Kelly T, He J. Genetic epidemiology of obesity. Epidemiol Rev 2007; 29:49–61.
16. Papoutsakis C, Dedoussis GV. Gene-diet interactions in childhood obesity: paucity of evidence as the epidemic of childhood obesity continues to rise. Per Med 2007; 4(2):133–146.
17. Fernandez JR, Casazza K, Divers J, et al. Disruptions in energy balance: does nature overcome nurture? Physiol Behav 2008; 94(1):105–112.
18. Racette SB, Deusinger SS, Deusinger RH. Obesity: overview of prevalence, etiology, and treatment. Phys Ther 2003; 83(3):276–288.

19. Carroll L, Voisey J, van Daal A. Mouse models of obesity. Clin Dermatol 2004; 22(4):345–349.
20. Lindgren CM, McCarthy MI. Mechanisms of disease: genetic insights into the etiology of type 2 diabetes and obesity. Nat Clin Pract Endocrinol Metab 2008; 4(3):156–163.
21. Ishihara S, Yamada Y. Genetic factors for human obesity. Cell Mol Life Sci 2008; 65(7–8):1086–1098.
22. Do R, Bailey SD, Desbiens K, et al. Genetic variants of FTO influence adiposity, insulin sensitivity, leptin levels, and resting metabolic rate in the Quebec family study. Diabetes 2008; 57(4):1147–1150.
23. Afridi AK, Khan A. Prevalence and etiology of obesity—an overview. Pak J Nutr 2004; 3(1):14–25.
24. Hill JO. Understanding and addressing the epidemic of obesity: an energy balance perspective. Endocr Rev 2006; 27(7):750–761.
25. Kumanyika SK. Environmental influences on childhood obesity: ethnic and cultural influences in context. Physiol Behav 2008; 94(1):61–70.
26. Iqbal O. Endocannabionoid system and pathophysiology of adipogenesis: current management of obesity. Per Med 2007; 4(3):307–319.
27. Zimmerman-Belsing T, Feldt-Rasmussen U. Obesity: the new worldwide epidemic threat to general health and our complete lack of effective treatment. Endocrinology 2004; 145(4):1501–1502.
28. Kelesidis T, Kelesidis I, Chou S, et al. Narrative review: the role of leptin in human physiology: emerging clinical applications. Ann Intern Med 2010; 152(2):93–100.
29. Weinsier RL, Hunter GR, Heini AF, et al. The etiology of obesity: relative contribution of metabolic factors, diet, and physical activity. Am J Med 1998; 105(2):145–150.
30. Kalra SP. Central leptin insufficiency syndrome: an interactive etiology for obesity, metabolic and neural diseases and for designing new therapeutic interventions. Peptides 2008; 29(1):127–138.
31. Cottrell EC, Ozanne SE. Early life programming of obesity and metabolic disease. Physiol Behav 2008; 94(1):17–28.
32. Patay BA. Obesity variants affect eating behavior in a predictable world: the FTO, MC4R, HBII-85 genes. Medscape. http://www.medscape. com/viewarticle/577822. Updated August 21, 2008. Accessed May 11, 2010.
33. Milewicz A, Jedrzejuk D. Climacteric obesity: from genesis to clinic. Gynecol Endocrinol 2006; 22(1): 18–24.
34. Yamada T, Katagiri H. Avenues of communication between the brain and tissues/organs involved in energy homeostasis. Endocr J 2007; 54(4):497–505.
35. Pasarica M, Dhurandhar NV. Infectobesity: obesity of infectious origin. Adv Food Nutr Res 2007; 52:61–102.
36. Cani PD, Delzene NM. The role of the gut microbiota in energy metabolism and metabolic disease. Curr Pharm Des. 2009; 15(13):1546–1558.
37. Ley RE. Obesity and the human microbiome. Curr Opin Gastroenterol 2010; 26(1):5–11.
38. Atkinson RL. Dhurandhar NV, Allison DB, et al. Viruses as an etiology of obesity. Mayo Clin Proc 2007; 82(10):1192–1198.
39. Dhurandhar NV, Kilkami PR, Ajinkya SM, et al. Screening of human sera for antibody against avian adenovirus. Obesity Res 1997; 5:464–469.
40. Arnold J, Janoska M, Kajon AE, et al. Genomic characterization of human adenovirus 36, a putative obesity agent. Virus Res 2010; 149(2):152–161.
41. Atkinson RL, Dhurandhar NV, Allison DB, et al. Human Adenovirus-36 is associated with increased body weight and paradoxical reduction of serum lipids. Int J Obes (Lond) 2005; 29(3):281–286.
42. Christakis NA, Fowler JH. The spread of obesity in a large social network over 32 years. N Engl J Med 2007; 357(4):370–379.
43. Levine JA, McCrady SK, Lanningham-Foster LM, et al. The role of free-living daily walking in human weight gain and obesity. Diabetes 2008; 57(3):548–554.
44. Pietrobelli A, Flodmark CE, Lissau I, et al. From birth to adolescence: Vienna 2005 European Childhood Obesity Group International Workshop. Int J Obes (Lond) 2005; 29(Suppl 2):S1–S6.
45. Lanningham-Foster L, Nysse LJ, Levine JA. et al. Labor saved, calories lost: the energetic impact of domestic labor-saving devices. Obes Res 2003; 11(10):1178–1181.

3 Health hazards of obesity

G. Michael Steelman

If obesity were only a cosmetic problem that would still be of significance in our society. Obesity is a disease with considerable social stigma (1–6) and obese individuals are subject to derision, discrimination, and prejudice, even from health care professionals (7–18).

But obesity is, in fact, one of our nation's biggest health care problems (no pun intended). Although there is some controversy about the number, it has been estimated that over 300,000 deaths per year in America are attributable to obesity (19), making it the second most frequent preventable cause of death (after tobacco use). It is linked to cardiovascular disease (CVD), diabetes mellitus (DM), and various types of cancer, as well as many other health problems (20).

This chapter reviews some basic information regarding some of the health hazards and comorbidities associated with obesity.

DIABETES MELLITUS TYPE II (DM II)

It is currently estimated that there are about 24 million Americans with diabetes (21), approximately 90% with type II. The medical and social costs of diabetes are significant, even in normal weight individuals. There is an even greater impact in those who are also obese (22). It has been projected that the number of Americans living with diabetes will nearly double in the next 25 years (by 2034) and that will result in medical costs of approximately $336 billion (23).

The etiology of DM II includes the development of insulin resistance and/or pancreatic beta cell dysfunction. One suggested pathway for the development of the disease is that insulin resistance is the primary abnormality and that beta cell dysfunction arises later as the pancreatic cells "burn out" in response to the increased demand placed on them as they attempt to maintain normoglycemia in the state of increasing insulin resistance (24). Thus, early in the course of the process, normal blood glucose levels are maintained by an increased supply of insulin.

Obesity contributes significantly to the development of insulin resistance; 80% to 95% of patients with DM II are obese, and most often demonstrate the android (apple-shaped) morphology, with an elevated waist–hip ratio (25,26).

In comparison to subcutaneous fat, visceral fat produces more compounds that are associated with the development of insulin resistance: angiotensin, interleukin-6, and plasminogen activator inhibitor-1, for example (21,27). It also releases less adiponectin ... an insulin-sensitizing compound. Visceral adiposity is associated with increased deposition of triglyceride in liver and skeletal muscle, and with subsequent insulin resistance in these tissues. It has been speculated that the triglyceride or metabolic byproducts may produce insulin resistance via the impairment of mitochondrial function (28).

In overweight individuals at high risk, the progression to frank diabetes can be abated with weight loss; glycemic control and attendant morbidity can be lessened in those with diabetes with as little as 5% to 10% reduction in weight (29,30). More drastic weight loss may, at times, eliminate diabetes altogether (31,32).

Medications used to treat diabetes often cause weight gain, especially insulin, the sulfonylurea drugs, and the thiazolidinediones. Metformin and incretin mimetics, like exenatide, are considered weight neutral and, also, less likely to cause hypoglycemia.

CARDIOVASCULAR DISEASE

Obesity has been identified as an independent risk factor of CVD, defined as including coronary heart disease (CHD), myocardial infarction (MI), congestive heart failure (CHF), hypertension, atrial fibrillation, and stroke (33,34). The Framingham Heart Study showed obesity to increase the age-adjusted relative risk of CVD to 1.46 and 1.64 in men and women, respectively, and the age-adjusted risk for hypertension was even higher (2.21 in men and 2.75 in women) (35). In a later follow-up study (36), the risk of CVD was 54.8% in normal weight, nondiabetic women versus 78.8% in their obese, diabetic counterparts. In men, the risk was 78.6% in the normal

Table 1 Cardiovascular System Manifestations Associated with Obesity

↑ Total blood volume
↑ Cardiac output
↑ Stroke volume
↑ (±) Heart rate
↑ LV filling and pressure (especially during exercise)
↑ LAH
↑ LVH (especially eccentric type)
↑ LV diastolic dysfunction
↑ Adipositas cordis (fatty heart)
↑ PR interval, QRS interval, QTc
↑ ↓ QRS voltage
↑ ST depression and other ST-T abnormalities
↑ False positive inferior MI on EKG

LV, left ventricular; LAH, left atrial hypertrophy; QTc, QT interval, corrected; EKG, electrocardiogram.

weight, nondiabetic compared to 86.9% in obese diabetic subjects. European studies (37,38) have shown such associations, as well, and abdominal obesity is recognized as a risk factor for CVD worldwide (39,40).

Obesity is associated with numerous structural and functional changes in the cardiovascular system, even in the absence of frank CVD. Some of these are shown in Table 1.

Venous insufficiency in the lower extremities can often be found in obese individuals. Pedal edema may be associated with several factors, including elevated ventricular filling pressure despite elevation of cardiac output (41,42), high volume lymphatic overload, increased intravascular volume, decreased mobility (leading to less pumping action of the calf and leg muscles), and increased venous valvular incompetence.

Obesity increases the risk of *CHF* (43–47). Each incremental increase of BMI of 1 unit has been estimated to increase the risk of CHF by 5% for men and 7% for women (45). Paradoxically, once CHF is present, patients with higher BMI have lower risk for hospitalization and death than patients with a healthy BMI (48–53).

Hypertension is strongly associated with obesity (54,55). The prevalence of hypertension is about six times more frequent in the obese and a majority of people with hypertension are overweight (56). A 10 kg higher weight is associated with a 3.0 mm higher systolic and a 2.3 mm higher diastolic blood pressure, with estimated increases of 12% risk for CVD and 24% risk for stroke (57).

An increase in BMI from <25 to >30 kg/m^2 is associated with an increased prevalence of hypertension from 15% to 40% (58). A prospective study of about 30,000 normotensive men and women (59) showed that an increase in BMI compared to baseline was associated with a 1.4-fold increase in the risk of hypertension.

Weight loss in obese patients is associated with a reduction in blood pressure. In 50% or more of individuals, blood pressure decreases an average of 1 to 4 mm Hg systolic and 1–2 mm Hg diastolic per kg of weight reduction (60–62).

The *sudden cardiac mortality* rate in both obese men and women has been estimated to be about 40 times higher than the rate in a matched nonobese population. This association is not newly found; Hippocrates is said to have stated, "Sudden death is more common in those who are naturally fat than in the lean" (63). Alterations in electrical activity of the heart may predispose the obese patient to various arrhythmias (64), especially in light of the structural changes often present in the heart of the severely obese individual. A 10% increase in weight decreases parasympathetic tone and increases heart rate while, conversely, heart rate declines during weight reduction (65). Heart rate variability, the fluctuation of heart rate around the mean heart rate, is associated with increased cardiac mortality (66–68) and improves with weight loss (69).

Atherosclerosis and CHD are associated with obesity. Postmortem examination of young people who died from homicide, suicide, or accidental injuries revealed that the extent of fatty

Table 2 Metabolic Syndrome

Diagnostic criteria (3 out of 5 of the following)	
Abdominal obesity (waist circumference)	$\geq$ 40″ in men, $\geq$ 35″ in women
Triglycerides	$\geq$ 150 mg/dL
HDL	$\leq$ 40 mg/dL for men, $\leq$50 mg/dL for women
Blood pressure	$\geq$ 130/80 mm Hg
Fasting glucose	$\geq$ 100 mg/dL

streaks and advanced lesions in the abdominal aorta and right coronary artery were associated with obesity and size of the abdominal panniculus (70–73).

Several studies (35,74–76) that have reported follow-up data over 20 years or more have well documented that obesity is an independent predictor of clinical CHD. Central fat distribution appears to be a greater factor for atherosclerosis than general fat distribution (77).

While obesity increases the risk of MI, reminiscent of the previous discussion regarding CHF, there is an inverse relationship between BMI and mortality in patients after an acute MI (78,79).

There is a correlation between obesity and the incidence of *stroke* (80–88). In fact, there is a 4% increase in the incidence of ischemic stroke and a 6% increase in the incidence of hemorrhagic stroke for every 1 unit increase of BMI. This relationship appears to be independent of the effect of hypertension, dyslipidemia, or diabetes (89). It is thought that the link may be related to the prothrombotic and proinflammatory changes that are associated with excess adiposity (90,91).

Metabolic syndrome (MetS) is a combination of several associated cardiovascular risk factors, including abdominal obesity, hypertension, elevated fasting glucose, increased triglycerides, and low high-density lipoprotein (HDL) levels. It was first described by Reaven (92) and is associated with an increased risk of mortality from CVD (93). Several sources have developed guidelines for the diagnosis of MetS. One set of diagnostic criteria is shown in Table 2. Weight reduction, even as little as 8 kg, has been shown to lower the prevalence of MetS significantly (94,95).

Weight reduction in obese patients can improve or prevent many of the obesity-related risk factors. Some of the benefits of weight loss on the cardiovascular system are listed in Table 3. At the same time, treatment of the obese patient with CVD is not without risks. The use of very low calorie diets (VLCD), liquid protein diets, and bariatric surgery has been associated with prolongation of the QT and QTc intervals and, subsequently, potentially life-threatening arrythmias (96–98). Nutritionally deficient diets may lead to increased predisposition to arrhythmias. Anorectic medications can potentially increase heart rate or blood pressure and are contraindicated in the face of unstable CVD (99). The use of such modalities is best left to those with special interest and training in their use in patients with CVD.

CANCER

Numerous studies have shown a correlation between obesity and the risk of developing or dying from cancer (100–104). The Million Women study (102) showed a significant increase in the incidence of cancer (at 5.4 years) and of cancer mortality (at 7 years). This was true for all cancers combined and specifically for leukemia, multiple myeloma, non-Hodgkin's

Table 3 Cardiovascular System Manifestations Associated with Weight Loss

↓ Total blood volume
↓ Cardiac output
↓ Stroke volume
↓ (±) Heart rate
↓ LV filling and pressure (especially during exercise)
↓ LV diastolic dysfunction
↓ PR interval, QRS interval, QTc

lymphoma, and cancer of the endometrium, esophagus, kidney, breast (in postmenopausal women), and colon/rectum (in premenopausal women). A prospective study (101) in the United States involving 900,000 subjects (cancer free at baseline) for more than 15 years, showed those with a BMI >39.9 had a 50% to 60% increase in overall cancer mortality and, more specifically, with higher death rates from cancer of the colon and rectum, gallbladder, liver, pancreas, kidney, esophagus, and multiple myeloma and non-Hodgkin's lymphoma.

Studies have shown an increase in the incidence and mortality rate of prostate cancer in association with obesity (103). Furthermore, the risk of high-grade nonmetastatic prostate cancer has been shown to be reduced as a result of weight reduction (103).

OSTEOARTHRITIS

Osteoarthritis (OA) is a common problem and leads to decreased mobility, lost productivity, chronic pain, and disability. Obesity has been shown to increase the risk of OA, especially in the knee and hip joints (105). OA of the knee, in turn, has been shown to reduce ambulatory capacity, exercise capacity, and quality of life (106–110).

In the Rotterdam Study (105), the progression of OA of the knee over a $6^1/_2$ year period was found to be over three times more likely in patients with BMI >27 kg/m^2. Data from a subset of elderly individuals without OA at baseline in the Framingham Heart Study (111) showed that the risk of developing knee OA over a 10-year period increased by 1.6 for each 5 unit increase in BMI.

Weight loss has been shown to significantly reduce the signs and symptoms of OA and improve functional capacity and quality of life in afflicted obese patients (112–117). A randomized study of 87 elderly adults with symptomatic OA of the knee showed those randomized to the weight loss intervention group lost 8.7% body weight (compared to no loss in the placebo group) and had significant improvement in functional status. A meta-analysis (112) of four trials (454 total patients) showed that modest weight loss (5%) was associated with lessened physical disability.

The possibility of improved pain, functional capacity, and quality of life may serve as a strong motivational factor to encourage weight reduction in appropriate patients.

NONALCOHOLIC FATTY LIVER DISEASE

Nonalcoholic fatty liver disease (NAFLD) affects 15% to 30% of the general population and up to 70% of patients with DM II (118). NAFLD is associated with obesity, hypertension, and dyslipidemia. It is a spectrum of disorders that ranges from steatosis and nonalcoholic steatohepatitis to, ultimately, cirrhosis and hepatocellular carcinoma (119). Studies (120,121) have shown that obesity is associated with NAFLD significantly and independently.

In one multivariate study (119), an increased BMI (>26.9) was shown to be the primary variable associated with NAFLD (odds ratio = 6.2). Another report (122) showed the prevalence of NAFLD in a group of Israeli people to be more common in men (38%) than women (21%) and independently associated with obesity (odds ratio = 2.9). A BMI > 30 and the lack of physical fitness were shown to be significantly and independently associated with NAFLD in a group of nonsmoking, healthy men (121).

Fortunately, weight loss may be beneficial for reducing the risk of NAFLD in obese patients (123).

OBSTRUCTIVE SLEEP APNEA

Obstructive sleep apnea (OSA) occurs in 2% to 3% of middle-aged females and 4% to 5% of middle-aged males, but its prevalence is >30% in obese patients and 50% to 98% for patients who are morbidly obese (124–126). Obesity is the most important risk factor for the development of OSA and the relative risk in obese patients is high (RR = 10) (127). Complications associated with OSA include pulmonary hypertension, right heart failure, stroke, hypertension, and cardiac arrhythmias (20).

One prospective study (125) showed a 32% increase in the apnea-hypopnea index and a sixfold increase in the odds of developing significant sleep-disordered breathing in association with a 10% weight gain during the study. Another study showed those with a 10 kg weight increase had an associated 2.5 to 5-fold increase in the risk of developing >15 respiratory events per hour (126).

Weight loss has been shown (128) to produce significant reduction in symptoms of OSA, including apnea, snoring, and daytime sleepiness.

GALLBLADDER DISEASE

An alliterative characterization of those at higher risk for gallbladder disease is that they are fat, forty, female, fertile, and flatulent. It is a common cause of hospitalization for women and significantly adds to overall health care costs (129).

A study (129) of more than one million English and Scottish women showed a strong association between gallbladder disease and obesity. After adjusting the data to account for other factors (age, socioeconomic status, etc.), subjects having a higher BMI were more likely to be admitted for gallbladder disease and to have longer hospital stays than their thinner counterparts. Twenty-five percent of hospital days for gallbladder disease were attributed to obesity.

The risk of gallbladder disease is also increased in men who are obese. In the Health Professions Follow-Up study of men originally free of gallbladder disease (130), those with a BMI > 28.5 kg/m^2 were at 2.5 times greater risk of having gallstones. Both overweight and obesity were associated with significant increase in the risk (OR = 1.86 and 3.38, respectively) of developing symptomatic gallstones in a study of Swedish twins (131).

MENTAL HEALTH ISSUES

The National Epidemiologic Survey on Alcohol and Related Conditions (132) showed that BMI was significantly associated with anxiety, mood, and personality disorders. The lifetime prevalence of major depressive disorder (MDD), specifically, was increased 1.5 to 2 fold among obese individuals compared to normal weight subjects. The odds ratio for a psychiatric disorder was similarly elevated in the study group.

The 2006 Behavioral Risk Factor Surveillance System (133) included data for more than 200,000 individuals. It showed that the prevalence of moderate or severe MDD increased from 6.5% to 25.9% with an increase in BMI from 25 to 35 kg/m^2. Similarly, the prevalence of obesity increased from 25.4% among those without MDD to 57.8% in those with moderate-to-severe MDD.

The nature of the relationship between MDD and obesity is unclear and may be multifactoral. Obese individuals are subject to ridicule, rejection, and other forms of bias and negative stereotyping in our society. Many psychotropic medications are associated with weight gain. Food, especially high carbohydrate and high fat items, is often used as to "comfort" in times of emotional need.

Weight loss may improve depression in many individuals. Some patients will benefit from a change in their psychotropic medications to alternatives that are more weight neutral. There has been a suggestion that an anorectic agent, such as phentermine or diethlypropion, may help alleviate the symptoms of depression (134). The clinician must work carefully with people who use their weight or food consumption as an important emotional defense mechanism (e.g., abuse victims). A nonjudgmental, compassionate physician functions as an extremely valuable part of a potentially life-changing pursuit of their obese patient, particularly in those whose weight is creating, or worsening, major social or emotional challenges.

FINAL THOUGHTS

Obesity is a medical condition with numerous comorbidities and deserves to be approached as a serious health threat. It has reached epidemic proportions and is continuing to increase in prevalence, and recent estimates place obesity-related health expenditures at $147 billion (135). The days of simply handing the patient a preprinted 1000-calorie diet plan with the admonition to "push away from the table" have passed. Overweight patients deserve competent, compassionate, and comprehensive treatment by medical personnel who are willing to take the time and have the patience to see them through a long-term treatment regimen.

REFERENCES

1. Allon N. The stigma of overweight in everyday life. In: Wolman BB, DeBerry S, eds. Psychological Aspects of Overweight: A Handbook. New York: Van Nostrand Reinhold, 1982:130–174.
2. Weiner B. Judgements of Responsibility: A Theory of Social Conduct. New York: The Guilford Press, 1955.
3. Pingitore R, Dugoni BL, Tindale RS, et al. Bias against overweight job applicants in a simulated employment interview. J Appl Psychol 1994; 79:909–917.
4. Roehling MV. Weight-based discrimination in employment: Psychological and legal aspects. Pers Psychol 1999; 52:969–1016.
5. Canning H, Mayer J. Obesity: An influence on high school performance? Am J Clin Nutr 1967; 20:352–354.
6. Hebl MR, Heatherton TF. The stigma of obesity: The differences are black and white. Pers Soc Psychol Bull 1997; 24:417–526.
7. Hebl MR, Xu J. Weighing the care: Physician's reactions to the size of a patient. Int J Obes 2001; 25:1246–1252.
8. Harvey EL, Hill AJ. Health professionals' views of overweight people and smokers. Int J Obes 2001; 25:1253–1261.
9. Maddox GL, Back K, Liederman V. Overweight as social deviance and disability. J Health Soc Behav 1968; 9:287–298.
10. Breytspraak LM, McGee J, Conger JC, et al. Sensitizing medical students to impression formation processes in the patient interview. J Med Educ 1977; 52:47–54.
11. Blumberg P, Mellis LP. Medical students attitudes toward the obese and morbidly obese. Int J Eat Disord 1985; 4:169–175.
12. Price JH, Desmond SM, Krol RA, et al. Family practice physicians beliefs, attitudes and practices regarding obesity. Am J Prev Med 1987; 3:339–345.
13. Bagley CR, Conklin DN, Isherwood RT, et al. Attitudes of nurses toward obesity and obese patients. Percept Mot Skills 1989; 68:954.
14. Peternelj-Taylor CA. The effects of patient weight and sex on nurses' perceptions: A proposed model of nurse withdrawal. J Adv Nurs 1989; 14:744–754.
15. Oberrieder H, Walker R, Monroe D, et al. Attitude of dietetics students and registered dietitians toward obesity. J Am Diet Assoc 1995; 95:914–916.
16. Young LM, Powelll B. The effects of obesity on the clinical judgments of mental health professionals. J Heath Soc Behav 1985; 26:233–246.
17. Ferrante JM, Piasecki AK, Ohman-Strickland PA, et al. Family physicians' practices and attitudes regarding care of extremely obese patients. Obesity (Silver Spring) 2009; 17:1710–1716.
18. Kaminsky J, Gadaleta D. A study of discrimination within the medical community as viewed by obese patients. Obes Surg 2002; 12:14–18.
19. Mokdad AH, Marks JS, Stroup DF, et al. Actual causes of death in the United States, 2000. JAMA 2004; 291:1238–1245.
20. Pi-Sunyer X. The medical risks of obesity. Postgrad Med 2009; 121(6):21–33.
21. Mafong D, Henry RR. Pathophysiology and complications of type 2 diabetes. Pract Diabetol 2009; 6:13–26.
22. Sullivan PW, Ghushchyan V, Ben-Joseph RH. The effect of obesity and cardiometabolic risk factors on expenditures and productivity in the Unites States. Obesity (Silver Spring) 2008; 16:2155–2162.
23. Huang ES, Basu A, O'Grady M, et al. Projecting the future diabetes population size and related costs for the U.S. Diabetes Care 2009; 32(12):2225–2229.
24. Weir GC, Laybutt DR, Kaneto H, et al. Beta-cell adaption and decompensation during the progression of diabetes. Diabetes 2001; 50(suppl 1):S154–S159.
25. Astrup A. Healthy lifestyles in Europe: Prevention of obesity and type II diabetes by diet and physical activity. Public Health Nutr 2001; 4(2B):499–515.
26. Perrini S, Leonardini A, Laviola L, et al. Biological specificity of visceral adipose tissue and therapeutic intervention. Arch Physiol Biochem 2008; 114:277–286.
27. Hevener AL, Febbraio MA; the Stock Conference Working Group. The 2009 Stock Conference Report: Inflammation, obesity, and metabolic disease [published online ahead of print December 11, 2009]. Obes Rev. DOI: 10.1111/j.1467-789X.2009.00691.x.
28. Abdul-Ghani MA, DeFronzo RA. Mitochondrial dysfunction, insulin resistance, and type 2 diabetes mellitus. Curr Diab Rep 2008; 8:173–178.
29. Knowler WC, Barrett-Conner E, Fowler SE, et al.; on behalf of the Diabetes Prevention Program Research Group. Reduction in the incidence of type 2 diabetes with lifestyle intervention or metformin. N Engl J Med 2002; 346:393–403.

30. Wadden TA, Berkowitz RI, Womble LG, et al. Randomized trial of lifestyle modification and pharmacotherapy for obesity. N Engl J Med. 2005; 353:2111–2120.
31. Dixon JB, Obrien PE. Health outcomes of severely obese type 2 diabetic subjects 1 year after laparoscopic adjustable gastric banding. Diabetes Care 2002; 25:358–363.
32. Buchwald H, Estok R, Fahrback K, et al. Weight and type 2 diabetes after bariatric surgery: Systematic review and meta-analysis. Am J Med 2009; 1222:248–256.
33. Must A, Spadano J, Coakley EH, et al. The disease burden associated with overweight and obesity. JAMA 1999; 282(16):1523–1529.
34. Klein S, Burke LE, Bray GA, et al.; American Heart Association Council on Nutrition, Physical Activity and Metabolism. Clinical implications of obesity with specific focus on cardiovascular disease: A statement for professionals from the American Heart Association Council on Nutrition, Physical Activity, and Metabolism: Endorsed by the American College of Cardiology Foundation. Circulation 1004; 110(8):2952–2967.
35. Wilson PW, D'Agostina RB, Sullivan L, et al. Overweight and obesity as determinants of cardiovascular risk: The Framingham experience. Arch Intern Med 2002; 162(16):1867–1872.
36. Fox CS, Pencina MJ, Wilson PW, et al. Lifetime risk of cardiovascular disease among individuals with and without diabetes stratified by obesity status in the Framingham heart study. Diabetes Care 2008; 31(8):1582–1584.
37. Balkau B, Deanfield JE, Despres JP, et al. International Day for the Evaluation of Abdominal Obesity (IDEA): A study of waist circumference, cardiovascular disease, and diabetes mellitus in 168,000 primary care patients in 63 countries. Circulation 2007; 116(7):1942–1951.
38. Wannamethee SG, Shaper AG, Walker M. Overweight and obesity and weight change in middle aged men: Impact on cardiovascular disease and diabetes. J Epidemiol Community Health 1005; 59(2):134–139.
39. Poierier P, Eckel RH. Obesity and cardiovascular disease. Curr Atheroscler Rep 2002; 4:448–453.
40. Poirier P, Eckel RH. The heart and obesity. In: Fuster V, Alexander RS, King S, et al., eds. Hurst's The Heart. New York: McGraw-Hill Companies, 2000:2289–2303.
41. deDivitiis O, Fazio S, Petitto M, et al. Obesity and cardiac function. Circulation 1981; 4:447–482.
42. Nakajima T, Fujioka S, Tokunaga K, et al. Correlation of intra-abdominal fat accumulation and left ventricular performance in obesity. Am J Cardio 1989; 64:369–373.
43. Kortelainen ML. Myocardial infarction and coronary pathology in severely obese people examined at autopsy. Int J Obes Relat Metab Disord 2002; 26:73–79.
44. He J, Ogden LG, Bazzano LA, et al. Risk factors for congestive heart failure in US men and women: NHANES I epidemiologic follow-up study. Arch Intern Med 2001; 161:996–1002.
45. Kenchaiah S, Evans JC, Levy D, et al. Obesity and the risk of heart failure. N Engl J Med 2002; 347:305–313.
46. Chen YT, Vaccarino V, Williams CS, et al. Risk factors for heart failure in the elderly: A prospective community-based study. Am J Med 1999; 10:605–612.
47. Wilhelmsen L, Rosengren A, Eriksson H, et al. Heart failure in the general population of men: Morbidity, risk factors and prognosis. J Inter Med 2001; 249:253–261.
48. Horwich TB, Fonarow GC, Hamilton MA, et al. The relationship between obesity and mortality in patients with heart failure. J Am Coll Cardiol 2001; 38:780–795.
49. Osman AF, Mehra MR, Lavie CH, et al. The incremental prognostic importance of body fat adjusted peak oxygen consumption in chronic heart failure. J Am Coll Cardiol 2000; 36:2126–2131.
50. Lissin LW, Gauri AJ, Froelicher VF, et al. The prognostic value of body mass index and standard exercise testing in male veterans with congestive heart failure. J Card Fail 2002; 8:206–215.
51. Davos CH, Doehner W, Rauchhaus M, et al. Body mass and survival in patients with chronic heart failure without cachexia: The importance of obesity. J Card Fail 2003; 9:29–55.
52. Lavie CJ, Osman AF, Milani RV, et al. Body composition and prognosis in chronic systolic heart failure: The obesity paradox. Am J Cardiol 2003; 91:91–894.
53. Mosterd A, Cost B, Hoes AW, et al. The prognosis of heart failure in the general population: The Rotterdam Study. Eur Heart J 2001; 22:1318–1327.
54. Johnson AL, Cornini JC, Cassel JC, et al. Influences of race, sex and weight on blood pressure behavior in young adults. Am J Cardiol 1975; 35:523–530.
55. Voors AW, Webber LS, Frerichs RR, et al. Body height and body mass as determinants of basal blood pressure in children: The Bogalusa Heart Study. Am J Epidemiol 1977; 106:101–108.
56. Stamler R, Stamler J, Riedlinger WF, et al. Weight and blood pressure: Findings in hypertension screening of 1 million Americans. JAMA 1978; 240:1607–1610.
57. National Institutes of Health. Clinical guidelines on the identification, evaluation, and treatment of overweight and obesity in adults: The evidence report. Obes Res 1998; 6(suppl 2):51S–209S.

58. Brown CD, Higgins M, Donato KA, et al. Body mass index and the prevalence of hypertension and dyslipidemia. Obes Res 2000; 8:605–619.
59. Dreyvold WB, Midthjell K, Nilsen J. Change in body mass index and its impact on blood pressure: A prospective population study. Int J Obes (Lond) 2005; 29(6):650–655.
60. Schotte DE, Stunkard AJ. The effects of weight reduction on blood pressure in 301 obese patients. Arch Intern Med 1990; 150:1701–1704.
61. Novi RF, Porta M, Lamberto M, et al. Reductions of body weight and blood pressure in obese hypertensive patients treated by diet. A retrospective study. Panminerva Med 1989; 31:13–15.
62. Staessen J, Fagard R, Amery A. The relationship between body weight and blood pressures. J Hum Hypertens 1988; 2:207–217.
63. Lavie CJ, Milani RV, Ventura HO. Obesity and cardiovascular disease. J Am Coll Cardiol 2009; 53(21):1925–1932.
64. Poirier P, Giles TD, Bray GA, et al. Obesity and cardiovascular disease: Pathophysiology, evaluation, and effect of weight loss; an update of the 1997 American Heart Association Scientific Statement on Obesity and Heart Disease from the Obesity Committee of the Council on Nutrition, Physical Activity, and Metabolism. Circulation 2006; 113:898–918.
65. Hirsch J, Leibel RL, Mackintosh R, et al. Heart rate variability as a measure of autonomic function during weight change in humans. Am J Physiol 1991; 261:R1418–R1423.
66. Kannel Wb, Kannel C, Paffenbarger RS Jr, et al. Heart rate and cardiovascular mortality: The Framingham Study. Am Heart J 1987; 113:1489–1494.
67. Seccareccia F, Pannozzo F, Dima F, et al. Malattie Cardiovascolari Aterosclerotiche Istituto Superiore di Sanita Project. Heart rate as a predictor of mortality: The MATISS project. Am J Public Health 2001; 91:1258–1263.
68. La Rovere MT, Bigger JT Jr, Marcus FI, et al. Baroreflex sensitivity and heart-rate variability in prediction of total cardiac mortality after myocardial infarction. ATRAMI (Autonomic Tone and Reflexes After Myocardial Infarction) Investigators. Lancet 1998; 351:478–484.
69. Poirier P, Hernandez TL, Weil KM, et al. Impact of diet-induced weight loss on the cardiac autonomic nervous system in severe obesity. Obes Res 2003; 11:1040–1047.
70. McGill HC Jr, McMahan CA, Herderick EE, et al. Origin of atherosclerosis in childhood and adolescence. Am J Clin Nutr 2000; 72:1307S–1315S.
71. Berenson GS. Bogalusa Heart Study: A long-term community study of a rural biracial (black/white) population. Am J Med Sci 2001; 322:267–274.
72. Enos WF, Holmes RH, Beyer J. Coronary disease among United States soldiers killed in action in Korea. JAMA 1953; 152:1090–1093.
73. McGill HC Jr, McMahan CA, Malcom GT, et al. Relation of glycohemoglobin and adiposity to atherosclerosis in youth. Pathobioliological Determinants of Atherosclerosis in Youth (PDAY) Research Group. Arterioscler Thromb Vasc Biol 1995; 15:431–440.
74. Rabkin SW, Mathewson FA, Hsu PH. Relation of body weight to development ischemic heart disease in a cohort of young North American men after a 26 year observation period: The Manitoba Study. Am J Cardiol 1977; 39:452–458.
75. Hubert HB, Feinleib M, McNamara PM, et al. Obesity as an independent risk factor for cardiovascular disease: A 26-year follow-up of participants in the Framingham Heart Study. Circulation 1983; 67:968–977.
76. Manson JE, Colditz GA, Stampfer MJ, et al. A prospective study of obesity and risk of coronary heart disease in women. N Engl J Med 1990; 322:882–889.
77. Fontaine KR, Redden DT, Wang C, et al. Years of life lost due to obesity. JAMA 2003; 289:187–193.
78. Dagenais GR, Yi Q, Mann JF, et al. Prognostic impact of body weight and abdominal obesity in women and men with cardiovascular disease. Am Heart J 2005; 149:54–60.
79. Kragelund C, Hassager C, Hildebrandt P, et al. TRACE study group. Impact of obesity on long-term prognosis following acute myocardial infarction. Int J Cardiol 2005; 98:123–131.
80. Abbott RD, Behrens GR, Sharp DS, et al. Body mass index and thromboembolic stroke in nonsmoking men in older middle age: The Honolulu Heart Program. Stroke 1994; 25:2370–2376.
81. Rhoads GG, Kagan A. The relation of coronary disease, stroke, and mortality to weight in youth and in middle age. Lancet 1983; 1:492–495.
82. Shinton R, Shipley M, Rose G. Overweight and stroke in the Whitehall study. J Epidemiol Community Health 1991; 45:138–142.
83. Rexrode KM, Hennekens CH, Willett WC, et al. A prospective study of body mass index, weight change, and risk of stroke in women. JAMA 1997; 227:1539–1545.
84. Lapidus L, Bengtsson C, Larsson B, et al. Distribution of adipose tissue and risk of cardiovascular disease and death: A 12 year follow up of participants in the population study of women in Gothenburg, Sweden. Br Med J (Clin Res Ed) 1984; 289:1257–1261.

85. Folsom AR, Prineas RJ, Kaye SA, et al. Incidence of hypertension and stroke in relation to body fat distribution and other risk factors in older women. Stroke 1990; 21:701–706.
86. Terry RB, Page WF, Haskell WL. Waist/hip ratio, body mass index and premature cardiovascular disease mortality in US Army veterans during a twenty-three year follow-up study. Int J Obes Relat Metab Disord 1992; 16:417–423.
87. Walker SP, Rimm EB, Ascherio A, et al. Body size and fat distribution as predictors of stroke among US men. Am J Epidemiol 1996; 144:1143–1150.
88. Pyorala M, Miettinen H, Lasko M, et al. Hyperinsulinemia and the risk of stroke in healthy middle-aged men: The 22-year follow-up results of the Helsinki Policemen Study. Stroke 1998; 29:1860–1866.
89. Kurth T, Gaziano JM, Berger K, et al. Body mass index and the risk of stroke in men. Arch Intern Med 2002; 162:2557–2562.
90. Rost NS, Wolf PA, Kase CS, et al. Plasma concentration of C-reactive protein and risk of ischemic stroke and transient ischemic attack: The Framingham study. Stroke 2001; 32:2575–2579.
91. Sriram K, Benkovic SA, Miller DB, et al. Obesity exacerbates chemically induced neurodegeneration. Neuroscience 2002; 115:1335–1346.
92. Reaven GH. Role of insulin in human disease. Diabetes 1988; 37:1595–1607.
93. Gao W; DECODE Study Group. Does the constellation of risk factors with and without abdominal adiposity associate with different cardiovascular mortality risk? Int J Obes 2008; 32(5):757–762.
94. Ilanne-Parikka P, Eriksson JG, Lindstrom J, et al.; Finnish Diabetes Prevention Study Group. Effect of lifestyle intervention on the occurrence of metabolic syndrome and its components in the Finnish Diabetes Prevention Study. Diabetes Care 2008; 31(4):805–807.
95. Phelan S, Wadden TA, Berkowitz RI, et al. Impact of weight loss on the metabolic syndrome. Int J Obes 2007; 31:1442–1448.
96. Sours HE, Frattali VP, Brand CD, et al. Sudden death associated with very low calorie weight reduction regimens. Am J Clin Nutr 1981; 34:453–461.
97. Isner JM, Sours HE, Pari AL, et al. Sudden unexpected death in avid dieters using the liquid-protein-modified-fast diet. Observations in 17 patients and the role of the prolonged QU interval. Circulation 1979; 60:1401–1412.
98. Drenick EJ, Fisler JS. Sudden cardiac arrest in morbidly obese surgical patients unexplained after autopsy. Am J Surg 1988; 155:720–726.
99. Shape Up America! and American Obesity Association. Guidance for Treatment of Adult Obesity. Bethesda, MD: Shape Up America!, 1996.
100. Thygesen LC, Grenbaek M, Johansen C, et al. Prospective weight change and colon cancer risk in male US health professionals. Int J Cancer 2008; 123(5):1160–1165.
101. Calle EE, Rodriguez C, Walker-Thurmond K, et al. Overweight, obesity, and mortality from cancer in a prospectively studied cohort of US adults. N Engl J Med 2003; 348(17):1625–1638.
102. Reeves GK, Pirie K, Beral V, et al.; Million Women Study Collaboration. Cancer incidence and mortality in relation to body mass index in the Million Women Study: Cohort study. BMJ 2007; 335(7630):1134.
103. Wright ME, Chang SC, Schatzkin A, et al. Prospective study of adiposity and weight change in relation to prostate cancer incidence and mortality. Cancer 2007; 109(4):675–684.
104. Rodriguez C, Freedland SJ, Deka A, et al. Body mass index, weight change, and risk of prostate cancer in the Cancer Prevention Study II Nutrition Cohort. Cancer Epidemiol Biomarkers Prev 2007; 16(1):63–69.
105. Reijman M, Pols HA, Bergink AP, et al. Body mass index associated with onset and progression of osteoarthritis of the knee but not of the hip: The Rotterdam Study. Ann Rheum Dis 2007; 66(2):158–162.
106. Creamer P, Lethbridge-Cejku M, Hochberg MC. Factors associated with functional impairment in symptomatic knee osteoarthritis. Rheumatology 2000; 39(5):490–496.
107. Jinks C, Jordan K, Croft P. Disabling knee pain—Another consequence of obesity: Results from a prospective cohort study. BMC Public Health 2006; 6:258.
108. Marks R. Obesity profiles with knee osteoarthritis: correlation with pain, disability, disease progression. Obesity (Silver Spring) 2007; 15(7):1867–1874.
109. Sutbeyaz ST, Sezer N, Koseoglu BF, et al. Influence of knee osteoarthritis on exercise capacity and qualify of life in obese adults. Obesity (Silver Spring) 2007; 15(8):2071–2076.
110. Tukker A, Visscher T, Picavet H. Overweight and health problems of lower extremities: Osteoarthritis, pain and disability. Public Health Nutr 2009; 12(3):359–368.
111. Felson DT, Zhang Y, Hannan MT, et al. Risk factors for incident radiographic knee osteoarthritis in the elderly: The Framingham Study. Arthritis Rheum 1997; 40(4):728–733.

112. Christensen R, Bartels EM, Astrip A, et al. Effect of weigh reduction in obese patients diagnosed with knee osteoarthritis: A systematic review and meta-analysis. Ann Rheum Dis 2007; 66(4):433–439.
113. Fransen M. Dietary weight loss and exercise for obese adults with knee osteoarthritis: Modest weight loss targets, mild exercise, modest effects. Arthritis Rheum 2004; 50(5):1366–1369.
114. Huang MH, Chen CH, Chen TW, et al. The effects of weight reduction on the rehabilitation of patients with knee osteoarthritis and obesity. Arthritis Care Res 2000; 13(6):398–405.
115. Messier SP, Loeser RF, Miller GD, et al. Exercises and dietary weight loss in overweight and obese older adults with knee osteoarthritis: The Arthritis, Diet and Activity Promotion Trial. Arthritis Rheum 2004; 50(5):1501–1510.
116. Miller GD, Nicklas BJ, Davis C, et al. Intensive weight loss program improves physical function in older obese adults with knee osteoarthritis. Obesity (Silver Spring) 2006; 14(7):1219–1230.
117. VanGool CH, Penninx BW, Kempen GI, et al. Effects of exercise adherence on physical function among overweight older adults with knee osteoarthritis. Arthritis Rheum 2005; 53(1):24–32.
118. Targher G, Arcaro G. Non-alcoholic fatty liver disease and increased risk of cardiovascular disease. Atherosclerosis 2007; 191(2):235–240.
119. Preiss D, Sattar N. Non-alcoholic fatty liver disease: An overview of prevalence, diagnosis, pathogenesis and treatment considerations. Clin Sci (Lond) 2008; 115(5):141–150.
120. Riquelme A, Arrese M, Soza A, et al. Non-alcoholic fatty liver disease and its association with obesity, insulin resistance and increased serum levels of C-reactive protein in Hispanics. Liver Int 2009; 29(1):82–88.
121. Church TS, Kuk JL, Ross R, et al. Association of cardiorespiratory fitness, body mass index, and waist circumference to nonalcoholic fatty liver disease. Gastroenterology 2006; 130(7):2023–2030.
122. Zelber-Sagi S, Nitzan-Kaluski D, Halpert Z, et al. Prevalence of primary non-alcoholic fatty liver disease in a population-based study and its association with biochemical and anthropometric measures. Liver Int 2006; 26(7):856–863.
123. Adams LA, Angulo P. Treatment of non-alcoholic fatty liver disease. Postgrad Med J 2006; 82(967): 315–322.
124. Resta O, Foschino-Barbaro MP, Legari G, et al. Sleep-related breathing disorders, loud snoring and excessive daytime sleepiness in obese subjects. Int J Obes Relat Metab Disord 2001; 25(5):669–675.
125. Peppard PE, Young T, Palta M, et al. Longitudinal study of moderate weight change and sleep-disordered breathing. JAMA 2000; 284(23):3015–3021.
126. Newman AB, Foster G, Givelber R, et al. Progression and regression of sleep-disordered breathing with changes in weight: The Sleep Heart Health Study. Arch Intern Med 2005; 165(20):2408–2413.
127. Pillar G, Shehadeh N. Abdominal fat and sleep apnea: The chicken or the egg? Diabetes Care 2008; 31(suppl 2):S303–S309.
128. Grunstein RR, Stenlof K, Hedner JA, et al. Two year reduction in sleep apnea symptoms and associated diabetes incidence after weight loss in severe obesity. Sleep 2007; 30(6):703–710.
129. Liu B, Balkwill A, Spencer E, et al.; Million Women Study Collaborators. Relationship between body mass index and length of hospital stay for gallbladder disease. J Public Health (Oxf) 2008; 30(2):161–166.
130. Tsai CJ, Leitzmann MF, Willett WC, et al. Prospective study of abdominal adiposity and gallstone disease in US men. Am J Clin Nutr 2004; 80(1):38–44.
131. Katsika D, Tuvblad C, Einarsson C, et al. Body mass index, alcohol, tobacco and symptomatic gallstone disease: A Swedish twin study. J Intern Med 2007; 262(5):581–587.
132. Petry NM, Barry D, Pietrzak RH, et al. Overweight and obesity are associated with psychiatric disorders: Results from the National Epidemiologic Survey on Alcohol and Related Conditions. Psychosom Med 2008; 70(3):288–297.
133. Strine TW, Mokdad AH, Dube SR, et al. The association of depression and anxiety with obesity and unhealthy behaviors among community dwelling US adults. Gen Hosp Psychiatry 2008; 30(2):127–137.
134. Meldman MJ. Diet medications as useful antidepressants. Am J Bariatric Med 2009; 24(1):234–235.
135. Finkelstein EA, Trogdon JG, Cohen JW, et al. Annual medical spending attributable to obesity: Payer-and service-specific estimates. Health Aff (Millwood) 2009; 28(5):w822–w831.

4 Evaluation of the obese patient

James T. Cooper

APPROACH TO THE PATIENT

The importance of how you interact with your patients who are obese cannot be emphasized enough. Your success or failure as a treating physician, or member of a treatment team, is often determined during the first encounter with the patient. The unspoken communication that you send to your patient can be stronger than the actual words spoken by you. An unconscious shrug of your shoulders, a smile that is taken as a smirk, a look of disbelief, or any of dozens of gestures and expressions can turn the patient off. This could happen in spite of your genuine desire to help the patient.

The first thing to understand about someone with a chronic obesity problem is that she (this applies to men as well, but the female pronoun will be used in this chapter exclusively) is usually accustomed to failure and rejection. You may be the latest in a long line of doctors who have all failed to be of help, for one reason or another, in the management of this person's dilemma. When you are successful, you will be the last and most effective therapist that she will ever need.

There is a widespread attitude among physicians that obesity is a self-induced condition that could be cured promptly if only each patient would exercise some self-control and just "push away from the table." Since alcoholism has been relatively destigmatized, obesity remains one of the only diseases that is perceived as a character weakness and an unwillingness to change and improve oneself.

Obesity is a disease that is difficult to treat successfully; therefore, doctors who cannot help their obese patients to become slim may turn to blaming the patient entirely for the failure. They may unconsciously reject the patient, just as many physicians have difficulties dealing with the terminally ill. The doctor's professional sense of omnipotence and omniscience can be threatened. Many doctors will send an obese patient off with a diet sheet, a pat on the shoulder, and perhaps a month's supply of anorectic agents, along with the admonition to "not come back until you lose 10 lb."

It is no wonder that the doctor who is successful in treating overweight patients soon has a crowded waiting room. Word soon gets out that this doctor, while not promising miracles, at least promises tolerance, understanding of the problem, and a sensible approach that will have a better than even chance at success.

The initial interview and history should be conducted in an atmosphere of understanding, respect, and kindness. The patient should not be patronized during this or any other visit to your office. This will turn off the flow of information that is so vital to your success with her. The sexual history and the food contact history are somewhat neglected in other medical work-ups, but could be quite productive when working with overweight patients. The food contact history does not have to be part of the initial work-up, but can be compiled and evaluated by the use of diaries and food contact interviews as treatment proceeds.

Many patients will be anxious when they first come to your office. Being in a strange office produces part of the anxiety, and part is related to the fact that you are going to "take food away" from them. In this type of setting, it is often best to be kind and patient with an obese patient. Even if you have to repeat or explain something two or three times because of anxiety-generated poor attention, be helpful and considerate of her feelings.

A good way to get a lot of data quickly is to have the patient fill out, when practical, the history form before you see her for the initial interview. There is even software now available so that people can do this before the clinic visit over the Internet. If there is difficulty with reading or writing on the patient's part, you might have to have one of your staff go through the questions with them. It is then important for you to take the completed form and review it with the patient. Make notes on the areas of the sheets where the answers were given, or on a separate place in the problem list that could be attached to the history. Many offices make use of yellow highlighter markers to point out the important positive responses in the body of the history. Notes in the doctor's handwriting are in black, for further information on positive responses, and in red when medications and/or allergies are mentioned.

You can then summarize the history by listing problems that are active and important to the present management of the patient. Medications and their frequency of use are listed. Impressions of the patient's apparent strengths and weaknesses are important to note at each visit. Sometimes you will be wrong, but a string of regular visits with the treatment team can often uncover most of the pressing problems that need to be addressed before each patient can learn to deal with her eating problem.

The description of the history and physical examination conducted on a beginning bariatric patient may seem familiar, but certain elements deserve special attention. Bariatrics, or medical weight control, could be considered a branch of internal medicine or family practice or gynecology. The bariatrician is a physician and should still practice medicine, including an excellent history, physical, and laboratory work-up, and proper follow-through. Anything less than excellent is not acceptable for this extremely neglected segment of the patient population, the obese. Of course, the history and physical procedures given here will need to be suited to your style of practice and to the patient's individual medical conditions.

THE HISTORY

The bariatric history has unique aspects that enable the bariatrician to identify underlying comorbidities and to develop an individualized treatment plan to optimize the patient's likelihood of success. The main purpose of the history is to understand what has happened in the past, and what is happening to this patient now. Without this "big picture" understanding, you can give all the diets to her that you want, and you will almost never produce lasting weight loss. Most practitioners use a standard medical history format.

The first task is to understand what the individual's goals and needs are in a weight loss program. Many practitioners use an open-ended question for this or questions pertaining to desired weight, monthly weight loss goal, clothes size. If it appears that the weight loss goals are not realistic, then work to make the goals become realistic will be needed. Special questions regarding the weight loss history, what has and has not worked are important to include. As bariatric surgery has been used for decades, some of your patients may even already have had some sort of surgical procedure for weight loss. Many malabsorptive procedures require ongoing nutritional and vitamin supplementation. Some sort of assessment of daily physical activity and/or exercise is needed.

The medical history will often reveal common conditions that accompany obesity like prediabetes (glucose intolerance), hypertension, type 2 diabetes, metabolic syndrome, insulin resistance, nonalcoholic fatty liver disease, hyperlipidemia, hypothyroidism, and obstructive sleep apnea. The review of systems will likely find lack of energy, some degree of shortness of breath, joint pains, snoring or spouse complaint of snoring. Sometimes there is a "positive review of systems" due to the multisystem effects of obesity.

It is important to state clearly that any information given to the clinic will be kept confidential and not shared with other doctors or insurance companies unless the patient specifically gives permission. This is also a good time to ask the patient to be candid and honest, as you are trying to work together toward the same goal of weight loss.

THE PHYSICAL EXAMINATION

In most disciplines of medical practice, the physical examination, or *laying on of hands*, can make or break a doctor–patient relationship. You can usually establish immediate rapport by meeting the patient prior to the physical examination and greeting her in a friendly manner. Most physicians have the patient fill out a history form, and then discuss the positive and significant answers with the patient prior to the physical examination. In my experience, it is better to go over the discussion of the history first with the patient fully clothed, and THEN conduct the physical examination after the patient changes into a gown. A careful look at the history will help you decide how you approach certain examinations conducted during the physical examination. Obtaining a comprehensive history and review of systems shows your genuine interest and makes it easier to spot and identify early problems that may impede progress.

Keep in mind that specific findings on the physical examination may be reflective of any medical problem, though the obese patient has a greater likelihood of having diabetes, vascular disease, skin problems, cancer, cataracts, and other medical comorbidities of obesity. I highly recommend that you have the patient change into a gown and to examine all body areas, just as you would on anyone else who gets a comprehensive examination from you. Again, your thoroughness will be rewarded by identifying problems in advance and your patients will be likely to refer their friends. Some clues about the weight gain can be obtained by inspecting the belt for new holes (rapid weight gain) or looking for the "well-worn" hole (slow weight gain). Some practitioners use their clinical judgment to abbreviate some parts of the examination as necessary.

Be sure that there is ample light in the room and that the patient is not too hot or too cold. I have observed that many heavy patients are extremely sensitive to cold. Be sure to have appropriate sized gowns and chairs that accommodate your patients (bariatric chairs, sofa, or chairs without arms). A blanket (for security or warmth) that the patient can get without getting off the table will be greatly appreciated. Proper instruments are those found in any standard examination room, but should include an ophthalmoscope, an otoscope, a gooseneck sinus illuminator, tongue blades, a stethoscope with a nonchill head, cotton balls, a dull safety pin, a reflex hammer, and a floor lamp with an aimable light beam.

The table should be wide and sturdy enough for an obese person. Some physicians have one that sits on "4 by 4" legs and is 42 in. wide and 72 in. long, with heavy and thick padding. It can hold patients who weigh over 600 lb. This design has to be custom made for your office, but costs less than the standard table. This type of table can also double as an extra pediatric examination table for those who see children too.

Pertinent negatives are as important as positive findings in order to show that this part of the physical examination was performed. Documenting each item properly will avoid confusion and prevent the overlooking of each important and possibly treatable item.

Skin

The complete dermal examination includes inspection of the axillae, the groin, and between the toes. Checking the intertriginous areas under the breast, under the abdominal panniculus if present, and in the groin and buttocks area is prudent. These areas are often the site of maceration, discoloration, and infection that could point out a diabetic condition in its early stages.

Acanthosis nigricans is a velvety black to light brown maculopapular lesion commonly found in the axillae, groin, or the side or rear of the neck. Acanthosis nigricans is associated with insulin resistance or type 2 diabetes mellitus, so its presence warrants testing for these conditions.

The scalp and hair can provide much information about the nutritional status of the patient, not to mention alerting you to the presence of psoriasis, seborrhea, and general dryness or oiliness of the skin. Hypothyroidism can lead to thinning of the lateral third of the eyebrows and general skin changes of dryness and scaliness. The area behind the neck and on the upper surface and posterior of the pinna may have had a lot of sun exposure and are good places to look for possible malignancies. Lesions and nevi on the palms of the hands and the soles of the feet should be looked for carefully. Acne may be a reflection of polycystic ovary syndrome or hypercortisolism. Hyperpigmentation can also occur with hypercortisolism.

The vascular flush area of the cheeks and the bridge of the nose should be carefully checked. Other similar areas are on the neck, the upper chest, the genital areas, and the flexor surface of the extremities. Often you may see vascular disturbances here that may tell you about systemic diseases, such as systemic lupus erythematosis.

Lipomas can be the cause of mechanical problems, or sebaceous cysts can be the source of infections in some cases. The nails can give valuable clues to systemic disease and should be checked on both hands and feet.

Eyes

A complete examination should include visual acuity, visual fields, ocular movements, a check of the external eye and the lids, and a funduscopic examination. Particular care should be taken to observe for cataracts, eyeground changes, and the state of the macula and optic nerve head in each eye. Check the intraocular pressure with a tonometer, or estimate the pressure through gentle tactile pressure. If you do not actually get a pressure measurement yourself, make sure the patient gets one on his or her next visit to an ophthalmologist. Pupillary light reflexes should be tested for, as well as accommodation changes in the pupils. Vertical nystagmus may reflect low magnesium levels.

Nose/Sinuses

The external shape of the nose may give clues to previous trauma. The mucous membranes should be checked for congestion, visible mucous (color if present), and possible erosions. A gooseneck light attached to your otoscope battery handle will enable you to look deep inside the mouth and direct your beam of light more accurately. In a totally dark examining room, it can be used to illuminate the frontal and maxillary sinuses. Place the head of the light above the infraorbital rim to see the maxillary sinuses and under the medial aspect of the supraorbital rim to see the frontal sinus areas. The hard palate and the forehead are observed to see if the sinuses illuminate.

Ears/Throat

The tongue should be checked for abnormalities of texture and color, not to mention looking for swelling and enlarged lymph nodes. A small hypopharynx is a risk factor for sleep apnea. Erosion of dental enamel and swollen parotid glands should raise the possibility of bulimia.

Neck

The thyroid, larynx, and lymph node chains should be visually inspected and palpated carefully. Goiters, nodules, and other thyroid pathology must be distinguished from a sometimes quite prominent pretracheal fat pad. A neck circumference of $\geq$17 in. in men and $\geq$16 in. in women increases the likelihood of the presence of obstructive sleep apnea. A buffalo hump fat pad suggests hypercortisolism.

Chest

A careful examination of the entire chest with inspection, palpation, percussion, and auscultation is carried out. Many overweight patients have early congestive heart failure and hypertension. Expect a decrease in vital capacity and tidal volume in extreme obesity. An increase in respiratory rate may be seen to maintain minute ventilation if the tidal volume is decreased.

Heart

Evidence of arteriosclerotic heart disease, hypertensive heart disease, and congestive heart failure would be of special interest in the examination. You should be no less thorough in a cardiac examination of an obese person than of anyone else, even though it can be difficult to move her around to conduct a complete examination, and sometimes difficult to hear heart tones.

Back

Examine the entire back, from the occipital area down to the coccyx. There is a lot of back pain in this type of patient, requiring palpation and light percussion over the vertebral area. Pilonidal sinuses and cysts are looked for, as well as old surgical scars in this lower spine area. Lightly percuss over the costophrenic angles where the kidneys are located.

Breasts

A breast examination in a massively obese female would seem to be an exercise in futility, but such is not the case—a breast examination can find abnormalities if one is careful and systematic. This means that if there is the slightest doubt, mammography and/or ultrasound studies should be considered. I recommend mammography on all obese women with a significant family history of breast cancer.

Abdomen

The abdomen of an overweight patient may have a large panniculus that overhangs the belly and pubic areas. It may be difficult or impossible to palpate the liver and spleen, but try your best. Check for ascitic fluid and hernias. Do the usual inspection, palpation, percussion, and auscultation that you would do on any other physical examination. The following gauge for the size of the pannus has been suggested: Grade 1 covers the pubic hairline but not the entire mons pubis, Grade 2 covers the entire mons pubis, Grade 3 extends to cover the upper thigh, Grade 4 extends to mid-thigh, and Grade 5 extends to the knee and beyond.

Anus/Rectum

Be especially careful in this examination for both men and women. It is difficult to conduct a careful rectal examination on a lot of overweight men and women, but I find two positions are more comfortable for them. The first position has the patient lying on his or her left side, facing away from the examiner. The patient takes the right hand and reaches around, lifting up his or her right buttock as much as possible. The examining finger is then well lubricated and the external and internal examination takes place. The second position I use places the male patient in the lithotomy position. The examination is carried out in the same way as a usual examination, except that you must palpate upward instead of downward to feel for the prostate.

Pelvic Examination

The pelvic examination is a necessary part of every obese patient's physical examination, unless another competent practitioner is following your female patient closely. The anterior abdominal fat is often quite thick and difficult to examine through. The size and texture of the uterine body and the adnexal structures can be obscured to a great degree by this heavy layer of fat. A complete examination should include the vulvar areas, and a rectovaginal palpation.

Extremities

At the time of physical examination, the color, turgor, and musculature of the arms and legs will often give you clues to other medical problems. Look for evidence of edema, passive congestion of the lower legs, pallor, cyanosis, clubbing, varicosities, and lymphedema. Many obese patients have poorly healing ulcers and scars on the lower legs, with atrophic and unhealthy skin that is thin, shiny, and full of darker pigmentation. Dry cracking heels may be from diabetes, hypothyroidism, or essential fatty acid deficiency.

Check for range of motion of all the joints from the digits to the hips and shoulders. Look for signs of arthritic swelling, particularly in the proximal and distal interphalangeal joints. Some physicians have noticed a fair number of patients with early or advanced Dupuytren's contracture. Tophi may indicate a history of gout. The pulses in all four extremities should be palpated on every patient.

Neurological Examination

A complete neurological examination includes tests for light touch, pain, proprioception, heat, and cold senses. All cranial nerves can be checked, including the olfactory senses with perfume, etc. Deep tendon reflexes are checked on all four extremities. Many doctors use the tips of two fingers, or the edge of the hand to elicit the reflexes. The hand is less threatening to a patient than a hammer and it is one less item to have to carry around to the hospital or keep in the examination room. The possibility of neuropathy from one or another problem peculiar to obesity (diabetes, etc.) makes a thorough job necessary. Particularly look for decreased sensitivity and signs of neuropathy in the lower extremities. Abnormal reflexes exhibiting a decreased relaxation time may suggest hypothyroidism or undertreatment with thyroid replacement. Hyperactive reflexes may indicate hypomagnesemia.

Mental Status

There are some observations of the mental state of the patient that are valuable during the physical and evaluation process. Orientation as to time, place, and purpose of the visit can be easily obtained. Overly friendly or hostile patients may be manifesting an underlying anxiety and acting out in their usual way. Any possible resentment of authority is noted and possibly discussed on the follow-up visit as an addressable problem that could slow down the weight loss. Dementia or delirium should raise the possibility of nutritional deficiencies, especially in the case of an individual who has had a prior surgical malabsorptive procedure.

Most of this part of the evaluation is obtained from the questions answered (or not answered) on the history. Careful and patient questioning on the part of the therapist can yield a good rapport that will permit the coverage of some potentially serious problems in the patient's lifestyle, family, work situation, or other areas of her environment.

OTHER MEASUREMENTS

Special considerations concerning the evaluation of an obese patient are discussed in this section. They include the use of proper blood pressure measurement technique, estimation of the extent of the obesity problem in each patient, the electrocardiogram, and the laboratory work needed to tailor treatment.

Blood Pressure

It is important to use an appropriately sized blood pressure cuff. If the cuff is too small, the blood pressure values obtained may be artificially elevated. The bladder length should wrap around more than two-thirds of the middle of the upper arm and the width should exceed the diameter of this point by 20%. An arm that is obviously above normal in size and circumference should be fitted with an adult thigh cuff in order to minimize distortions in measurement of the blood pressure.

Waist Circumference

The waist circumference and/or waist-to-hip ratio (WHR) are easily obtained and usually reproducible. The waist is measured at the level of the umbilicus, but without pulling the tape too tight. The hips are measured at the widest point. Divide the waist measurement by those of the hips to get the WHR. A waist circumference greater than 40 in. in men or 35 in. in women or a WHR greater than 1.0 for men or 0.8 for women is a sign of central obesity (android type or "apple shape") and higher likelihood of insulin resistance, metabolic syndrome, and other comorbidities. A WHR less than those figures indicates the gynecoid type of obesity (pear-shaped) that is less likely to be associated with the comorbidities.

The therapist who is just starting out would do well to measure the patient with a number of methods before deciding which way, or combination of ways to use. Remember to take a good look at the patients when they are disrobed. Note the relative lack or presence of muscle mass and the degree of fatness visible when the examination is being performed. The WHR will give an indication if the body shape has central obesity (android—apple shape) or lower body obesity (gynecoid—pear shape).

SEVERITY OF OVERWEIGHT OR OBESITY

Obesity is defined as an excess of total body fat—not just excess weight. For example, there are differences between a sedentary accountant who weighs 235 lb and a football player who weighs the same, even if the height is the same. Obviously, the less active accountant may have a greater percentage of his body composed of fat versus the football player with a much heavier mass of muscle tissue.

The most widely used measurement of degree of fatness in the body is the body mass index (BMI). A BMI of 24 or under is considered normal, a BMI of 24 to 27 shows a modest degree of obesity, a BMI of 27 to 30 is borderline significant obesity, and a BMI over 30 is medically significant obesity. To calculate the BMI, the weight in pounds is converted into kilograms (pounds $\times$ 0.454), the height in inches is changed into meters (inches $\times$ 0.0254). The BMI is then calculated by dividing the weight in kilograms by the square of the height in meters. The BMI can be calculated by the following formula as well: BMI $=$ 703 (weight in pounds)/(height in inches)^2. Though imperfect, the BMI does correlate well with body fat, morbidity, and mortality.

An estimate of body composition (fat mass and fat-free mass) can be obtained using bioelectrical impedance analysis (BIA). For this determination, a machine is used to introduce an imperceptible electrical current through the body and measure its conduction. The total body mass is divided into two compartments: nonconductive (fat mass) and conductive (fat-free mass: water, muscle, other tissues). Based on the amount of electrical impedance, the relative size of the different compartments can be determined. The advantages of BIA are that it is safe, rapid, easy to use, and inexpensive. Disadvantages are that it is affected by hydration status, fasting, and recent exercise and there are some difficulties applying its use to athletes, children, and the elderly. Using percent body fat, obesity is defined as >25% body fat for men and >30% body fat for women.

Here is a simple, but not always accurate, rule of thumb to estimate "normal" weight. For women, they should weigh 100 lb for being 5 ft tall and an additional 5 lb for each additional inch of height. For men, it is 106 lb for the first 5 ft and an additional 6 lb for each additional inch above. In both sexes you can vary by 10%. If frame size is small, you can subtract up to 10% and if frame size is larger, you add an additional 10%.

Skinfold thickness measurement is used at many centers, but presents some real challenges to accuracy and reproducibility. A good caliper, such as the Lange caliper, is more accurate than most. This type of precision caliper exerts the same amount of pressure at any point on its scale, thereby eliminating a major error in measuring the skinfold thickness.

THE ELECTROCARDIOGRAM

After years of reading ECGs from obese patients, what is remarkable to me is the relative lack of electrical pathology seen, even on massively obese patients. We still should look for abnormalities in rate, rhythm, axis, hypertrophy and evidence of old infarctions. Dale Dubin, in his excellent book on reading of ECGs, reminds us to check the rate and rhythm, evidence of incomplete or complete heart blocks, premature beats, QRS and T vectors, atrial or ventricular hypertrophy, and evidence of ischemia, injury, or infarction. We also look for ST or T elevation or depression and significant Q waves, QT interval, and other abnormalities indicating imbalance of potassium or calcium.

It is best to carefully do all 12 leads, plus any extra ones that are thought necessary. Care should be taken in placing the electrodes on the chest, particularly in light of the mechanical difficulties when the breasts are extremely large in size and overlay or obscure the points where the precordial leads are placed.

The examination table, such as the one recommended earlier in this chapter, should be wide enough to hold even the largest patient you might see. It is unprofessional to see a doctor or technician attempt to do an ECG when the patient has arms, legs, buttocks, back, and shoulders hanging off both sides of the table. This instability produces a nightmare of artifacts and prevents an accurate and usable tracing in many cases. Where suction cups are not used to make contact on the limb leads, it might be good to have long enough bands, or large enough clamps, to fit around the wrists and ankles of the patient.

Common indications for an EKG include: coronary risk factors, diabetes mellitus, hypertension, coronary artery disease, family history of cardiovascular disease, diuretic use, consideration of anorectic medication use. Additional cardiovascular evaluations and risk estimates may be required, depending on the degree of obesity of the patient and other factors.

THE LABORATORY EVALUATION

Laboratory tests are performed to identify metabolic problems and to tailor therapy. A fasting period of at least 10 hours prior to the drawing of the initial blood work is needed for greater accuracy in lipid measurements. Some patients will deliberately fast prior to the physical examination to impress the doctor with how "little" they weigh. A usual fasting blood profile consists of a complete blood cell count, a thyroid profile, 20 or so other tests, and a complete lipid profile that includes triglycerides, total cholesterol, HDL, and LDL. Clean-voided, midstream urine is obtained when fasting blood is drawn. If a fasting glucose of 100 or more is detected, you may want to subsequently obtain an oral glucose tolerance test of at least 2 hours duration, with determinations at 30, 60, 90, and 120 minutes following ingestion of the test meal. Fasting insulin levels should be obtained if insulin resistance is suspected. It is important that the results of every test performed be discussed with the patient, even if all the tests are within the normal range.

THE PROBLEM-ORIENTED SUMMARY

When all the history, physical, laboratory, and other data are obtained, these are put into a problem list and a differential diagnosis is created. For example, is there a possibility of a hormonal cause of obesity that requires further testing? This type of problem-oriented medical record is assembled and updated on each visit. Medication of a chronic or acute nature is documented on a separate sheet inside the front cover of the medical chart. In our office, the medications are written in red ink for more rapid spotting. When a medication is discontinued or changed a note is made to that effect (e.g., insulin discontinued and metformin 500 mg daily begun on 10-01-09). The problem-oriented summary becomes the foundation for a more thorough follow-up system for this patient. The time taken to systematically set up such a system pays dividends later in more efficient management of the patient. While the details of the work-up will vary from patient to patient, the completeness of your evaluation marks you as a caring and competent physician and helps you build valuable rapport with your patient.

BIBLIOGRAPHY

Bickley LS, ed. Bates' Guide to Physical Examination and History Taking. 10th ed. New York: Lippincott Williams & Wilkins, 2008.

Dubin, D. Rapid Interpretation of EKG's, 6th ed. Tampa, Florida: Cover Publishing Inc., 2000.

Orient JM. Sapira's Art & Science of Bedside Diagnosis. New York: Lippincott Williams & Wilkins, 2009.

Ross EJ, Linch DC. Cushing's Syndrome—Killing disease: Discriminatory value of signs and symptoms aiding early diagnosis. Lancet 1982; 2:646–649.

Simel DL, Rennie D. The Rational Clinical Examination: Evidence-Based Clinical Diagnosis. New York: McGraw-Hill, 2009.

5 Dietary treatment of the obese individual

Mary C. Vernon, Eric C. Westman, and James A. Wortman

INTRODUCTION

Overweight and obesity are high priority areas for primary care practitioners because they are associated with many comorbidities. Unfortunately, treating obesity can also be frustrating for the practitioner for want of effective therapies. We started using low-carbohydrate diets for the treatment of obesity and found that they could be just as effective as medication therapy (1). Over the past five years, numerous randomized, controlled trials have shown that low-carbohydrate diets lead to weight loss and cardiometabolic risk factor improvements (2–4).

The underlying principle by which the low-carbohydrate ketogenic diet works is the metabolic state of nutritional ketosis (5–7). When carbohydrate consumption is less than approximately 50 g per day, the body uses fatty acids and ketone bodies as its major metabolic fuels (8,9). However, when carbohydrate consumption is high, fatty acids and glucose are the major metabolic fuels. This metabolic change from using glucose to ketones has to occur to some extent for any method of adipose tissue loss to be effective, because lipolysis leads to an increase in ketone body production. One of the major hormonal changes that occurs with carbohydrate restriction is a reduction in serum insulin levels to approximately basal levels. The alteration of the insulin/glucagon ratio leads to a reduction in glycolytic/lipogenic activity and an enhancement of fatty acid/ketone utilization. In this chapter, we describe several methods that exploit nutritional ketosis, and discuss how to implement a diet in a medical outpatient practice.

WHAT IS HEALTHY NUTRITION DURING WEIGHT LOSS?

Before starting a discussion of optimal diets for weight loss, a discussion of what nutrient inputs are needed for the body's proper structure and function is appropriate. A balanced diet is one that meets all of the minimal requirements for essential nutrients, including amino acids, fatty acids, vitamins, minerals, and vitamin-like substances (Table 1). Although minimal requirements are set by governmental advisors for the general population to prevent nutritional deficiencies, the nutritional requirements during weight loss are different from the nutritional needs of the otherwise healthy individual. An optimal diet during weight loss provides all of the nutrients in a way that maintains optimal health (which may include changes in body composition) during the adipose tissue loss process. Because carbohydrates are simply a source of energy, if energy needs are otherwise met, there is no dietary need for carbohydrate intake. Because certain amino acids in protein are not made by the human body, and dietary protein is used for structure (muscle, bone connective tissue) and provides more than just an energy source, this macronutrient is indispensable. Likewise, essential fatty acids are required for optimal health. It is very important to keep in mind that there may be differences in requirements based on individual variation.

Water

Water has so many uses in the body and is so essential for human life that it must be consumed daily for optimal function. A few of the important functions that water performs are dissolving nutrients to make them accessible to cells, assisting in moving nutrients through cells, keeping mucous membranes moist, lubricating joints, evaporating for body temperature regulation, and removing waste from the body. For most people, the daily water losses are about six cups (1.5 L) of urine, two cups (0.5 L) of sweat, and one cup (0.25 L) from breathing. In sum, about nine cups (2.25 L) are required for most people each day, but the body has many regulatory systems to allow for a wide variation in water intake. Interestingly, about 20% of the water is obtained from the water in food and is generated from metabolic processes. For practical purposes, the general recommendation to "drink when you are thirsty" will suffice during the weight loss process.

Table 1 Essential Human Nutrients

- Vitamins: A, B1 (thiamine), B2 (riboflavin), B3 (niacin), B5 (pantothenic acid), B6 (pyridoxine), B7 (biotin), B9 (folic acid), B12 (cyanocobalamin), C (ascorbic acid), D, E, K
- Minerals: calcium, phosphorus, magnesium, iron
- Trace minerals: zinc, copper, manganese, iodine, selenium, molybdenum, chromium
- Electrolytes: sodium, potassium, chloride
- Amino acids: histidine, isoleucine, leucine, lysine, methionine, phenylalanine, threonine, tryptophan, valine
- Essential fatty acids: linoleic, α-linolenic

Protein

Protein is the major structural component of the human body. Dietary protein is the source of amino acids to provide the "building blocks" to make the proteins, and when used for energy, burned in a bomb calorimeter, contains 4 kcal/g. Protein is required in the human diet because there are nine essential amino acids that the body cannot manufacture by itself ("essential" means that the body is unable to synthesize the nutrient). While maintenance dietary protein needs are estimated to be from 0.7 to 1.0 mg/kg/day, 1.2 to 1.5 g/kg lean body weight of dietary protein is needed for preservation of lean body mass and physical performance during weight loss (10). Picking the value of 1.5 g/kg/day, for adults with reference weights ranging from 60 to 80 kg, this translates into total daily protein intakes 90 to 120 g/day. When expressed in the context of total daily energy expenditures of 2000 to 3000 kcal/day, about 15% of an individual's daily energy expenditure (or intake if the diet is eucaloric) needs to be provided as protein. If calories are severely limited then protein needs should be determined on a gram per kilogram basis. During weight loss, especially if strenuous exercise is a component of the process, more dietary protein may be advantageous.

Fat Requirement

Fat is a major component of cell structure and hormones, and is the body's primary source of energy containing 9 kcal/g when burned in a bomb calorimeter. Fat is required in the human diet because there are two essential fatty acids. A "tolerable upper limit intake level" is not set for total fat because there is no known level of fat at which an adverse effect occurs. Dietary fat may enhance fatty acid oxidation, and thus high-fat diets may be desirable to achieve the goal of dietary treatment of the obese individual. The optimal type of fat to eat during weight loss is not known, although recent evidence indicates that in the absence of carbohydrate intake (20 g or less/24 h) high-fat diets lead to lower levels of bloodstream saturates than in those eating a low-fat diet (11). (This may not be the case in calorie-restricted, low-fat diets.)

Carbohydrate Requirement

Carbohydrates are a source of energy containing 4 kcal/g when burned in a bomb calorimeter, and some single carbohydrates (monosaccharides) are used in physiologic compounds such as glycoproteins and mucopolysaccharides. While some dietary carbohydrates contain vitamins and minerals, there is no requirement for carbohydrate in the human diet because metabolic pathways exist within the body to make carbohydrate from dietary protein and fat. Dietary and endogenously created carbohydrate is stored as glycogen or converted to and stored as fat.

Source of Energy

To achieve lipolysis and increased fat oxidation in the dietary treatment of the obese individual, an important goal is to maximize fat as the major fuel source—fat from the diet and from adipose tissue stores. Carbohydrate then becomes a fuel source of much less importance because ketones (a metabolic product of lipolysis) can substitute for glucose in most tissues. Because carbohydrate use as a fuel is linked with lipogenesis, lipolysis and fat mobilization are reduced or halted when carbohydrate is a dominant fuel source. For optimal lipolysis and adipose tissue mobilization, keeping carbohydrate as an energy source to a minimum is preferable.

Table 2 Indications for Medical Nutritional Program

- Overweight or obesity (body mass index > 27 kg/m^2)
- Type 2 diabetes mellitus
- Metabolic syndrome
- Hyperlipidemia
- Polycystic ovarian syndrome
- Nonalcoholic fatty liver disease
- Gluten hypersensitivity (celiac disease)
- Seizure disorder refractory to medication
- Obesity-related comorbidities: sleep apnea, hyperinsulinemia, hypertension, asthma, GERD, irritable bowel syndrome

Essential Vitamins and Minerals

Dietary vitamins and minerals are required in small amounts and are found in food naturally. A few of the functions of vitamins include hormonal signaling and acting as mediators of cell signaling, regulators of cell and tissue growth and differentiation, precursors for enzymes, catalysts and coenyzmes, and substrates in metabolism. Vitamins and minerals are now available in inexpensive pill and liquid form, and a "multivitamin" is recommended during weight loss, as a safety net.

USING NUTRITIONAL KETOSIS AS DIET THERAPY FOR OBESITY

The rationale of the dietary treatment of the obese individual is to alter the hormonal milieu to direct the body's metabolism away from fat storage and toward fat mobilization and oxidation (Table 2). Body systems can be directed toward fat oxidation in many ways, for example, through carbohydrate restriction or caloric restriction. Caloric restriction is usually achieved at least in part by carbohydrate restriction. Nutritional ketosis is a metabolic state in which fat and ketones are the major fuel sources to generate adenosine triphosphate (ATP) while glycolysis is minimized. Although often misconstrued as harmful or unhealthy, nutritional ketosis is not known to cause any short or long-term adverse consequences. In fact, many indigenous populations living on very low-carbohydrate diets were likely in chronic nutritional ketosis. Nutritional ketosis produces a relatively low level of ketone elevation above populations eating carbohydrate-containing diets, but is not associated with a reduction in pH or a significant metabolic acidosis (12). Frequently, nutritional ketosis is confused with diabetic ketoacidosis—the metabolic state during which the absence of insulin leads to very high levels of ketones, elevated blood glucose, dehydration, and a low blood pH.

When an individual is adapted to nutritional ketosis, fatty acids and ketones become the major energy sources (Figure 1). Fatty acids are an excellent fuel source and can be utilized for energy by most tissues, including cardiac and skeletal muscle. Ketone bodies (β-hydroxybutyrate and acetoacetate) contain 4 kcal/g (when burned in a bomb calorimeter) and can be utilized by all cells except those that do not have mitochondrial fat oxidation enzymes (erythrocytes, cornea, lens, retina) or sufficient oxygen to support oxidative metabolism (renal medulla). During nutritional ketosis, it is estimated that the daily glucose need can be as low as 30 g/day because fatty acids and ketones are available for muscle and central nervous system use (5). Glucose becomes less important as a fuel source, with ketones substituting for glucose in most tissues that would otherwise use glucose. Glucose is manufactured through a process called gluconeogenesis, which occurs in both the liver and kidney. While the liver is the major gluconeogenic organ, capable of producing up to approximately 240 g of glucose per day when insulin levels are low, the kidneys may produce up to 20% of daily glucose needs (13,14). Precursors for gluconeogenesis come mainly from amino acids in the diet.

As ketosis is desirable, some clinical programs use urinary ketone strips to verify adherence and the presence of the lipolytic state, colloquially known as "being in ketosis." However, there can be significant subject-to-subject variability in urinary ketone response even when subjects eat uniform diets. Type 2 diabetes can also reduce the likelihood of urinary ketones. Most studies of the low-carbohydrate ketogenic diet (LCKD) have observed that the level of

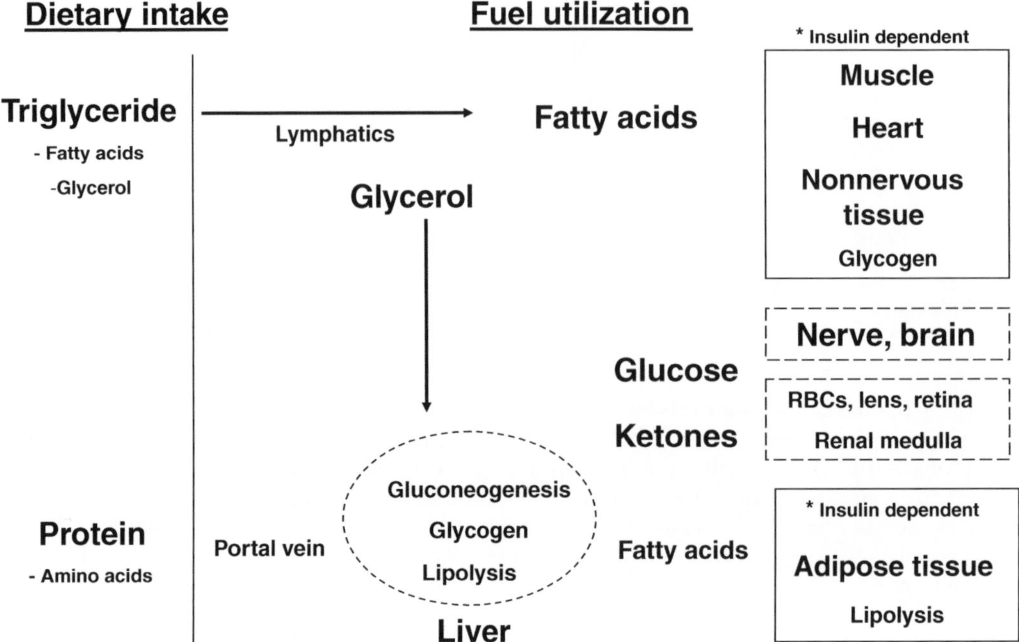

Figure 1 Fat oxidation is linked to lipolysis.

ketosis (urine and blood levels) decreases with time. It is unclear whether this effect is a result of increased efficiency at utilizing ketone bodies for energy or a decrease in the production of ketone bodies over time (presumably from adding carbohydrates back into the diet). However, this effect was also observed in one inpatient study that closely controlled carbohydrate intake at 21 g over two weeks and measured urine ketones on a daily basis (15).

Nutritional ketosis enhances adipose tissue loss in several ways. First, a reduction in insulin facilitates lipolysis at the adipose tissue via hormone-sensitive lipase. This reduction in insulin also leads to inhibition of metabolic pathways of lipogenesis (fat production) in many sites throughout the body (16). A diet that uses nutritional ketosis can also be regarded as a diet that lowers endogenous insulin production.

Nutritional Ketosis and Sodium Regulation

During nutritional ketosis, the traditional thinking about the need to limit sodium in the diet does not apply. It is actually important to provide 2 to 3 g of dietary sodium during nutritional ketosis, for patients who do not have salt-sensitive conditions like congestive heart failure. The reason for this is that the prior higher levels of serum insulin promote sodium and water retention, and after dietary changes that decrease the serum insulin while there is an increase in renal sodium excretion (17). This is one of the factors leading to the diuresis that occurs during the first few weeks of nutritional ketosis. Urinary ketone bodies can also act as an osmotic diuretic and glycogen loss leads to water loss because water is stored with glycogen to keep the glycogen in aqueous form (3 g of water are stored with every gram of glycogen). Presumably, when the glycogen is utilized, the water is released, and if insulin is low, this water also becomes part of the initial diuresis.

Carbohydrate restriction has many similarities to the metabolic state of starvation (no nutritional intake) (8). The main similarities are that there is no (or little) intake of exogenous carbohydrate, and there is a shift from the use of fatty acids and glucose as fuel toward the use of fatty acids and ketones as fuel. During starvation, however, endogenous sources (muscle protein, glycogen, and fat) are used as energy supplies resulting in significant loss of

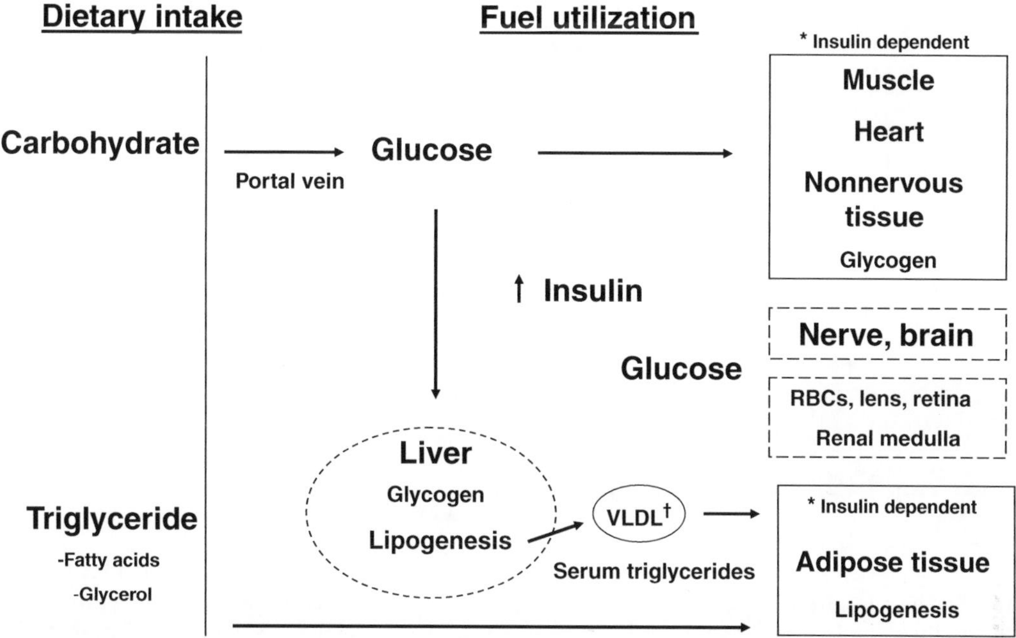

Figure 2 Glycolysis is linked to lipogenesis.

muscle mass. However, under conditions of nutritional ketosis (carbohydrate restriction but not caloric restriction), exogenous sources of protein and fat provide energy, along with endogenous glycogen and fat if caloric expenditure exceeds caloric intake. When sufficient dietary protein is provided, a very low-carbohydrate diet with nutritional ketosis may preserve lean body mass even during loss of adipose mass (11). Unlike starvation, glucose levels are sustained despite the lack of carbohydrate intake under low-carbohydrate conditions. So, the important differences between starvation and nutritional ketosis are that during nutritional ketosis, serum glucose levels are maintained, and breakdown of endogenous protein (muscle mass) is minimized.

METHODS FOR ATTAINING NUTRITIONAL KETOSIS

Carbohydrate Restriction

Dietary carbohydrate is the primary insulin secretagogue (Figure 2). Because pancreatic insulin secretion is stimulated by the glucose/amino acid ratio in the portal vein and in response to an increase in blood glucose, a powerful way to lower insulin levels is to reduce dietary carbohydrate. When the dietary intake of carbohydrate is reduced to less than 50 g/day, most individuals excrete ketones in the urine, leading to the descriptive name of "ketogenic diet." Several popular diets have used the recommendation of very low levels of carbohydrate (<20 g/day) in the early stages of the diet to enhance lipolysis. The presence of urinary ketones is an indicator of an increase in fat oxidation. Several research groups have referred to this approach as a "very low-carbohydrate ketogenic diet" (VLCKD) or "low-carbohydrate ketogenic diet". When dietary carbohydrate is low (20 g/day), insulin secretion remains low—close to basal levels—and fat "burning" (lipolysis) and protein "burning" (gluconeogenesis) occur as glucagon levels rise. A "low-carbohydrate diet" is one that contains 50 to 150 g per day, and is not typically associated with nutritional ketosis. When dietary carbohydrate is present in sufficient amounts for stimulating insulin secretion, fat storage will occur. This may even be true in situations where total energy intake is limited resulting in fat storage and lean tissue breakdown. The dietary carbohydrate signals fat deposition, while the need for gluconeogenesis in energy

Table 3 Metabolic Changes Comparing Low-fat to Low-Carbohydrate Diets

		Low fat				Low carbohydrate			
References	**Duration**	**Weight**	**LDL**	**Trig**	**HDL**	**Weight**	**LDL**	**Trig**	**HDL**
Brehm (29) ($n = 42$)	6 mo	−3.9 kg	−5%	+2%	+8%	−8.5 kg	0%	−23%	+13%
Samaha/ Stern (31, 32) ($n = 132$)	6 mo	−1.9 kg	+3%	−4%	−2%	−5.8 kg	+4%	−20%	0%
	12 mo	−3.1 kg	−3%	+2%	−12%	−5.1 kg	+6%	−29%	−2%
Foster (30) ($n = 63$)	6 mo	−5.3 kg	−3%	−13%	+4%	−9.7 kg	+4%	−21%	+20%
	12 mo	−4.5 kg	−6%	+1%	+3%	−7.3 kg	+1%	−28%	+18%
Yancy (33) ($n = 119$)	6 mo	−6.5 kg	−3%	−15%	−1%	−12.0 kg	+2%	−42%	+13%
Shai (3) ($n = 272$)	24 mo	−3.3 kg	−5%	−2%	+16.3%	−5.5 kg	−3%	−13%	+22%

limited diets results in lean tissue utilization. In general, the low-carbohydrate diet will raise high-density lipoprotein (HDL)-cholesterol, lower triglycerides, and have little effect on low-density lipoprotein (LDL)-cholesterol (Table 3). The average weight loss over 6 to 12 months in clinical trials ranged from 5.1 to 12.2 kg, although in private clinical settings larger amounts of weight loss have been reported. Examples of popular carbohydrate-restricted programs include the Atkins Diet, South Beach Diet, and Protein Power Plan.

Calorie Restriction

In calorie-restricted diets, calories are explicitly limited and instruction is given to either count calories or to follow a diet protocol that is low in calories. Calorie and fat reduced diets and balanced deficit diets generally do not achieve nutritional ketosis because they contain sufficient carbohydrate to prevent ketogenesis. While calorie-restricted diets will lead to weight loss, they do not lead to the same pattern of cardiometabolic risk reduction or lean tissue sparing as low-carbohydrate diets. In general, the 30% fat calorie-restricted diet will lower LDL-cholesterol, modestly impact triglycerides, and modestly raise HDL-cholesterol. The average weight loss in clinical trials over 6 to 12 months ranged from 1.5 to 6.4 kg (Table 3). Examples of popular calorie-restricted diet programs include Weight Watchers, Jenny Craig, and Nutrisystem.

Combination of Calorie Restriction and Carbohydrate Restriction (VLCD)

Very low-calorie/low-carbohydrate diets (VLCD), also referred to as "supplemented fasting," are diets that provide between 300 and 800 kcal per day. VLCDs provide enough protein to meaningfully reduce lean tissue wasting and supply essential minerals and vitamins along with varying amounts of carbohydrates and fats. There are two general classes of VLCD: one consisting of common foods with dietary supplements of minerals and vitamins; the other consisting of a defined formula providing all nutrients as beverages, soups, and/or bars taken three to five times per day. The food-based VLCD consists mostly of lean meat, fish, and poultry; whereas the formula VLCD usually requires the addition of carbohydrate as sugar or modified starch to enhance palatability. The food-based VLCD provides a modest dose of fat inherent in the food choices, whereas fat is not always provided in the defined formula diets.

Upon initiation of a VLCD, through the natriuresis of fasting (insulin-reduction) and the mobilization of liver and muscle glycogen, with its associated intracellular water release, up to 10 lb of total weight loss in the first week is possible. Along with the water loss, the adipose tissue loss may total 2 to 3 lb, plus 1 or 2 lb of lean body mass as the body adapts to nutritional ketosis. By the end of the second week of a VLCD, the patient's fluid and electrolyte status stabilizes and, given adequate protein and minerals, the loss of lean body mass is minimized. Then, the average weekly weight loss ranges from 1.5 lb/wk for the shorter person with little

Table 4 Causes of Dizziness During the First 2 Weeks

Low blood pressure due to overmedication	Reduce medication
Low blood glucose due to overmedication	Reduce medication
Fluid shifts from diuresis	Discontinue diuretic
	Add or increase bouillon (salt)
Other common illnesses	Treat as indicated

Troubleshooting

- First take a diet history, then take a routine medical history
- Is the patient strictly following the allowed foods? Are adequate salad greens and nonstarchy vegetables being consumed?
- Too much sucralose, nutrasweet, or sugar alcohols may cause diarrhea
- Overmedication or undermedication?
- Nondiet-related events can occur, such as adverse effects of medications

activity to 3 lb/wk for a taller and/or more active person. The total weight loss achievable with a VLCD varies greatly depending on a number of factors such as initial weight, the degree of support provided to the patient, and the duration of diet use. The average weight loss in clinical trials over a 50-week period ranged from 6.2 to 19.9 kg (16).

Side Effects

There are two groupings of side effects based on whether they occur early or late in the process. VLCDs (400–800 kcal/day) probably have a higher incidence of side effects than carbohydrate restriction using food (1200–1500 kcal/day) due to the lower caloric intake. During adaptation to carbohydrate restriction and nutritional ketosis, the most common side effects are weakness, fatigue, and lightheadedness (Table 4). Although there is a modest reduction in peak aerobic performance in the first week or two of a VLCD, orthostatic symptoms occurring during normal daily activities are the result of the combination of diet-induced natriuresis and an inadequate sodium intake. These symptoms can be prevented by the addition of 2 to 3 g/day of sodium (taken as bouillon or broth, for example) in all patients not requiring continued diuretic medication, along with attention to adequate dietary potassium.

After the first few weeks of adaptation to carbohydrate restriction, the most common side effects are constipation and muscle cramps. The constipation may result in part from the lower fiber content of dietary intake, but is also exacerbated by dehydration. If increasing fluid intake to a minimum of 2 L/day does not resolve the constipation, then 1 teaspoon of milk of magnesia at bedtime, bouillon supplementation or a carbohydrate-free fiber supplement can be used. Muscle cramps can occur either early or late in treatment, and are more common in people with a history of diuretic medication use or prior heavy ethanol consumption. In almost all cases, the muscle cramps respond promptly to supplementation with 1 teaspoon of milk of magnesia at bedtime or 200 mEq/day of slow-release magnesium chloride, suggesting prior depletion of this essential mineral as the root cause. Hypokalemia is another potential cause that should not be overlooked.

In patients with a history of gout, an attack of this acute arthritis can be induced during the adaptation period. The mechanism for this effect of ketogenic diets is the competition between β-hydroxybutyrate and uric acid for excretion in the renal tubule. This process induces a transient rise in serum uric acid in the first few weeks of a VLCD, during which time those patients prone to gout are at risk of an attack. With the subsequent adaptation to nutritional ketosis, however, the renal handling of uric acid returns to normal and the risk of an acute attack subsides. This can be managed by prophylaxis with allopurinol in selected patients with a history of gout, or by treatment of the acute event with a nonsteroidal anti-inflammatory drug (NSAID) or colchicine. Chronic nutritional ketosis may actually prevent gout because metabolic syndrome is one of the predisposing factors for gout, and nutritional ketosis improves all of the components of metabolic syndrome.

During the weight loss process, mobilization of adipose cell cholesterol results in transient increases in both serum cholesterol and increased biliary excretion of cholesterol. Cholestasis is best prevented by >20 g of fat/day in the nutritional intake. Given the typical individual net oxidation of 150 to 200 g/day of body fat, this modest dietary fat intake does not significantly impact the rate of weight loss. Additionally, patients deemed high risk because of prior history of or existing gallstones can be treated prophylactically with ursodeoxycholic acid. Later onset side effects can include dry skin, hair loss, and loss of normal menstrual cycles in women, or resumption of normal menstrual cycles in amenorrheic women. Hair loss is telogen effluvium and is treated symptomatically or by reassurance of its self-limited nature. Some practitioners have reported that fatty acid (omega 3) supplementation decreases the telogen effluvium.

Excessive Weight Loss

After the first week, weight loss exceeding an average of 1.5 kg/wk is a medical concern, and warrants evaluation of potential inappropriate diuretic use or nonadherence to the prescribed diet. Patients need to understand that speeding weight loss by not consuming the prescribed nutrients sacrifices lean body mass and function, possibly increasing the risk of fluid and electrolyte imbalance and lean tissue loss.

FLUIDS AND ELECTROLYTES

The water loss associated with nutritional ketosis has been called the "natriuresis of fasting" and was for many years only thought to be a result of the osmotic effects of ketones in the distal tubule. Another likely mechanism for an increase in sodium excretion is the increase in the phospholipid arachadonic acid (ARA). Because ARA is the precursor of prostaglandin E2 (PGE2), an increase in ARA leads to an increase in PGE2. An increase in PGE2 causes an excretion of sodium, leading to water loss. If uncompensated sodium loss occurs, sodium depletion elicits aldosterone secretion, which then increases potassium excretion. This may lead to hypokalemia that has the attendant risk of muscle wasting and cardiac arrhythmias.

An examination of populations that lived on very little dietary carbohydrate may give insights into the healthiest long-term use of a diet low in carbohydrate. The Inuit people of the Arctic lived much of the year on coastal ice (which is partially desalinated sea water), and much of their food consisted of soup made with meat in a broth from this brackish source of water. When they went inland to hunt, they traditionally added caribou blood (also a rich source of sodium) to their soup. With these empirically derived techniques, the Inuit culture had adapted the available resources to optimize their intakes of both sodium and potassium. When meat is baked, roasted, broiled, or when it is boiled but the broth discarded, potassium initially present in the meat is lost, making it more difficult to maintain potassium balance in the absence of fruit and vegetable intake. Using bouillon as a sodium supplement, the optimal amount of daily sodium intake of 3 to 5 g can be ensured. If dietary potassium supplementation is appropriate, "Lite salt" may be used as well.

TREATMENT OF THE MAJOR COMORBIDITIES OF OBESITY

The major comorbidities of obesity that generally improve with weight-loss treatment are diabetes mellitus, metabolic syndrome (which includes hypertension and hypertriglyceridemia), and gastroesophageal reflux disorder. The management of obesity in patients who are medicated for these comorbidities is more complicated because of the need to monitor, reduce, and eliminate medications.

Diabetes Mellitus

Carbohydrate restriction can have a potent effect on glycemic control of diabetes mellitus initially and can, in many cases, result in remission of type 2 diabetes. While large scale clinical trials regarding carbohydrate restriction are lacking, there are five case series involving 229 patients showing that the low-carbohydrate diet has a potent effect on type 2 diabetes mellitus and obesity (19–22). Among patients with type 1 diabetes, carbohydrate restriction generally leads to a reduction in the daily insulin dose requirement and may lead to a reduction in hypoglycemic events.

Metabolic Syndrome

Successful adipose tissue loss will improve the components of the metabolic syndrome. The Adult Treatment Panel III (ATP III) of the National Cholesterol Education Program (http://www.nhlbi.nih.gov/guidelines/cholesterol/atp3upd04.htm) definition of metabolic syndrome includes any three or more of the following: (a) waist circumference: >102 cm in men, >88 cm in women, (b) serum triglycerides >150 mg/dL, (c) HDL-cholesterol: <40 mg/dL in men, < 50 mg/dL in women, (d) blood pressure >130/85 mm Hg, (e) serum glucose: >110 mg/dL. Carbohydrate-restricted diets have a greater effect on improving these aspects of the metabolic syndrome than fat-restricted diets (23).

GERD

Practitioners using carbohydrate-restricted diets have noted the resolution of heartburn symptoms in their patients for some time. This observation has been supported by recent research: first in a case series of five individuals noting improvement of their heartburn symptoms, and then a subsequent, more detailed study (24,25). In the second study, eight obese individuals with gastroesophageal reflux disorder (GERD) were instructed to follow a diet containing fewer than 20 g/day of carbohydrates. One day prior to the initiation of the diet, participants completed the GSAS-ds (a GERD-specific questionnaire) and underwent dual channel 24-hour pH probe testing. After removal of the pH probe, participants initiated the diet. Three to six days later, a second pH probe was performed and the GSAS-ds was administered again. Outcomes included changes in GSAS-ds scores, percent total time with a pH < 4 in the distal esophagus, and the Johnson–DeMeester score (a score based on the pH probe measurements). All individuals showed an improvement in the severity of their symptoms, with the mean GSAS-ds score decreasing from 1.28 prior to the diet to 0.72 afterwards ($P = 0.0004$). Participants had a significant decrease in the Johnson–DeMeester score (mean of 34.7 before the diet vs. 14.0 afterwards, $P = 0.023$). Participants also exhibited a significant decrease in the percent time with a pH < 4 (5.1 before the diet vs. 2.5 afterwards, $P = 0.022$). The authors concluded that the initiation of a very low-carbohydrate diet in obese patients with GERD significantly reduces distal esophageal acid exposure and improves the symptoms of GERD. Further research is needed to identify mechanisms.

Irritable Bowel Syndrome

After anecdotal reports of improvement in IBS symptoms after consuming low-carb diets, a prospective study was performed to determine whether this observation was robust (26). Patients with moderate to severe diarrhea-predominant IBS were provided a two-week standard diet, then four weeks of a very low-carbohydrate (20 g carbohydrate/day) diet. A responder in symptoms was defined as having adequate relief of gastrointestinal symptoms for two or more weeks during the low-carbohydrate phase. Of the 17 participants enrolled, 13 completed the study and all 13 were responders. Seventy-seven percent reported adequate relief for all four weeks of the low-carbohydrate diet phase. The frequency of stools decreased and the consistency of the stool improved from diarrheal to normal form. Pain scores and quality of life measures significantly improved, also. The authors concluded that a very low-carbohydrate diet can provide adequate relief of IBS.

CLINICAL CONSIDERATIONS

If your patient is otherwise healthy, and not taking diabetes or hypertensive medication, it is possible that all you need to do is to recommend, or give permission to your patient to follow a low-carbohydrate popular diet book. Most of these books combine dietary advice with supportive and motivational writing to instruct individuals in lifestyle modification. At a minimum, check underlying organ function using blood tests at baseline (Table 5). Even this type of patient often has improved outcomes with physician support and monitoring.

If your patient is taking medication, then closer evaluation and follow-up is recommended after instruction (Table 6). Many clinical practices have their patients return for a follow-up visit after one week of diet change to monitor self-reported adherence and to check adherence by using urinary ketones and food diaries. If your patient is taking diabetic or antihypertensive

Table 5 Medical Evaluation Prior to a Medical Nutritional Program

- Complete medical history
- Physical examination (including waist measurement, blood pressure, pulse and body composition measurement if available)
- Complete blood count, serum chemistries, fasting serum lipid profile or lipid subfraction test
- Serum thyroid function tests (T3, T4, TSH)
- Electrocardiogram if heart disease present or high risk for heart disease
- HgbA1C, hs-CRP, c-peptide
- Vitamin D
- Hormonal evaluation tailored to patient including sex steroid status testosterone, estrogen, progesterone, LH/FSH: consider if cortisol or DHEAS needed
- Pelvic sonogram or hepatic sonogram to evaluate PCOS or NASH, cholelithiasis
- 24-h urine for creatinine clearance and quantitative urinary albumin or other measure such as creatinine/albumin
- 3–5 h glucose tolerance test with insulin levels at each blood draw
  - No need for a glucose tolerance test in known diabetics
  - C peptide may indicate hyperinsulinemia and the presence of endogenous insulin production

TSH, thyroid stimulating hormone; hs-CRP, highly sensitive C-reactive protein; LH, leutinizing hormone; FSH, follicle stimulating hormone; PCOS, polycystic ovary syndrome; NASH, non-alcoholic steatohepatitis.

medication, then frequent medical monitoring is necessary for medication adjustment. Follow-up clinic visits may be scheduled at one- to two-week intervals, or more frequently if needed.

Patients taking medications for certain conditions require more attention, as many medications will need to be adjusted or discontinued due to the potent effect of nutritional ketosis (Table 7). Common medications that may result in iatrogenic problems if doses are not adjusted include diuretics, antihypertensives, and hypoglycemics (both oral and injectable hypoglycemics). Thus, hypoglycemics and antihypertensives may require rapid tapering (days to weeks) to avoid hypoglycemia and hypotension. Patient self-monitoring can be done using simple worksheets for patients to monitor their own food intake, glucose levels, or blood pressures can be very helpful during this initial phase, when medication adjustment is required. If the patient is taking vitamin K antagonists for anticoagulation, then more frequent monitoring may be needed if there has been a change in intake of leafy greens or other foods containing vitamin K.

Some medications create problems with the treatment of obesity because they inhibit lipolysis or increase appetite. Niacin and beta blockers block lipolysis via lipoprotein lipase and a

Table 6 Follow-up Medical Evaluation

- Focused history (symptoms, hunger level) and physical examination (heart, lungs, waist, peripheral edema), review of medical problems
- Vital signs (blood pressure, pulse)
- Serum chemistry panel (electrolytes, renal function, liver function)
- Fasting serum lipid profile
- Serum thyroid function tests (T3, T4, TSH)
- HgBA1C, c-peptide, hs-CRP, fasting, and random serum glucose
- If muscle cramps then check serum K^+, Mg^+, and supplement with magnesium
- Repeat of any previously abnormal values
- Medication review

Table 7 Medication Management

Insulin

- If the insulin is long acting, stop the insulin in the evening before starting the diet
- If the total daily dose of insulin is <20 units, stop the insulin in the morning (or night before if long acting) before the diet is started. Stop exenatide on the first day of the diet
- Decrease all other insulin doses by half on the first day of the diet. When the fasting blood glucose is <200 mg/dL, decrease insulin dose by 1/3 to 1/2. Repeat until the insulin dose is below 10 units, then discontinue insulin
- Instruct the patient to call if the blood glucose is above 250 mg/dL, or if the blood glucose is <100 mg /dL

Oral hypoglycemic medication

- Stop all oral diabetic medication except metformin the day the diet is started
- Continue metformin until the fasting blood glucose <100 mg/dL
- Instruct the patient to call if the blood glucose is above 250 mg/dL (16 mmol/L) to see if any additional intervention is required

Diuretics

- If the patient is normoglycemic, it is ok to stop the diuretic as soon as the patient has urinary ketones (usually some time within the first week)
- If the patient has elevated blood sugars, observe blood pressure. If blood pressure begins to drop, consider tapering diuretic first. If patient has edema, taper as tolerated by blood pressure and edema, allowing a few days for equilibration of edema
- Once the patient is off the diuretic and free of edema, begin 2 bouillon servings daily as needed up to every 4 hours to treat orthostatic symptoms, fatigue, and headache

Other antihypertensives

- When the patient is no longer taking the diuretic, begin to taper the beta blocker as tolerated as long as normal blood pressure maintained, unless beta blocker is used for rhythm control
- When the patient is off the diuretic and beta blocker, consider tapering the ARB or ACE if blood pressure is low, the patient has evidence or symptoms of orthostatic hypotension, the blood sugar is normal and proteinuria absent

ARB, angiotensin receptor blocker; ACE, angiotensin converting enzyme.

reduction in sympathetic activity, respectively. Psychiatric medications, especially antipsychotic medications, and subcutaneous insulin injections are common offenders.

Hypertension

For patients taking antihypertensive medications, wean diuretics as soon as the patient measures positive for urinary ketones, as the natriuresis of ketosis will cause diuresis. If symptoms of dizziness, light-headedness or orthostatic hypotension occur, other antihypertensive medications should also be reduced with continued monitoring of the blood pressure. Supplementation with bouillon may be helpful to reduce symptoms during the first few weeks. (Drinking 1 g of sodium in the form of bouillon can improve symptomatic hypotension within a few minutes.) Check serum electrolytes, including calcium and magnesium and replace deficits if salt supplementation does not relieve these symptoms. Even if serum magnesium is normal, a trial of magnesium supplementation may ameliorate fatigue and cramping.

Blood pressure monitoring at home or at the clinic is required because a reduction in blood pressure frequently occurs soon after the initiation of the diet. Taper or discontinue the antihypertensives if home or clinic blood pressures are less than 110 mm Hg systolic. If the blood pressure is systolic 130 mm Hg or below or diastolic 70 mm Hg or below, consider initiating taper. Due to their effect on inhibiting lipolysis, decrease beta blockers first, followed by calcium channel blockers and then angiotensin converting enzyme inhibitor (ACE) or angiotensin II receptor blocker (ARB). Until microalbuminuria is resolved, a low dose of renal protective medication may be continued if the patient does not become hypotensive. In diabetic patients, continue a low dose ACE or ARB until blood glucoses are normal and urinary microalbumin is normal. Consider the use of prophylactic potassium citrate if there is a history of kidney stones (27).

Most patients with hypertension have been told to *restrict* their sodium intake in the past, and will probably continue to restrict sodium out of habit even after instruction to not be concerned about the sodium. It is very important during carbohydrate restriction to have adequate sodium intake to counteract the natriuresis that occurs because of the cessation of the hyperinsulinemia-induced sodium retention that accompany high-carbohydrate diets.

Type 2 Diabetes Mellitus

Oral Hypoglycemics

For patients taking oral hypoglycemic medications stop all oral hypoglycemic agents except metformin on the day that the diet begins. Patients with diabetes should monitor home glucoses once (fasting a.m. value will be the highest of the day) or twice daily. Because these meals do not raise the blood glucose, it no longer matters if the home glucoses are before or after meals. Because short-term hyperglycemia poses less immediate risk than hypoglycemia, the glucoses are allowed to go up to 200 to 250 mg/dL during the weight loss process. Restart oral hypoglycemic of choice if the blood glucose is >250 mg/dL after the first three days. If a downward trend in serum glucose is noted, continue to observe the patient without reintroducing the medication. Individuals with untreated type 2 diabetes should have fasting blood sugar values near normal within a few weeks of nutritional ketosis if they have intact insulin secretion. Metformin can be discontinued when the blood glucoses remain <100 mg/dL.

Injectable Hypoglycemics

Because injectable hypoglycemics (insulin or exenatide) introduce the risk of severe hypoglycemia, it is recommended to discontinue these medications as quickly as tolerated. For patients with type 2 diabetes taking insulin, if the daily insulin use is less than 20 units per day, discontinue the insulin on the first day of the lifestyle change. In other patients, reduce the insulin or other injectable hypoglycemic by 50% at diet initiation. (Again, short-term hyperglycemia poses less immediate risk than hypoglycemia.) Patients should self-monitor their glucose several times a day and record the results for reporting to their health care provider. When the fasting glucose is less than 200 mg/dL, decrease the insulin or exenatide dose by another 50%. Consider changing to short-acting insulin preparations because longer acting preparations do not allow flexible dosing when serum glucose levels are falling rapidly. Insulin is then discontinued when the daily dose is 10 to 20 units, depending upon the individual's response. CAUTION: some individuals may have a dramatic reduction in blood glucoses with the initiation of *nutritional ketosis*, and *may* become hypoglycemic if the injectable hypoglycemic agent is not reduced or discontinued rapidly.

Hyperglycemic individuals may not demonstrate urinary ketones as quickly as normoglycemic individuals. As a result, the absence of urinary ketones does not accurately reflect adherence among patients with diabetes. When treating hyperglycemic patients, even if the preprandial glucose levels are similar to baseline, the next measurement of HgbA1c will probably be lower than before because there are no large postprandial rises in glucose on the LCKD.

Other Medical Conditions

Other medical conditions that require consideration include congestive heart failure, gout, hyperchylomicronemia (triglycerides > 1000 mg/dL), or history of calcium oxalate renal stones. Patients with heart failure may need to limit sodium and water consumption. Patients with a history of gout may be placed on prophylactic allopurinol prior to diet initiation or a prescription for colchicine or NSAID may be provided as well for the patient to initiate if needed. Patients with a history of calcium oxalate renal stones may reduce the risk of subsequent stones by taking potassium citrate supplements. GERD medications may be eliminated on a trial basis at any time—resume if the GERD recurs. After significant weight loss, continuous positive airway pressure (CPAP) therapy for sleep apnea may be discontinued if upon retesting, apnea and hypoxia are resolved. Some practitioners repeat a sleep study to document resolution of the sleep apnea. While we have observed many patients with severe hypertriglyceridemia

(>6500 mg/dL) improve with a low-carbohydrate diet, the current diet recommendation for these patients is a low-fat diet, due to the possibility of the rare condition of severe hyperchylomicronemia. A high-fat diet in the presence of chylomicronemia may lead to pancreatitis (28). If the hypertriglyceridemia is chylomicron in origin, then a low-carbohydrate, high-fat diet is contraindicated. Test for this by asking your laboratory to measure for the presence of chylomicrons if the fasting serum triglycerides are >500 mg/dL. Careful clinical monitoring will show rapid decreases in serum triglycerides if the elevation is due to hyperinsulinemia. Triglyceride values will begin to decrease in a few days.

Areas of the body that have a substantial loss of weight may require plastic surgery for removal of the stretched skin.

Instructions on When to Call the Clinic

While some mild symptoms of fatigue may occur during the keto-adaptation phase, if your patients are taking medications these symptoms can also occur due to overmedication by antihypertensive or hypoglycemics. Instruct your patient to call the clinic if they experienced symptoms such as dizziness, light-headedness, or muscle cramping. Home monitoring of glucose and/or blood pressure is recommended. Home glucose monitoring is highly recommended if the patient is taking insulin or taking multiple hypoglycemic agents. If fatigue or muscle cramping occurs, recommend 1 bouillon cube dissolved in hot water every four hours as needed. If symptoms persist, then bring the patient back to the clinic for measurement of serum electrolytes. Potassium or magnesium supplementation can be added if serum measurements are abnormally low. Because potassium and magnesium are intracellular electrolytes, serum levels are a poor indicator of total body depletion. For example, a history of muscle cramps and hyper-reflexia on physical exam is highly suggestive of magnesium deficiency. As a preventive treatment for muscle cramping and constipation, a slow release magnesium preparation like Slo-Mag or 1 teaspoon of milk of magnesia at bedtime is helpful. For patients who are taking insulin or other injectable hypoglycemic agents, we instruct patients to call the doctor on call when the glucoses go below 100 mg/dL.

HOSPITAL MANAGEMENT OF A PATIENT IN NUTRITIONAL KETOSIS

Many hospitals do not have a standard low-carbohydrate selection, even though foods that are low-carbohydrate are available at the hospital. Choosing to not eat the carbs on the plate is an option. Stating that there is an allergy to wheat, milk, and fruit may lead to a discussion of personal dietary selections. The patient may order multiple portions of protein and fat.

In regard to intravenous therapy during hospitalization, if the hospital has a pharmacy capable of making total parenteral nutrition (TPN), use 3% amino acids, 30 mEq of sodium, 20 mEq of potassium, 15 mMol of phosphorus, 20 mEq of magnesium, and run 2 L per day by peripheral vein after the first few liters of normal saline. If a customized TPN prescription is not available, use normal saline (without glucose or dextrose). Since about half of the water becomes intracellular, this can lead to hypernatremia after a few liters. Serum electrolytes, magnesium, and phosphorus should be measured daily. Oral fluid resuscitation should use bouillon and sugar-free gelatin. Small amounts of sugar substitutes or sugar-free beverages may be used for palatability.

REFERENCES

1. Vernon MC, Mavropoulos J, Transue M, et al. Clinical experience of a carbohydrate-restricted diet: Effect on diabetes mellitus. Metab Syndr Relat Disord 2003; 1:233–237.
2. Nordmann AJ, Nordmann A, Briel M, et al. Effects of low-carbohydrate vs low-fat diets on weight loss and cardiovascular risk factors: A meta-analysis of randomized controlled trials. Arch Intern Med 2006; 166(3):285–293.
3. Shai I, Schwarzfuchs D, Henkin Y, et al. Weight loss with a low-carbohydrate, Mediterranean, or low-fat diet. N Engl J Med 2008; 359(3):229–241.
4. Lim SS, Noakes M, Keogh JB, et al. Long-term effects of a low carbohydrate, low fat or high unsaturated fat diet compared to a no-intervention control. Nutr Metab Cardiovasc Dis 2009 Aug 17 [epub ahead of print].
5. Phinney SD, Horton ES, Sims EAH, et al. Capacity for moderate exercise in obese subjects after adaptation to a hypocaloric, ketogenic diet. J Clin Invest 1980; 66:1151–1161.

6. Phinney SD, Bistrian BR, Evans WJ, et al. The human metabolic response to chronic ketosis without caloric restriction: Preservation of submaximal exercise capability with reduced carbohydrate oxidation. Metabolism 1983; 32:769–776.
7. Phinney SD, Bistrian BR, Evans WJ, et al. The human metabolic response to chronic ketosis without caloric restriction: Physical and biochemical adaptation. Metabolism 1983; 32:757–768.
8. Westman EC, Mavropoulos J, Yancy WS, et al. A review of low-carbohydrate ketogenic diets. Curr Atheroscler Rep 2003; 5(6):476–483.
9. Westman EC, Feinman RD, Mavropoulos JC, et al. Low-carbohydrate nutrition and metabolism. Am J Clin Nutr 2007; 86(2):276–284.
10. Layman DK. Dietary guidelines should reflect new understandings about adult protein needs. Nutr Metab (Lond) 2009; 6:12.
11. Volek JS, Fernandez ML, Feinman RD, et al. Dietary carbohydrate restriction induces a unique metabolic state positively affecting atherogenic dyslipidemia, fatty acid partitioning, and metabolic syndrome. Prog Lipid Res 2008; 47:307–318.
12. Yancy WS Jr, Olsen MK, Dudley T, et al. Acid-base analysis of individuals following two weight loss diets. Eur J Clin Nutr 2007; 61(12):1416–1422.
13. Harber MP, Schenk S, Barkan AL, et al. Alterations in carbohydrate metabolism in response to short-term dietary carbohydrate restriction. Am J Physiol Endocrinol Metab 2005; 289:E306–E312.
14. Allick G, Bisschop PH, Ackermans MT, et al. A low-carbohydrate/high-fat diet improves glucoregulation in type 2 diabetes mellitus by reducing postabsorptive glycogenolysis. J Clin Endocrinol Metab 2004; 89:6193–6197.
15. Boden G, Sargrad K, Homko C, et al. Effect of a low-carbohydrate diet on appetite, blood glucose levels, and insulin resistance in obese patients with type 2 diabetes. Ann Intern Med 2005; 142:403–411.
16. Volek JS, Sharman MJ, Love DM, et al. Body composition and hormonal responses to a carbohydrate-restricted diet. Metabolism 2002; 51:864–870.
17. Quinones Galvan A, Natali A, Baldi S, et al. Effect of insulin on uric acid excretion in humans. Am J Physiol 1995; 268:E1–E5.
18. Tsai AG, Wadden TA. The evolution of very-low-calorie diets: An update and meta-analysis. Obesity (Silver Spring) 2006; 14:1283–1293.
19. O'Neill DF, Westman EC, Bernstein RK. The effects of a low-carbohydrate regimen on glycemic control and serum lipids in diabetes mellitus. Metab Syndr Relat Disord 2003; 1:291–298.
20. Yancy WS Jr, Vernon MC, Westman EC. A pilot trial of a low-carbohydrate, ketogenic diet in patients with Type 2 Diabetes. Metab Syndr Relat Disord 2003; 1:239–243.
21. Westman EC, Yancy WS Jr, Mavropoulos JC, et al. The effect of a low-carbohydrate, ketogenic diet versus a low-glycemic index diet on glycemic control in type 2 diabetes mellitus. Nutr Metab (Lond) 2008; 5:36.
22. Vernon MC, Kueser B, Transue M, et al. Clinical experience of a carbohydrate-restricted diet for the metabolic syndrome. Metab Syndr Relat Disord 2004; 2:180–186.
23. Gardner CD, Kiazand A, Alhassan S, et al. Comparison of the Atkins, Zone, Ornish, and LEARN diets for change in weight and related risk factors among overweight premenopausal women: The A TO Z Weight Loss Study: A randomized trial. JAMA 2007; 297(9):969–977.
24. Yancy WS Jr, Provencale D, Westman EC. Improvement of gastroesophageal reflux disease after initation of a low-carbohydrate diet: Five brief case reports. Altern Ther Health Med 2001; 7:120–122.
25. Austin GL, Thiny MT, Westman EC, et al. A very low carbohydrate diet improves gastroesophageal reflux and its symptoms: A pilot study. Dig Dis Sci 2006; 51:1307–1312.
26. Austin GL, Dalton DB, Hu Y, et al. A very low-carbohydrate diet improves symptoms and quality of life in diarrhea-predominant irritable bowel syndrome. Clin Gastroenterol Hepatol 2009; 7:706–708.
27. Pak CY. Pharmacotherapy of kidney stones. Expert Opin Pharmacother 2008; 9:1509–1518.
28. Buse J, Riley KD, Dress CM, et al. Patient with gemfibrozil-controlled hypertriglyceridemia that developed acute pancreatitis after starting ketogenic diet. Current Surgery 2004; 61:224–226.
29. Brehm BJ, Seeley RJ, Daniels SR, et al. A randomized trial comparing a very low carbohydrate diet and a calorie-restricted low fat diet on body weight and cardiovascular risk factors in healthy women. J Clin Endocrinol Metab 2003; 88:1617–1623.
30. Foster GD, Wyatt HR, Hill JO, et al. A randomized trial of a low-carbohydrate diet for obesity. N Engl J Med 2003; 348:2082–2090.
31. Samaha FF, Iqbal N, Seshadri P, et al. A low-carbohydrate as compared with a low-fat diet in severe obesity. N Engl J Med 2003; 348:2074–2081.
32. Stern L, Iqbal N, Seshadri P, et al. The effects of low-carbohydrate versus conventional weight loss diets in severely obese adults: One-year follow-up of a randomized trial. Ann Intern Med 2004; 140:778–785.
33. Yancy Jr WS, Olsen MK, Guyton JR, et al. A low-carbohydrate, ketogenic diet versus a low-fat diet to treat obesity and hyperlipidemia: A randomized, controlled trial. Ann Intern Med 2004; 140:769–777.

6 The role of physical activity in the treatment of the obese individual

Deborah Bade Horn

INTRODUCTION

Obesity in America has been increasing over the last 25 years, and only recently there is conflicting evidence that the epidemic problem may or may not be stabilizing. The National Center for Health Statistics published a brief indicating that National Health and Nutrition Examination Survey (NHANES) data for 2005 to 2006 suggest the prevalence of obesity was not significantly different than it was in 2003 to 2004 (1). In contrast, in a more recent analysis of the Behavioral Risk Factor Surveillance System (BRFSS) data, researchers reported on the Robert Wood Johnson Foundation web site (www.rwjf.org/childhoodobesity/product.jsp?id=45050) that obesity rates increased "in 23 states and did not decrease in a single state." The difference may come from two sources: (*i*) the use of two different datasets and (*ii*) the latter analysis looked at trends between three-year time intervals instead of individual year to year changes. If the obesity epidemic is indeed leveling off, it may be partially the result of increased physical activity. Physical activity levels in the United States have improved slightly over the last two decades. The percentage of Americans who report participating in no leisure-time physical activity has decreased from 31% in 1989 to 24% in 2007 (www.cdc.gov/brfss/). Because physical activity can affect caloric expenditure and therefore energy balance, it plays an important role in the comprehensive approach to weight management and the obesity epidemic.

The Centers for Disease Control (CDC) evaluates physical activity participation in America through the BRFSS survey via state health departments. The survey is a self-reported telephone survey and thus is subject to "recall and social-desirability bias." Following the US Department of Health and Human Services (USDHHS) release of the new 2008 Physical Activity Guidelines for Americans, the CDC reanalyzed BRFSS data from 2007 to determine the number of Americans sufficiently active to achieve health benefits. The CDC analysis found that 64.5% of surveyed participants were meeting the new guidelines as defined by the USDHHS. Interestingly, when the same responses were applied to the Healthy People 2010 recommendations, only 48.8% of respondents were meeting recommended guidelines. The CDC attributes the difference to two factors: (*i*) the newer HHS guidelines allow for an accumulation of physical activity over the entire week as opposed to the previously prescribed number of minutes per day and a prescribed number of days per week, and (*ii*) the newer guidelines offer an option of varied intensities that can be combined together to meet the requirements. When the analyzed data was reduced to obese participants over the age of 18, only 57% met the HHS guidelines. Similarly, when this subset was applied to the Healthy People 2010 recommendations, only 41% of obese individuals were meeting guidelines (www.cdc.gov/brfss/).

Additionally, the new HHS guidelines indicate that the amount of physical activity required to achieve health benefit and reduced risk of disease may be much less than the amount of exercise needed to affect change in weight or prevent weight gain and weight regain (2). Unfortunately, as reported above, overweight and obese individuals are less likely to meet even the minimum recommendations for physical activity. Finally, research is discovering that the physical activity required to affect weight change or weight maintenance may be highly variable from individual to individual (3,4)

This chapter reviews the concept of physical activity, the multiple sets of guidelines available for consideration, and the role that physical activity can play in preventing weight gain, achieving weight loss, and sustaining long-term weight maintenance after significant weight loss. Included is a practical approach to physical activity in overweight and obese individuals from exercise prescription to special needs in the bariatric population. While public health experts, scientists, and clinicians agree that physical activity plays a key role in weight management, the recommended message to the patient is not always consistent and therefore can be confusing. The goal of this chapter is to review the currently available guidelines and tools, and to assist clinicians as they initiate a dialogue regarding daily physical activity with their overweight and obese patients.

PHYSICAL ACTIVITY VERSUS EXERCISE

While the two terms are often used interchangeably, physical activity and exercise are not synonymous. Physical activity is a larger umbrella term than can include exercise and all other nonrest activities; it is defined as "movement produced by skeletal muscle and that results in energy expenditure" (5). Total energy expenditure (EE) is composed of resting energy expenditure (REE), the thermic effect of meals (TEM), and energy expenditure from physical activity (EEPA). (EE = REE + TEM + EEPA) (6). EEPA is energy expenditure from all physical activity accumulated throughout the day. Examples of energy expenditure from physical activity include walking from the car to the office, swimming, exercise class, walking the dog, household chores, gardening, and playing with one's children. Some researchers choose to categorize physical activity into transportational, occupational, and leisure-time activities.

Exercise is more specific. It is a subset of physical activity or EEPA. Exercise is "planned, structured, and repetitive and has a final or an intermediate objective, the improvement or maintenance of physical fitness" (5). Examples can include jogging, rowing, cycling, lunchtime exercise class, yoga, or dance class. In the preceding categories, it would fall under leisure-time activities.

Most of the current literature on physical activity and weight loss is reported as exercise. Research subjects are commonly asked to complete a specific physical activity, for a prescribed amount of time, with the ultimate goal to measure some aspect of improved health outcomes. Researchers choose prescribed or predetermined exercise intentionally because it is difficult to quantify and/or instruct individuals to increase their overall daily physical activity—when activities and intensities could vary widely between study participants and dilute the potential results. As physical activity and weight management research evolves, increasing the component of physical activity that is built into otherwise fixed daily responsibilities may provide an opportunity to achieve recommended levels of physical activity without dedicating as much time specifically to exercise (see section "Novel Approaches to Increasing Physical Activity"). Smaller amounts of "exercise" could potentially provide the cardiorespiratory benefits needed, while larger bouts of nonexercise physical activity may be able to contribute significantly to EE and maintenance of a healthier weight.

PHYSICAL ACTIVITY AND PREVENTING INITIAL WEIGHT GAIN: TRUE PRIMARY PREVENTION

Overall health benefit and reduced risk of diseases related to a sedentary lifestyle were the focus of the original 1995 ACSM/CDC guidelines for physical activity: at least 30 minutes per day of moderate-intensity physical activity most, preferable all, days of the week. The primary American College of Sports Medicine (ACSM) recommendation to the U.S. public has since been revised, but it is still directed at general health benefits and risk prevention, not the specific treatment or prevention of obesity. How much physical activity does it take to reduce the risk of becoming overweight or obese? The most recent 2009 ACSM position stand suggests that 150 to 250 minutes per week of physical activity (an EE of 1200-2000 kcal) should provide a stable weight profile, but this will of course depend upon an individual's caloric intake (7). Less than 150 minutes per week of physical activity is not adequate to prevent age-related increases in weight. Furthermore, the amount of physical activity needed to maintain a healthy body weight may vary throughout life.

Minor weight fluctuations are normal based on hydration status, hormonal changes, clothing, time of day, and other factors. Therefore, prevention of weight gain or weight "stability" may actually be a range of absolute weights. Although still a debated topic, weight stability has been defined as a <3% change in body weight over time (8). Thus, while 150 minutes of physical activity per week may be sufficient to lower the risk of diseases like diabetes, coronary artery disease, and hypertension, more than 150 minutes per week will be necessary in most people to maintain actual weight stability over a lifetime—which in turn also affects the risk of these same diseases. The relationship between physical activity, weight, and risk of disease may result in a continuum of risk or rather risk reduction based on the amount of physical activity participation.

PHYSICAL ACTIVITY AND WEIGHT LOSS

"Calories in = calories out" is an equation often discussed in weight loss interventions and treatment. However, changes in energy intake versus EE are not equally effective at weight loss or prevention of weight gain. Exercise or physical activity as a sole intervention is less effective than diet alone or diet plus exercise in producing weight loss in short-term studies (7,9,10). Exercise alone has a widely variable affect and achieves only 3% to 23% of the weight loss that can be achieved by dieting alone, and only 2% to 20% of the weight loss that can be achieved with dieting plus exercise (9,10). The length of an intervention or time spent on an attempt at weight loss may play a role in the overall contribution of physical activity to the outcome of weight loss. Studies with a longer follow-up time of 12 to 18 months found that exercise was associated with better weight loss results (4,11).

The ACSM position stand recently concluded that weight does indeed demonstrate a dose response to physical activity. Modest overall weight loss, defined as 2 to 3 kg or 4.4 to 6.6 lb, would require 150 to 225 minutes of physical activity per week. Additionally, 225 to 420 minutes of physical activity per week can yield greater weight loss at 5 to 7.5 kg (7). Put in the context of a patient's typical expectations, the amount of physical activity required to achieve a 1 to 2 lb weight loss per week without dietary changes is likely prohibitive in the daily schedules of most individuals (see section "Novel Approaches to Increasing Physical Activity"). The estimated time commitment necessary to produce this affect is between 1.3 and 2.75 hours per day (12). The current body of research indicates that exercise or physical activity combined with decreased calorie intake, rather than physical activity alone or calorie restriction alone will produce the greatest change in weight and more quickly meet an individual's weight loss expectations. Therefore, physical activity should be paired with adjusted caloric intake to achieve optimal weight loss.

PHYSICAL ACTIVITY AND WEIGHT MAINTENANCE OR PREVENTION OF WEIGHT REGAIN

Once an individual has reached their maintenance or goal weight, the role of physical activity versus caloric intake shifts. Returning to the calorie balance equation, increased EE, or "Calories Out," contributes more significantly to weight maintenance or the prevention of weight regain. Regular physical activity is associated with long-term weight loss maintenance (13–15). Predicting the amount or type of physical activity that will optimize this weight loss maintenance has yet to be accomplished. The National Weight Control Registry (NWCR), which is described in more detail below, reported that the majority of individuals, who have successfully maintained a significant weight loss, report high levels of physical activity (3). Unfortunately, most of the data on weight maintenance and physical activity is by self-report and often includes retrospective categorization of participants in to high, medium, and low active groups. A minimum threshold of required physical activity to allow for weight maintenance or prevention of weight regain has yet to be truly determined. Theoretically, an individual could reduce caloric intake to the point that no physical activity is needed to maintain weight. However, this individual would not benefit from the many health improvements and reduced risk of chronic diseases afforded by an active lifestyle.

The NWCR is a self-reported database of individuals that have lost at least 13.6 kg or approximately 30 lb and maintained that loss for at least one year. A recent NWCR data analysis found that on average its participants were completing 60 to 75 minutes of moderate-intensity physical activity or 35 to 45 minutes of vigorous activity per day (3). This data was, in part, used to help determine the new USDHHS guidelines on weight loss maintenance and physical activity. It is important to note that these are participation averages; the range of reported amount of activity from individual to individual was actually quite broad. Fifteen percent of entrants in the registry reported very low levels of physical activity: levels even lower than those recommended simply for general health benefits (<30 minutes per day). And yet, they reported successful maintenance of weight loss. Alternatively, some participants reported very high levels of physical activity, greater than 90 minutes per day. However, overall the registry participants are still engaging in more daily physical activity than the average American. Approximately one-half of the entrants "meets or exceeds 60 min/day of moderate-intensity physical activity" and "one-third meet or exceeds 90 min/day of physical activity" (3).

Several studies have demonstrated that like the NWCR participants, individuals who do more physical activity experience better weight maintenance. Jakicic et al. found that individuals participating in more than 200 minutes of moderate-intensity physical activity per week tend to be more successful at weight maintenance (4). More recently, individuals who had lost more than 10% of their body weight after two years reported 275 minutes per week of physical activity (16). The 2009 ACSM position stand by Donnelly et al., rates the evidence for PA prevention of weight regain as a category "B" based on National Heart Lung and Blood Institute (NHLBI) categories of level of evidence.

In order to more accurately prescribe physical activity to an individual, randomized control trials that include randomization to physical activity levels for weight maintenance are needed. Few studies exist and the range of actual EE in low, medium, and highly active groups in the available studies is so broad that a clinically significant conclusion regarding a threshold or minimum recommendation regarding amount of physical activity for maintaining a weight loss is difficult to determine. After reviewing these and other studies, the ACSM position stand concluded that on average, weight maintenance is likely to require approximately 60 minutes of moderate-intensity physical activity per day or about 420 minutes per week. This is almost three times the amount of physical activity recommended for "health benefits" regardless of weight status.

The importance of preventing weight regain is often underestimated. Unfortunately many individuals cycle through major weight fluctuations from weight gain, to weight loss, to weight maintenance, to weight regain. Fluctuating weight has been associated with increased risk of cardiovascular disease and all-cause mortality (17,18). A successful weight loss attempt needs to be carefully monitored and supported to avoid these increased risks. Physical activity, nutritional, behavioral, and pharmacologic tools all need to be optimized. Weight loss alone is not the ideal goal. The ultimate and optimal goal is weight loss followed by successful weight maintenance.

A REVIEW OF THE CURRENT RECOMMENDATIONS

As previously mentioned, physical activity guidelines in the United States have been recently updated. These guidelines are geared at both health benefits in the general U.S. population as well as weight loss/weight maintenance efforts. Confusion related to physical activity guidelines is predominately secondary to two problems: (*i*) multiple sets of guidelines exist from various different public health and specialty organizations and (*ii*) failure to differentiate between physical activity recommendations for overall health benefit versus recommendations specific to preventing weight gain, assisting in weight loss, and managing weight maintenance.

The 2008 USDHHS published their "Physical Activity Guidelines for Americans" for individuals aged six years and older. Previously, HHS did not publish separate physical activity guidelines, but instead offered recommendations within the Dietary Guidelines for Americans that were published jointly by HHS and the U.S. Department of Agriculture (USDA). This was an opportunity to provide both nutritional and physical activity recommendations to the United States from a single source.

The HHS guidelines recommend 150 minutes per week of moderate-intensity physical activity, in at least 10 minutes blocks, to gain the basic health benefits associated with physical activity. This is consistent with ACSM /American Heart Association guidelines. These health benefits include decreased mortality and decreased risk of obesity-related comorbidities: heart disease, stroke, diabetes, and some cancers (17,18). While the basic HHS guidelines do not give specific recommendations for obesity treatment, the second level recommendations indicate that "additional and more extensive health benefits" are provided by increasing moderate-intensity physical activity to 300 minutes per week (HHS website).

The HHS physical activity guidelines advisory committee recognized that 150 to 300 minutes of physical activity per week may be necessary to avoid the 1% to 3% average yearly weight gain in most Americans. The committee also found that without dietary changes, approximately 45 minutes per day of moderate physical activity would be needed to obtain at least a 5 % weight loss over the long term. This is greater than 300 minutes per week of physical activity as well.

Finally, in patients who have already lost weight, even more physical activity may be necessary. To prevent weight regain after successful weight loss, HHS guidelines recommend that individuals need to participate in approximately 60 minutes of walking or 30 minutes of jogging daily (or an equivalent physical activity). This amounts to 420 minutes per week of moderate-intensity physical activity or 210 minutes of more vigorous physical activity. However, the summary recommendations simply indicate that greater than 300 minutes may be necessary (HHS website).

The above recommendations may be surprising, given that physical activity guidelines put forth by the ACSM and the CDC in 1995 were much lower. Originally, the ACSM/CDC recommendation was that adults "should accumulate 30 minutes or more of moderate intensity exercise on most, preferably all, days of the week" (19). This is the "sound bite" or "mantra" that Americans can typically recall. Unfortunately, these guidelines are specific to the amount of physical activity necessary to improve health and reduce risk of disease. They were not written with the intention of weight control. These recommendations were also revised in 2007. Although the baseline recommendation is still 150 minutes per week, the new guidelines are more specific. They recommend 30 minutes of moderate intensity, specifically cardiovascular, exercise five days per week and strength training an additional two days per week. The new ASCM guidelines are in conjunction with the American Heart Association (AHA), not the CDC, and are again the recommendations to "maintain health and reduce the risk of chronic disease" without any specific intent of weight change. Beyond basic health benefit, the ACSM/AHA recommendations go on to indicate that "to lose weight or maintain weight loss, 60 to 90 minutes of physical activity may be necessary" (20).

In 2009, the American College of Sport Medicine released an updated Position Stand that offered more specific recommendations regarding: "Appropriate physical activity intervention strategies for weight loss and prevention of weight regain for adults" (7). The new ACSM position stand found that there was "A" level evidence, as defined by the National Heart, Lung, and Blood Institute, to support that 150 to 250 minutes of exercise per week are needed to prevent initial weight gain in most adults. The level of evidence is not as strong for the amount of physical activity needed for weight loss and weight maintenance. The amount of activity required for "substantial weight loss" (5–7.5 kg) is 225 to 420 minutes per week. This is up to 60 minutes all days of the week for 11 to 16.5 lb. ACSM rates the level of evidence associated with this statement to be category "B."

Finally, the amount of activity required for preventing weight regain after weight loss appears even less clear. The position stand indicates that correctly designed studies are lacking to allow for definitive comment. However, the available information indicates that 200 to 300 minutes of exercise per week is likely necessary (7).

The recent revision of the ACSM guidelines and the development of the new HHS guidelines were triggered by increasing research and observational data that suggest that weight management in general requires more physical activity than was originally prescribed for overall health. This issue was discussed and identified by many national and international organizations prior to the publication of both new sets of guidelines. The increased physical activity requirement for weight management was previously suggested by many other groups including the International Association for the Study of Obesity Stock Conference report in 2002, the Institute of Medicine Committee on Dietary Reference Intakes report in 2002, the researchers from the NWCR, and many others. Although some differences remain, these two new sets of guidelines are consistent in that they recognize a much larger volume of physical activity is necessary when weight management is the key treatment variable.

VOLUME VERSUS INTENSITY OF PHYSICAL ACTIVITY AND WEIGHT

In addition to deciphering the physical activity guidelines, individuals trying to address weight control often ask whether it is more important to focus their efforts on a higher volume of physical activity at a lower intensity or a lower volume of physical activity at a higher intensity. In other words, are calories burned equivalent, which would allow an individual to reduce their total time requirement by increasing their physical activity intensity?

Physical activity intensity can be described in terms of metabolic equivalents or METs. The amount of oxygen consumed or metabolic work done during quiet sitting is defined as "at rest," and equal to 1 MET. Physical activity intensity has been classified as light, <3 METs; moderate,

3 to 6 METs; and vigorous, >6 METs (19). The reference to light, moderate, and vigorous are therefore specific and the previously discussed guidelines specifically refer to these levels of intensity. Researchers have quantified 605 activities based on their MET requirement in the "Compendium of Physical Activities" (21). The compendium, while initially developed for researchers, is useful to clinicians as well. Clinically, it can assist a health care provider in prescribing appropriate physical activity choices for their patients. A similar compendium has been developed specifically for youth (22). Table 1 provides a few examples at each level.

It is important to note that the compendium offers absolute intensity levels and does not take into account variations in weight, body mass index, or body composition. Researchers have demonstrated that the compendium values underestimate the energy cost or met level of weight bearing physical activity in overweight and obese individuals and overestimate the MET level of nonweight bearing physical activity (23) (see "Exercise Clearance" below for further discussion). Still, the compendium is useful as a guide and can help health care providers begin the conversation about level and intensity of physical activity, which then must be translated into an individualized exercise prescription.

The Cochrane review on "Exercise for Overweight or Obesity" from 2006 looked at physical activity intensity, volume, and changes in weight. The review examined the pooled effect of many studies. The authors reported that, in four randomized controlled trials, exercising at greater than 60% of VO_2 max is more effective at promoting weight loss than exercising at less intense levels (1.5 kg), when there were no dietary changes (24). Interestingly, when dietary changes were added to the analysis, exercise still contributed a modest amount to weight loss, but the intensity of exercise was no longer a factor. In other words, the effects of moderate-intensity physical activity were similar to those of vigorous physical activity when calorie restriction was added to the intervention. Keep in mind that the exercise involved in these pooled studies was on average three to five days per week and ranged dramatically from 10 to 60 minutes in duration. This wide range in volume and frequency of physical activity across individuals may have made it impossible to tease out significant differences. Given what is currently understood about physical activity and weight loss/maintenance, this volume of physical activity may have been sufficient in subjects at the high end of frequency and duration (i.e., high volume), but insufficient at the low end, to demonstrate significant results when combined with the known larger effect of diet.

Similarly, Jakicic et al. found no difference in weight loss when total volume of EE was kept constant but intensity ranged from moderate to vigorous over the course of 12 months (4). There is some evidence to suggest that physical activity intensity may have very specific benefits to individual comorbid conditions of obesity. For example, increased exercise intensity was found to reduce fasting serum glucose to a greater extent than lower intensity exercise (24). However, overall, the current literature suggests that sufficient volume of physical activity is more important in achieving weight loss or weight maintenance goals, and intensity of physical activity can be left to individual choice, ability level, and optimized to decrease risk of injury.

PHYSICAL ACTIVITY AND COMORBID CONDITIONS OF OBESITY

Physical activity is not only helpful in the long-term treatment of obesity, but it also has a positive effect on many comorbid conditions of obesity. Physical activity is inversely related to all-cause mortality (25–27). In adults, exercise decreases overall risk of early death, heart disease, hypertension, stroke, diabetes, hyperlipidemia, metabolic syndrome, colon and breast cancer, anxiety, depression, and falls (2). Physical activity also improves bone density, sleep quality, and cardiorespiratory endurance. In children, it results in improved metabolic health biomarkers, bone health, body composition, cardiorespiratory fitness and muscular fitness, and decreased anxiety and depression (2).

EXERCISE TESTING FOR EXERCISE CLEARANCE

The risk of an acute cardiac event during exercise from underlying coronary artery disease (CAD) is increased in obese individuals, because obesity itself a risk factor for CAD. Overweight and obese individuals also tend to carry multiple risk factors for CAD beyond their elevated BMI. These individuals have an increased incidence of metabolic syndrome, diabetes, impaired fasting glucose, dyslipidemia, and hypertension. However, the risk of an acute cardiac event is

Table 1 Energy Levels Required to Perform Some Common Activities

<3 METs	3–5 METs	5–7 METs	7–9 METs	>9 METs
Washing	Cleaning windows	Easy digging in garden	Sawing wood	Carrying load up stairs
Shaving	Raking	Hand lawn mowing	Heavy shoveling	Climbing stairs quickly
Dressing	Power lawn mowing	Climbing stairs slowly	Climbing stairs	Shoveling heavy snow
Desk work	Carrying objects (15-30 lbs)	Carrying objects (30-60 lbs)	Carrying objects (60–90 lbs)	
Washing dishes				
Driving auto				
Light housekeeping				
Golf (cart)	Golf (walking)	Tennis (singles)	Canoeing	Handball
Knitting	Dancing (social)	Basketball, football	Mountain climbing	Ski touring
Hand sewing	Tennis (doubles)	Snow skiing (downhill)		
Walking (2 mph)	Level walking (3–4 mph)	Level walking (4.5–5.0 mph)	Level jogging (5 mph)	Running >6 mph
Stationary bike	Level biking (6–8 mph)	Bicycling (9–10 mph)	Bicycling (12 mph)	Walking uphill (5 mph)
Very light calisthenics	Light calisthenics	Swimming, breast stroke	Swimming, crawl	Rope jumping
			Rowing machine	Bicycling (>12 mph)

lower in individuals with CAD that participate in regular physical activity than in those who do not (28,29). The AHA states that maintaining regular physical activity may reduce the risk of exercise-related cardiac events during heavy exertional activities (28). Individuals who were active four or more times per week had a much lower relative risk of an adverse event than those who were physically active less than four times per week (29). Although, no specific testing is identified, the AHA statement also recommends both preparticipation screening and avoidance of certain exercises in high-risk patients.

The ACSM provides a set of "Guidelines for Exercise Testing and Prescription" (30). Under these guidelines, ACSM recommends diagnostic exercise testing in patients based on an initial assessment of their CAD risk factors. Risk factors include: (*i*) family history of MI before 55 in 1st degree male relative or before 65 in 1st degree female relative, (*ii*) smoking with in the last six months, (*iii*) hypertension, (*iv*) abnormal lipids, (*v*) impaired fasting glucose—greater than 100 mg/dL, (*vi*) obesity—BMI greater than or equal to 30, and (*vii*) sedentary lifestyle. Exercise testing is recommended in asymptomatic patients with "moderate risk of CAD" who plan to participate in physical activity that is >75% of their maximal heart rate. Moderate risk is defined as any man ≥ 45 years and woman ≥ 55 years OR two or more the risk factors listed above. Physical activity that is >75% of the patient's maximal heart rate is considered vigorous. However, in the overweight or obese population this could correlate with activities that are defined as "moderate intensity" according to absolute MET level. As discussed previously, the compendium of MET levels will underestimate an obese individual's relative intensity during land-based activities.

If the fitness level of an individual is low due to deconditioning, exercises that would normally be considered at the high end of "moderate" physical activity (5–6 METs) would actually be "vigorous" physical activity for this individual (>6 METs). For example, walking at a 4.0 mph pace on a level firm surface is considered 5.0 METs. This would be classified as moderate physical activity in absolute terms. However, if an overweight or obese individual is deconditioned, this same intensity of walking may actually be a vigorous activity when their individual capacity is taken into account. This scenario can occur frequently in obese patients and directly affects exercise prescription for these individuals. A detailed algorithm to determine whether or not screening is needed prior to the initiation of an exercise regimen is available in the ACSM guidelines (30).

Exercise testing overweight and obese patients may also require modifications to the testing protocols and the testing equipment. For example, most overweight and obese patients require either a large or even more often a thigh-sized blood pressure cuff. A blood pressure cuff that is too small can elicit an inaccurately elevated reading. Orthopedic limitations may require accommodation by adjusting the type of exercise testing equipment utilized for the test. Some clients will require arm or leg ergometry instead of a standard treadmill test due to lower extremity arthritis or other orthopedic pathology. Finally, the actual stress test protocol may need to be adjusted. Some overweight and obese patients have such a low fitness capacity that a lower initial workload (measured in METs) and smaller increases in workload increments per stage of the testing protocol are required. The ACSM guidelines for exercise testing recommend that the initial workload may need to be decreased to 2 to 3 METs and the workload increments reduced to 0.5 to 1.0 METs in obese patients (30).

Because of severely decreased functional capacity and orthopedic issues, overweight and obese individuals often cannot complete an "adequate" stress test. In other words, functional limitations often result in an inadequate test because the patient fails to reach 85% of their maximal predicted heart rate. While this suboptimal result cannot rule out cardiac ischemia at higher levels of physical activity, it does provide the individual and the medical provider a level of reassurance within the scope of the individual's current functional capacity. This type of result is typically interpreted as "negative and inadequate." Maximal heart rate measured during the test can be used to calculate a targeted heart rate training range during prescribed physical activity. It is unlikely that individuals will exert themselves to a greater extent during a regular workout than they would have during their exercise stress test.

In addition to standard treadmill exercise stress testing, sometimes testing with imaging modalities is required. In the overweight and obese population, a few additional details must be considered. Nuclear imaging may be not be possible secondary to table weight limitations for the CT scanner. Most standard tables have a 350 lb weight limit. Nuclear imaging may require two consecutive days of testing secondary to the increased body mass. Stress echocardiograms can also be utilized, but may be affected by body habitus interference that can diminish the quality of the study.

In general, overweight and obese individuals are more likely to require exercise testing than the general population because they tend to have related comorbidities that increase their risk for CAD. As functional capacity increases with decreased weight, improved cardiorespiratory fitness, and typically improved orthopedic limitations, repeat cardiac testing should be considered to obtain an "adequate" test at 85% of predicted maximal heart rate. Exercise testing will not only provide reassurance for an individual's safety to participate in physical activity, but it can also help guide exercise prescription. During weight loss and weight maintenance, exercise testing data can provide a measure of maximal functional capacity in METs and these levels can guide submaximal exercise prescription.

EXERCISE OR PHYSICAL ACTIVITY PRESCRIPTION

An exercise prescription should include the five fundamentals of physical fitness regardless of BMI. The fundamentals include: cardiovascular endurance, muscular strength, muscular endurance, flexibility, and body composition. Eventually, a comprehensive exercise program should address and improve all five fundamentals. In order to build this program, individuals need instructions that are clear, simple, and based on measurable goals. These instructions come in the form of an exercise or physical activity prescription.

At a minimum, prescriptions should cover the four components of physical activity that are outlined with the acronym FITT: (*i*) frequency, (*ii*) intensity, (*iii*) time, and (*iv*) type. Initially, individuals should be assessed for their current level of physical activity participation. This will directly affect the volume and intensity of exercise prescribed. Then, to meet the requirements of FITT, a prescription should indicate how often, how hard, how long, and what kind of exercise will be done. FITT should be completed for the four activity-related fundamentals of physical fitness described above (cardio, strength, muscular endurance, and flexibility.)

Optimally, exercise or physical activity prescriptions should include a few additional key components. Motivational interviewing techniques and stages of change research have demonstrated the importance of assessing an individual's readiness for change. The prescription and goals from someone in contemplation about exercise will be very different from an individual who is in the action or maintenance stage of change. It is important to discuss appropriate and realistic goals. The prescribing provider will need to strategize with the individual about techniques to handle lapses and relapses into sedentary habits. Ideally the written prescription will have a place for the health care provider and the individual patient to sign. This allows the prescription to become a contract that is no longer passive, but instead active and engages the commitment of the individual. A copy of the prescription should be retained in the patient record for review and modification at follow-up visits.

Finally, consider exposing the individual to the concept of "Optimal Default." In the United States today, we have successfully engineered most physical activity out of our lives. Overweight and obese individuals need to find ways to reincorporate as much physical activity back into their activities of daily living (ADLs) as possible in an effort to accumulate the large volumes of physical activity described previously as required for success. Examples can be simple and/or creative: take the stairs, change your mode of transportation from passive (driving) to active (walking or cycling), park farther away, fidget more, initiate active hobbies, meet friends for a walk instead of a coffee, consider a standing or walking workstation. If an individual's original physical activity plan for the day, week, or year runs into a barrier, have a default (not just a back up plan) that creates increased physical activity.

SPECIAL CONSIDERATIONS IN EXERCISE PRESCRIPTION

Equipment Modifications

Overweight and obese individuals can require specialized exercise equipment. Strength training equipment is now available to allow appropriate access for obese individuals to enter and exit the equipment. Cardiovascular equipment like treadmills, elliptical trainers, and recumbent bicycles are available that have increased maximal weight limits. Recumbent bicycles often have larger more comfortable and appropriate seating. Upright stationary bicycles often do not come with appropriate seating for the overweight and obese patient, but the seat is often easily removable and an alternative wider seat can be attached. Physiology balls come in a variety of maximum static and dynamic weight capacities. These should be evaluated carefully based on an individual's needs. Physiology balls also come in varying shapes. Different shapes can increase or decrease the balance challenge requirement to help develop core strength skills safely in the obese and sedentary population. In general, equipment to be used by obese clients, especially those in class III obesity or higher, requires clarification of weight limits.

Personal equipment and attire should also be considered carefully. Aqua belts need to have adequate buoyancy support. Athletic footwear often needs to be increased in shoe width to accommodate increased fat deposition and/or lower extremity swelling from lymphedema. Individuals with large anterior fat deposition in the form of a pannus often require careful attention to skin care during physical activity. Clothing that is developed to pull moisture away from the body can help minimize candidal infections and skin breakdown in dependent skin folds. Waistbands need to be comfortable and nonrestrictive. Tight clothing in the lower torso can lead to meralgia paresthetica (numbness of the anterior leg), which although unlikely to cause harm can be uncomfortable and become a barrier to physical activity participation.

Monitoring Physical Activity in the Overweight or Obese Patient

Using tools to monitor physical activity can help determine an individual's compliance with and response to a weight loss or weight maintenance program. Tracking individual progress can also assist with patient motivation. Individuals can use physical activity recall surveys, physical activity logs, pedometers, or accelerometers to keep track of their physical activity participation.

Physical activity surveys can be completed at regular intervals and reviewed by the patient and the medical provider. Surveys ask the individual to look back and estimate their physical activity participation/compliance. They are typically quick but can be affected by the patient's ability to recall information correctly, termed "recall bias." Physical activity logs if done daily can be more accurate, but still depend on the subjective assessment of the individual. Because they are done more frequently, they are more labor intensive. Online programs can ease some of the burden and provide ongoing feedback to the individual that is often useful and motivational.

Direct measurement of physical activity is the best option for monitoring participation. However, there are obstacles to direct measurement in the overweight and obese population. Physical activity measurement devices may be less accurate in the obese population. Previous studies have demonstrated conflicting results. Initially, researchers reported that pedometers, used to measure step counts, were less accurate in overweight and obese individuals (31,32). Other studies have reported that pedometer accuracy was unaffected by BMI (33,34). A more recent investigation by Crouter et al. suggests that the type of pedometer may play a role in whether or not BMI classification, waist circumference, and position of the pedometer (due to increased abdominal fat) affect the accuracy of the results. In general, when an inaccuracy was found, it was typically an underestimation of actual steps (35).

Accelerometers, electronic motion sensors that detect changes in acceleration, can also be used to track physical activity. Accelerometers provide more in depth information regarding physical activity than pedometers, which only count number of steps. Accelerometers record frequency, intensity, and duration of physical activity. Few studies exist that have looked at accelerometer use specifically in the adult overweight or obese population (36–38). A recent study found that the amount of time an overweight or obese individual must wear an accelerometer to get a reliable estimation of physical activity is probably less than originally expected. The researchers reported that six hours of monitored time per day for four days was sufficient to reliably estimate moderate to vigorous physical activity participation (36). In a nonresearch setting, using pedometers/accelerometers can provide individuals with immediate objective daily feedback on whether or not their physical activity intentions are consistent with their daily actions, and more importantly their weight management goals. Overall, monitoring may be useful in individuals who find physical activity less enjoyable or struggle with compliance for any reason. Monitoring can serve as a trigger to improve regular participation.

Mobility Issues and Physical Activity in the Overweight/Obese Population

Physical activity in overweight and obese individuals is directly affected by underlying mobility issues. Obesity leads to increased functional limitations and disabilities with age in both men and women. These deficits range from mild to severe and include activities of daily living and instrumental activities of daily living (39). Degenerative joint disease, previous total joint replacements, and previous or active injuries may affect participation in physical activity. Weight bearing exercises with increased impact, such as a moderate to high impact group exercise classes, jogging, and treadmill walking or running often need to be avoided or restricted until a substantial amount of weight is lost. Mobility in the overweight and obese population is frequently affected by spinal pathology and/or pain, lower extremity pain or dysfunction, and balance deficits.

For example, obesity is associated with increased rates of osteoarthritis in the knee. The risk of osteoarthritis of the knee is 6.8 times greater in the obese population than in the lean population (40). Additionally, obese individuals with osteoarthritis of the knees are 9.8 times more likely to experience deterioration in physical function than lean individuals with no arthritis (41). Body mass is a major determinant of decreased mobility, termed "mobility disability" in 55 to 74 year old adults. Angleman et al. measured mobility disability using a timed eight foot walk and self-reported difficulty with variables like walking 100 yards, getting up from a chair after extended time spent sitting, and climbing several flights of stairs without rest. Increased body mass was related to decreased mobility. The authors reported that waist circumference was found to be the best predictor for obesity-related mobility disability (42).

Overweight or obese status also leads to an abnormal gait secondary to multiple biomechanical changes including: forefoot positioning, shortened stride, and rear-foot motion (43). Obese individuals are five times more likely to experience heel pain and plantar fasciitis than nonobese individuals (44). These are just select examples of many orthopedic issues that affect physical activity and exercise prescription in overweight or obese individuals.

In older adults with a BMI greater than 30 kg/m^2, obesity is also related to decreased balance regardless of overall strength (45). Obese individuals report an increased fear of falling (46). The odds of sustaining an injury, including those from falls, is increased 15% in the overweight population and 48% in class III obese patients (BMI $\geq$ 40) compared to normal weight individuals (47).

Finally, adipose tissue itself can be a physical barrier to effective movement. It can actually obstruct an exercise position or movement. Abdominal adipose tissue, including a large pannus, can prevent full hip flexion in either the seated or supine position. This makes stretching the ileotibial band, medial gluteus muscle, hamstrings, and low back difficult. These body areas are amongst those commonly injured in newly active individuals if not stretched adequately in a comprehensive exercise plan. A large dependent pannus can also severely limit land-based physical activity due to uncomfortable tissue movement, rubbing, and skin tension. This may occur with treadmill, elliptical, stationary bicycle, and recumbent exercise equipment in addition to free motion land movement. Evaluating individuals for mobility deficits or barriers is essential in the process of successful exercise prescription and long-term physical activity participation.

Resources for Physical Activity Prescription

There are many resources available as examples for physical activity prescription. The American Academy of Family Physicians provides an excellent provider toolkit that includes an exercise prescription pad, BMI calculators, a physician primer, and tools for patients as the embark on increased physical activity as a medical management approach to their weight and weight-related comorbidities. The toolkit is part of the AAFP initiative called Americans in Motion or AIM. The "AIM to Change Toolkit" can be found on the AAFP website at www.aafp.org. The National Heart Lung and Blood Institute also has helpful resources that are targeted and family/community-based resources. These resources can be found under the "We Can" program on the www.nhlbi.nih.gov/health website. Finally, the Centers for Disease Control and Prevention (CDC) are always expanding and adding to their physical activity enhancing resources (go to www.cdc.gov). Finally, understanding the continuum of "Stages of Change" can be useful when helping patients increase their level of physical activity by giving information and direction that is stage specific.

The goals for physical activity and exercise prescription in the obese population go beyond the contribution to energy expenditure (EE) and weight loss and or weight maintenance. Physical activity prescription in this population needs to include goals regarding mobility associated with activities of daily living, reduced pain, increased overall flexibility, improved strength, and decreased risk of fall. All of these considerations are in addition to typical calorie expenditure and improved cardiovascular health expectations.

Novel Approaches to Increasing Physical Activity

Increasing physical activity in the United States, as one of many methods to treat overweight and obese individuals, will require a matrix of solutions to support the differences between people and their varied living environments. Health care providers, public health specialists, researchers, exercise specialists, policy makers, and entrepreneurs are all introducing novel approaches to increasing EE through physical activity. Some approaches include environmental changes like innovative city planning and developmental models to increase pedestrian activities. Others are more behaviorally focused including mass marketing approaches like the CDC's VERB campaign to increase physical activity in children. Policy changes are slow in coming but are starting to appear. Americans now have the ability to claim their health club or wellness center membership dues as a tax deduction. Similarly, many larger U.S. companies offer partial payment for health club memberships and employee bonuses for voluntarily meeting or improving upon basic physical fitness criteria.

Perhaps one of the more creative recent solutions recently revolves around a concept called NEAT—nonexercise activity thermogenesis. Although the acronym is novel, the underlying premise reverts back to the idea that not all physical activity that contributes to EE is in the form of exercise. Looking back at the earlier equation for total EE, EE = REE + TEM + EEPA, nonexercise activity thermogenesis is equal to total EE from physical activity minus exercise (EEPA−energy expenditure from exercise = NEAT). EEPA accounts for approximately 30% of total daily EE. Unlike resting EE or the thermic effect of food, it is largely modifiable and appears to be highly variable from person to person. Researchers estimate that EE from physical activity that does not include intentional exercise may vary by up to 2000 kcal per day. Highly active individuals expend three times more energy per day than inactive individuals (48).

In considering a solution to the obesity epidemic, how could an inactive individual be converted to highly active individual if their day does not allow for dedicated time to exercise? Consider that the average American spends 1000 to 2000 hours at work per year. Researchers believe that this extensive time spent sitting may play a key role in the development of and solution to obesity. Could physical activity be constructed and introduced such that it occurs simultaneously and without interrupting an individual's work day? A major determinant in answering this question depends on how a given individual's work day is constructed. For a commercial airline pilot, it would be difficult to redesign a cockpit to allow for increased physical activity. However, for the majority of workers in America that spend a large component of their day sitting at a desk, there may be a relatively simple solution. Researchers have been examining the possibility of increasing daily physical activity by transitioning workers from a sedentary "chair dependent" work environment to an active work environment.

One proposed solution is to replace an individual's chair-dependent workstation (i.e., a desk) with an active workstation that employs a treadmill or bicycle. However, the goal is not to exercise. Recall that exercise has a purpose—to increase or maintain physical fitness. The goal of an active workstation is not to improve or maintain cardiovascular fitness, but to increase EE throughout the day by making sedentary work tasks slightly active. For example, in an exercise bout, an individual might walk at a speed of approximately 4 mph. When walking at a treadmill workstation, an individual would walk at less than 2 mph. The MET level for walking at less than 2 mph is 2.0. This would be classified as light physical activity. In comparison, walking at 4 mph is a MET level of 5.0, which is moderate-intensity physical activity. The goal of an active workstation is not to exercise; the goal is to increase EE while completing normal work tasks. Research by Levine et al. suggests that increasing standing or ambulating time by 2.5 hours per day could result in an additional 350 kcal per day of energy output. Thus, approximately every 10 work days an individual could loose 1 lb without any other behavioral changes. This could amount to 20 to 25 lb over the course of a year (49).

Table 2 Reincorporating Physical Activity into Activities of Daily Living

Take the stairs
Change your mode of transportation from passive (driving) to active (walking or cycling)
Park farther away from stores
Fidget more
Start an active hobby (bring fun into activity)
Meet friends for a walk instead of coffee or food
Consider a standing or walking workstation (desk)
Increase active family time: backyard Olympics, front yard baseball, family room dancing
Plan active vacations: check out walking, cycling, and hiking vacations in United States and Europe
Take on a new sport: great for your brain and your weight

Keep in mind, this type of increased EE has been shown to improve weight over time, but it will not provide the cardiovascular benefits of more moderate or vigorous physical activity. However, it may play a significant role in decreasing the suggested volume of 300 minutes of physical activity per week (discussed earlier in the review of guidelines) to a more manageable volume of exercise during nonwork leisure time hours.

Many other approaches to increasing EE throughout the day can be considered. Maximizing pedestrian activity whenever possible by: parking farther away from a destination when driving, bicycling for transportation, utilizing the stairs instead of elevators or escalators, or avoiding horizontal people movers like those found in airports. Have patients consider a "wake-up" walk on their lunch hour. See Table 2 for suggestions.

Even personal time can become more physically active without necessarily spending time at the gym. Recreational activities can incorporate more movement. Spending time as a family can be transitioned away from sedentary activities such as television or movies and refocused on active options such as backyard Olympics, family oriented 3k and 5k fun walks or runs, or block party baseball with the neighbors. Consider active vacations that can be individually developed, but are also now available through travel agencies. Companies now specialize in walking, hiking, cycling, kayaking, climbing, and many other active adventure vacations. Encourage your patients in creative problem solving. There are infinite ways to increase physical activity throughout the day.

SUMMARY

In summary, physical activity is a vital component to both weight and health management. Armed with scientific evidence behind the most recent guidelines, tools for patient assessment, and a thorough physical activity prescription, medical providers can facilitate the patient transition to a more active life. Get to know the local resources available including recreational and athletic facilities, physical activity trainers, exercise physiologists, community experts, and physical therapists. These resources will help guide the patient as they are preparing for the transition. Finally, keep in mind that advances in technology have engineered almost all physical activity out of everyday life. In order to aid in weight loss and succeed at weight maintenance, individuals will need to re-engineer physical activity back into their lives—perhaps in new and creative ways—and participate in traditional exercise.

REFERENCES

1. Ogden CL, Carroll MD, McDowell MA, et al. Obesity among adults in the United States—no change since 2003–2004. NCHA data brief no 1. Hyattsville, MD: National Center for Health Statistics, 2007.
2. US Department of Health and Human Services. 2008 Physical Activity Guidelines for Americans. United States Department of Health and Human Services. www.health.gov/paguidelines/guidelines/summary.aspx. Accessed May 27, 2010.
3. Catenacci VA, Odgen LG, Stuht J, et al. Physical activity patterns in the national weight control registry. Obesity (Silver Spring) 2008; 16(1):153–161.
4. Jakicic JM, Marcus BH, Gallgher KL, et al. Effect of exercise duration and intensity on weight loss in overweight sedentary women. JAMA 2003; 290:1323.

5. Caspersen CJ, Powell KE, Christenson GM. Physical activity, exercise, and physical fitness: Definitions and distinctions for health-related research. Public Health Rep 1985; 100(2):126–131.
6. Tataranni PA, Larson DE, Snitker S, et al. Thermic effect of food in humans: Methods and results from use of a respiratory chamber. Am J Clin Nutr 1995; 61:1013–1019.
7. Donnelly JE, Blair SN, Jakicic JM, et al.; American College of Sports Medicine. American College of Sports Medicine Position Stand. Appropriate physical activity intervention strategies for weight loss and prevention of weight regain for adults. Med Sci Sports Exerc 2009;41:459–471.
8. Stevens J, Truesdale KP, McClain JE, et al. The definition of weight maintenance. Int J Obes 2006; 30:391–399.
9. Hagan RD, Upton SJ, Wong L, et al. The effects of aerobic conditioning and/or calorie restriction in overweight men and women. Med Sci Sports Exerc 1986; 18:87–94.
10. Wing RR, Vendetti EM, Jakicic JM, et al. Lifestyle intervention in overweight individuals with a family history of diabetes. Diabetes Care 1998; 21:350–353.
11. Jakicic JM, Winters C, Lang W, et al. Effects of intermittent exercise and use of home exercise equipment on adherence, weight loss and prevention of weight regain for adults. JAMA 1999; 282:1554–1560.
12. Jakicic JM, Otto A. Treatment and prevention of obesity: What is the role of exercise? Nutr Rev 2006; 64(2):S57–S61.
13. Hill JO, Hyatt HR. Role of physical activity in preventing and treating obesity. J Appl Physiol 2005; 99:765–770.
14. Fogelholm M, Kukkonen-Harjula K. Does Physical activity prevent weight gain: A systematic review. Obes Rev 2000; 1:95–111.
15. Jakicic JM. The role of physical activity in the prevention and treatment of body weight gain in adults. J Nutr 2002; 132:3826S–3829S.
16. Jakicic JM, Marcus BH, Lang W, et al. Effect of exercise on 24-month weight loss maintenance in overweight women. Arch Intern Med 2008; 168:1550–1559; discussion 1559–1560.
17. Diaz VA, Mainous AG III, Everett CJ. The association between weight fluctuation and mortality: Results from a population based cohort study. J Community Health 2005; 30(3):153–165.
18. Blair SN, Shaten J, Brownell K, et al. Body weight change, all-cause mortality, and cause-specific mortality in the Multiple Risk Factor Intervention Trial. Ann Intern Med 1993; 1:119(7, pt 2) 749–757.
19. Pate RR, Pratt M, Blair SN, et al. Physical activity and public health: A recommendation from the Centers for Disease Control and Prevention and the American College of Sports Medicine. JAMA 1995; 273:402–407.
20. Haskell WL, Lee I, Pate RR, et al. Physical activity and public health: Updated recommendation for adults from the American College of Sports Medicine and the American Heart Association. Med Sci Sports Exerc 2007; 39(8):1423–1434.
21. Ainsworth BE, Haskell WL, Whitt MC, et al. Compendium of physical activities: An update of activity codes and MET intensities. Med Sci Sports Exerc 2000; 32(suppl 9):S498–S516.
22. Ridley K, Ainsworth BE, Olds TS. Development of a compendium of energy expenditures for youth. Int J Behav Nutr Phys Act 2008; 10(5):45.
23. Howell W, Earthman C, Reid P, et al. Doubly labeled water validation of the Compendium of Physical Activities in lean and obese college women (Abstract). Med Sci Ssport Exerc 1999; 31:S142.
24. Shaw K, Gennat H, O'Rourke P, et al. Exercise for overweight or obesity. Cochrane Database Syst Rev 2006; 18(4):CD003817.
25. Paffenbarger RS, Hyde RT, Wing AL, et al. Physical activity, all-cause mortality, and longevity of college alumni. N Engl J Med 1986; 314:605–613.
26. Paffenbarger RS, Hyde RT, Wing AL, et al. The association of changes in physical activity level among other lifestyle characteristics with mortality among med. N Engl J Med 1993; 328:538–545.
27. Lee IM, Rexrode KM, Cook NR, et al. Physical activity and coronary heart disease in women. JAMA 2001; 285:1447–1454.
28. Thompson PD, Franklin BA, Balady GJ, et al. Exercise and acute cardiovascular events placing the risks into perspective: A scientific statement from the American Heart Association Council on Nutrition, Physical Activity, and Metabolism and the Council on Clinical Cardiology. Circulation 2007; 115(17):2358–2368.
29. Giri S, Thompson PD, Liernan FJ, et al. Clinical and angiographic characteristics of exertion-related acute myocardial infarction. JAMA 1999; 282(18):1731–1736.
30. Whaley MH (ed.). ACSM Guidelines for Exercise Testing and Prescription. 7th Edition. Preparticipation Health Screening and Risk Stratification: Preparticipation Screening Algorithm. Philadelphia: Lippincott, Williams, and Wilkins 2006.
31. Melanson EL, Knoll JR, Bell ML, et al. Commercially available pedometers: Considerations for accurate step counting. Prev Med 2004; 39:361–368.

32. Shepherd EF, Toloza E, McClung CD, et al. Step Activity monitor: Increased accuracy in quantifying ambulatory activity. J Orthop Res 1999; 17:703–708.
33. Swartz AM, Bassett DR Jr, Moore JB, et al. Effects of body mass index on accuracy of an electronic pedometer. Int J Sports Med 2003; 24:588–592.
34. Elsenbaumer KM, Tudor-Locke C. Accuracy of pedometers in adults stratified by body mass index category. Med Sci Sports Exerc 2003; 35:S282.
35. Crouter SE, Schneider PL, Bassett DR Jr. Spring-levered versus piezo-electric pedometer accuracy in overweight and obese Adults. Med Sci Sports Exerc 2005; 37(10):1673–1679.
36. Jerome GJ, Young DR, Laferriere D, et al. Reliability of RT3 accelerometers among overweight and obese adults. Med Sci Sports Exerc 2009; 41:110–114.
37. Fogelholm M, Hiiloskorpi H, Laukkanen R, et al. Assessment of energy expenditure in overweight women. Med Sci Sports Exerc 1998; 30:1191–1197.
38. Jacobi D, Perrin AE, Grosman N, et al. Physical activity-related energy expenditure with the RT3 and TriTrac accelerometers in overweight Adults. Obesity 2007; 15:950–956.
39. Houston DK, Stevens J, Cai J, et al. Role of weight history on functional limitations and disability in late adulthood: The ARIC Study. Obes Res 2005; 13:1793–1802.
40. Coggon D, Reading I, Croft P, et al. Knee osteoarthritis and obesity. Int J Obes Relat Metab Disord 2001; 25(5):622–627.
41. Ettinger WH, Davis MA, Neuhaus JM, et al. Long-term physical functioning in persons with knee osteoarthritis from NHANES I: Effects of comorbid medical conditions. J Clin Epidemiol 1994; 47(7):809–815.
42. Angleman SB, Harris TB, Melzer D. The role of waist circumference in predicting disability in periretirement age adults. Int J Obes 2006; 30: 365–373.
43. Messier SP. Obesity and osteoarthritis: Disease genesis and nonpharmacologic weight management. Med Clin North Am 2009; 93(1):145–159.
44. Riddle DL, Pulisic M, Pidcoe P, et al. Risk factors for plantar fasciitis: A matched case-control study. J Bone Joint Surg Am 2003; 85(5):872–877.
45. Jadelis K, Milller ME, Ettinger WH, et al. Strength, balance, and the modifying effects of obesity and knee pain: Results form the Observational Arthritis Study in Seniors (OASIS). J Am Geriatr Soc 2001; 49(7):884–891.
46. Austin N, Devine A, Dick I, et al. Fear of falling in older women: A longitudinal study of incidence, persistence, and predictors. J Am Geriatr Soc 2007; 55(10):1598–1603.
47. Finkelstein EA, Chen H, Prabhu M, et al. The relationship between obesity and injuries among US adults. Am J Health Promot 2007; 21(5):219–224.
48. Black AE, Coward WA, Cole TJ, et al. Human energy expenditure in affluent societies: An analysis of 574 doubly-labelled water measurements. Eur J Clin Nutr 1996; 50:72–92.
49. Levine JA, Vander Weg MW, Hill JO, et al. Non-exercise activity thermogenesis: The crouching tiger hidden dragon of societal weight gain. Arterioscler Thromb Vasc Biol 2006; 26:729–736.

7 Behavioral modification

Erin Chamberlin-Snyder

Behavior and lifestyle changes are necessary for weight loss and maintenance (1). This chapter will discuss the importance of behavioral evaluation that includes interviewing and other methods of assessing patients' desire to change. Goal setting and self-monitoring (food/behavior diary) are integral to treatment, and specific practical hints/resources will be included for the clinician to use in his/her office (2). The types of behavioral therapies (3) will be reviewed and examples applied to the obese/overweight patient. Emotional factors, along with the hormonal and neurochemical processes, play a large role in disordered eating patterns. Current research studies are exploring the influence of the neurotransmitters on the limbic system of the human brain and the implications this influence has for behavior modification in the obese or overweight patient.

In the past, self-defeating lifestyle choices (i.e., self-restraint in food choices or self-discipline with exercising) were viewed as a lack of personal willpower. Even if clients lose weight initially, shaming or negative approaches rarely result in long-term success with weight maintenance. Now, in light of the findings of research on hunger hormones, neurotransmitters, and the effect of genetics, as well as the environment, it is evident that treatment of obesity requires behavior modification, as well as nutrition education, increase in physical activity, medical evaluation and, sometimes, pharmacotherapy (4,5).

Food programs should serve as a template to be adjusted on an individual basis, based on information from the patient's food/behavior diary and ongoing weight loss success. Following a "DIE-T" elicits a negative emotion when an alternate "unhealthy" choice is made (1). Individual tailoring of a food plan according to patient goals, family commitments, and work situations works best, but it takes homework on the part of the patient and time devoted by the medical bariatric team.

Exercise or increased physical activity normalizes neurotransmitters (such as serotonin [5-HT] and norepinephrine [NE]), optimizes cardiovascular health, increases muscle mass, and improves metabolism of nutrients, leading to a lower chance of weight regain. This important lifestyle change is the subject of another chapter and should be noted as a critical change necessary in most obese people.

In the past, most behavioral programs focused on participants changing diet and exercise (6). Personality and behavior tests were often used (6,7). Several assessment tools have since been developed to evaluate a wide range of specific behaviors, including disordered eating and thinking that may be present in a bariatric patient (9–10). As medical bariatricians, our expertise lies not only in the evaluation of genetic and physical causes of comorbid illnesses but also in the medical treatment of obesity, along with supplying huge doses of patient education and emotional support. Some clinicians provide the education piece in group sessions. The groups themselves can provide some emotional support to the patient and are a more efficient use of clinician time. On the other hand, individualized lifestyle suggestions are most appreciated and may be more likely to be internalized by the patient (11).

During the initial evaluation, use a patient history form which includes questions related to current lifestyle and questions that illuminate whether a patient has insight to causes of their excess weight and self-defeating actions. Spend time learning various factors in the person's life that may have contributed to weight gain (4).

A number of useful forms that help with this task are presented in Appendix B. For example, the American Society of Bariatric Physicians' patient history form/template is an excellent resource, designed specifically for medical bariatric evaluations. The Weight Loss Questionnaire, Assessment of Patient Readiness Form, and Food and Activity Diary (also available on the American Medical Association Web site) (12) were developed by bariatric medicine specialists, including leaders of the American Society of Bariatric Physicians and diplomates of the American Board of Bariatric Medicine. The Quality of Life Assessment (from LEARN) can be completed by the patient at the initial consultation and utilized at various points during the follow-up office visits. The Diet Readiness Test Questionnaire (from LEARN) gleans information from the patient that may indicate their insight into behaviors needing to be changed (13).

Goal setting should take place at the initial visit. Include a "weight loss goals list" for the patient to complete and encourage the goals to be specific (personal), measurable (precise), time framed (present), and realistic (possible) (14,15). The goals should be positive and include short-term, intermediate, and long-term goals. The patient's goal (wish) list is a very useful tool to use during follow-up appointments when discussing success reached and behaviors yet to be modified. Information gathered on the history form will prove invaluable in assessing the patient's baseline regarding the necessary behavioral changes to be addressed. Self-monitoring is integral to the success of weight loss, as well as long-term maintenance of healthier weight (13,15).

A food diary kept by the patient will also give clues as to the understanding of why food choices are made. Several examples of food, activity, and behavior diaries are included in Appendix B and can be adapted to fit the individual needs and preferences of the clinician and patient. Depending on the food program chosen by the patient and clinician to meet the patient's specific metabolic and weight loss needs, a column for amounts, calories, and grams of carbohydrates, proteins, or fats to be recorded should be included. We ask our patients to record physical activity so that we can estimate their macronutrient needs. Also, if a suboptimal food choice is made, we ask the patient to write down why that food was chosen. This enables the patient to gain insight to his or her actions/behaviors. Some of the reasons listed include habit, environment, mood, addiction, and lack of interpreting hunger cues (physiologic) (15), convenience, lack of boundary setting, advertising, and lack of portion or dietary knowledge (9). The patient may not know the "why" and, in fact, an automatic response, or "mindless eating," may be discovered by the patient (16). Later, emotional antecedents may be identified and the patient encouraged to develop strategies to deal proactively with similar high-risk situations in the future.

The transtheoretical model of change (17) includes five stages of change; precontemplation, contemplation, preparation, action, and maintenance (see Table 1). Relapse was added to later versions of this model; the concepts of "spiral of change" (19) and "contemplation ladder" (20) were added to suggest that a patient may relapse from any given stage to a previous stage. Although the majority of patients may come to your office ready for preparation and action, they may still be in precontemplation or contemplation about changing a certain behavior (e.g., dining out frequently) in order to lose weight. Each of the stages is applicable to each self-defeating behavior and takes varied amounts of time to extinguish, depending on the individual. The clinician can determine what stage the patient is in by asking open-ended questions *and listening to the answer*. For example, precontemplation can be discovered by asking the patient whether they want to change (e.g., "My wife/husband made me come here. I don't see a problem"). At this stage, the clinician should give the client information and advise about the positive health reasons to make a change. When a patient is in contemplation ("I would like to lose weight, but I don't believe I can lose or keep it off"), the clinician should accept ambivalence and avoid argument. Even patients who enter at the preparation stage need your help with short-term, intermediate, and long-term goal setting and to design a plan individualized to their goals (which may not necessarily be the same as your goals for the patient).

In the action stage, the clinician assists patients find their own solution by reviewing their eating cues and discussing patient recognition of triggers and consequences of actions chosen/taken. A helpful technique is to use the "ask-tell-ask" method (e.g., "Why do you think you chose fast food? You could choose to pack your lunch. Do you think you could pack a lunch four out of five work days?").

Maintenance of healthier weight improves with ongoing support that results from periodic visits with the clinician or a trained staff member of the bariatric office (21– 23) Increasing the length of the treatment phase (though not necessarily the time spent at each visit) improves weight loss and maintenance (9) Provide a supportive environment so that patients can create their own strategies for combating threats (i.e., plan a, b, and, c) (21). Long-term contact with providers, whether by phone, in person, in groups, or through the Internet, improves maintenance of a healthy weight (24). Social support studies show that weight loss/maintenance

Table 1 Applying the Stages of Change Model to Assess Readiness

Stage	Characteristic	Patient verbal cue	Appropriate intervention	Sample dialogue
Precontemplation	Unaware of problem, no interest in change	"I'm not really interested in weight loss. It's not a problem."	Provide information about health risks and benefits of weight loss	"Would you like to read some information about the health aspects of obesity?"
Contemplation	Aware of problem, beginning to think of changing	"I know I need to lose weight, but with all that's going on in my life right now, I'm not sure I can."	Help resolve ambivalence; discuss barriers	"Let's look at the benefits of weight loss, as well as what you may need to change."
Preparation	Realizes benefits of making changes and thinking about how to change	"I have to lose weight, and I'm planning to do that."	Teach behavior modification; provide education	"Let's take a closer look at how you can reduce some of the calories you eat and how to increase your activity during the day."
Action	Actively taking steps toward change	"I'm doing my best. This is harder than I thought."	Provide support and guidance, with a focus on the long term	"It's terrific that you're working so hard. What problems have you had so far? How have you solved them?"
Maintenance	Initial treatment goals reached	"I've learned a lot through this process."	Relapse control	"What situations continue to tempt you to overeat? What can be helpful for the next time you face such a situation?"

Source: Adapted from Ref. 18. With permission from American Medical Association.

is better when a patient utilizes like-minded friends rather than a "significant other" as their support system (25). Self-help for patients can include written media, radio, television (26,27), visual and audio (CDs/MPs/iPod) media, and, of course, the Internet More recent studies are exploring the use of the Internet as a tool to reach those who are homebound to increase availability of information, treatment, and maintenance support (28,29).

It is important to teach the patient to recognize danger signals that old behaviors are returning and suggest strategies for the mind games other people in their lives might play (e.g., "You have lost so much weight/worked so hard, you DESERVE to eat (poorly) when you are with us, your overweight family/friends/coworkers"). When a patient relapses into old self-defeating behaviors, a regain in weight is often the only sign. The clinician should reinforce "the positive" by praising previous success (e.g., "You did it before, you can do it again"). Rather than becoming frustrated about the relapse, the clinician should be welcoming the patients' return for help and assist them in learning what antecedent event lead *up to the relapse*. Then, you can help patients develop the skills necessary to maintain their success and prevent a future relapse (30).

The "stages of changes" model serves as a guide but has limitations (31) in that matching specific interventions to certain stages has not proven to facilitate change as well as motivational interviewing (MI) (32).

The standard modes of treatments include MI, interpersonal therapy (IT), behavioral therapy, cognitive therapy, cognitive behavioral therapy, and, more recently, maintenance-tailored therapy. The older technique of operant conditioning (Pavlov's dogs) is not as applicable to humans for producing desired behavior changes, but might help explain the patient how past emotions and stored memories may have an influence on undesired behaviors. I know I always salivate when thinking about a warm yeast donut (33).

MI is a directive, client-centered counseling style for eliciting behavior change by helping clients to explore and resolve ambivalence (34) Physicians who use MI in preventative health and chronic disease visits improve patients' efforts at weight loss (35). Also individual MI results in more weight loss and maintenance (36,37). The goal is to increase intrinsic motivation by encouraging the patient to think about change rather than impose an external demand by telling the patient what to do. Collaboration instead of confrontation is of key importance. Through open-ended questions, the clinician can discover the patient's own perceptions, goals, and values. Rather than acting as an authority that assumes the patient lacks knowledge, the clinician provides resources to facilitate the patient's realization of the benefits of changing a self-defeating behavior, as opposed to the probable outcome of not changing (38). A similar approach has been described by the acronym, GRACE (39): **G**enerate a gap, **R**oll with resistance, **A**void arguments, **C**an do, and **E**xpress empathy.

MI can be employed at each patient encounter when a clinician notes a positive behavior is lacking (e.g., no exercise) or damaging (e.g., eating out frequently) (40). Specific phrases have been suggested to use in the framework of MI (41). To generate a gap, you, as a clinician, can point out discrepancy between patients' goals and their present behavior by refreshing their awareness of their stated reasons for change (refer back to the patients' own written goal list). Roll with resistance; listen attentively; and acknowledge patients' feelings, attempts to cope, and their right to choose or reject change. It may be helpful to say, "I know how you feel, I have felt the same way, and this is what I found." You, personally, may not have had the same issue as the patient, but you can empathize by saying "I had a hard time changing (insert self-defeating behavior)." A simple statement that "Nothing will ever change until YOU decide to change" may assist patients in acknowledging the discrepancy between the continued self-defeating behavior and achievement of their goals.

Show empathic warmth by asking open-ended questions. Avoid arguments; remember, "He that complies against his will, is of the same opinion still" (Samuel Butler, 1612–1680). We are not called to this profession to argue with patients about their choices. Can do; a better strategy is to emphasize the patient's strengths and encourage hope for success. Express empathy, offer more information when the patient requests it, acknowledge that "change is difficult," and provide a supportive atmosphere for your patient (35,39).

Many studies have shown that IT can lead to weight normalization (17,42). IT has a more individualized, focused approach to emotional triggers and reframing of previous experiences.

Because of the high prevalence of depression as a coexisting condition with obesity, it is recommended that a depression screen (such as Beck's Depression Inventory) be performed on initial examination (43). You may prefer to refer the patient to a skilled psychiatrist and/or psychotherapist for more in-depth counseling, especially if the patient has a past personal history of emotional, physical, or sexual abuse. Remember the Osler motto, "Do no harm." Several other approaches to behavioral modification are available and can be used within your practice, particularly if you or a staff member/colleague has some psychotherapy training. But some simple brief interventions, focused on one behavior change per visit, can be implemented by a well-trained clinician within the constructs of brief follow-up visits.

Behavioral therapy is designed to reinforce or extinguish a behavior. It is based on principles of learning and is intended to alter lifestyle through action/behavior changes. Positive reinforcement is the most effective therapeutic tool (9). This can be verbal praise ("I knew you could do it"), tangible/visual recognition of success (certificates, buttons, before and after pictures on bulletin board) (1), pointing out the improvement of a comorbid condition as a result of the weight loss ("Your knee pain is down to a level 3 from your previously stated level of 9 on a scale of 1–10"), or showing patients an indirect positive to their behavior changes ("You saved $200 this month by not dining outside your home"). You can refer patients back to their goal list to point out the positive achievements ("You are able to play with your grandchildren longer now that your knees are less painful" or "You can buy new smaller/better fitting clothes").

Negative reinforcement is generally not as effective as positive reinforcement but may work as a form of mini-intervention if the patient continues to deny harm from the behavior, and the consequences are high (e.g., "The usual course of uncontrolled diabetes mellitus is renal failure, probable dialysis treatments, and possible loss of eyesight or amputation of a limb. Do you want to boat/fish/travel [per patient's goals] in your retirement years?"). Some earlier approaches utilized increased exposure to the action/behavior/food, sometimes along with aversive association (6). This is a strong approach and better implemented by a clinician with intervention/addiction training. Yet, as primary care providers and medical bariatricians, we often develop the repertoire, albeit after months and years of clinical experience, to take an aggressive interventional approach such as this to save the life of a patient.

Cognitive therapy includes techniques to alter ineffective thinking. The patient is encouraged to change habits over time, since it takes an average of 21 days to establish a habit and 2 years to make the habit more permanent (1). Reframing the patient's thoughts regarding a behavior may include clinician's statements, such as, "Eating a relative's sugar-loaded treat is not necessarily a sign of love for them." You can assist the patient with phrases to use as tools in those situations ("I am full, but may I please have the recipe"). Presenting alternatives to the patient may widen their perspective. An example would be suggesting they might take two bites of a treat instead of a whole portion. Visualization, as practiced by successful athletes who create an image of themselves successfully attaining their goal (e.g., making a free throw) just before they actually attempt it, is a helpful practice. You can encourage your patient to visualize behaving as a leaner person when they find themselves in challenging situations.

Cognitive behavioral therapy combines both behavior changes with cognitive understanding to enable the patient to identify the environmental and emotional triggers for their self-defeating actions/behaviors. Suggestions and tools are given to the patient to modify the nature of antecedent events that trigger unwanted eating behavior or the response to them, so the patient is better equipped to *choose* the action they wish to take. *Avoidance* of trigger foods or situations that lead to unwanted eating provides an important strategy for the patient. Encourage your patient to substitute a noncaloric, pleasurable reward instead of food. "Pleasure," like beauty, is in the eye of the beholder and is the key characteristic of a substitute behavior. Doing work, such as washing the laundry or running on the treadmill, is unlikely to activate the pleasure centers of the brain's limbic system, like the patient's trigger food does. Again, this is where the patient goal/desire list may help identify pleasurable, substitute behaviors. Success is more likely if the patient plans for a food-centered event by eating a healthy snack prior to the event or having a "good choice" food available by bringing it with him or her. A diary that records food intake, associated emotions, and information, such as "why did I eat that," promotes self-recognition of mindless eating (18), identifies triggers for behaviors, and assists the patient in devising strategies to eliminate or modify reactions to antecedent events.

Success is best accomplished by taking a tailored approach that addresses the patient's specific challenges (44,45). Whether a patient needs to implement more effective time management (e.g., using a day planner, taking a time management course, or reading a self-help book) to help him or her create time for fun physical activity and healthy meal planning, or needs help developing healthy boundaries in interactions with others, the most successful approach by the clinician is assisting the patient to explore his or her own values/thoughts preceding an emotion that produces his or her response/behavior.

Emotional stimulation involves three types of responses: behavioral, physiologic, and psychological. Behavioral actions can be verbal, displaying, or passive aggression.

Current data suggests biologic factors such as hunger/antihunger hormones may be more powerful than other natural reinforcing factors, such as having more energy (9). Recent theory has suggested that mechanisms involving the disregulation or misinterpretation of cues to the limbic system, as well as the possibility of addiction to behavior-induced neurotransmitters, may explain the difficulty humans have in achieving and maintaining a healthy weight (46– 51).

Physiologic responses can lead to an increase in the fight-or-flight hormone epinephrine (due to a relative cell hypoglycemia) (16) or a modulation/activation of the dopamine (DA) receptors, causing changes in appetite, thirst, sexual desire, or other pleasure centers in the limbic system of the human brain. Treating certain foods (or behaviors) as an addiction may work for some patients, but the physiologic hunger must be addressed also, whether this is done pharmacologically or by reinforcing the proper amounts of micro- and macronutrient intake and balancing those nutrients with an enjoyable form of physical activity. A food addiction questionnaire (Appendix B) may be an illuminating tool (52). Food addiction has been studied, and fasting potentiates the consumption of food and self-administration of drugs and, even, sucrose solutions (53). Addiction treatment would start with avoidance of stimulus and adding cues in the environment to prompt a new behavior. Do not buy trigger foods, plan ahead for healthier choices to be readily available, change your routine to avoid stimulus (e.g., drive a different way home to bypass your favorite fast food restaurant). Some patients benefit from applying the concepts of 12 steps of Overeaters Anonymous, including avoiding getting too hungry, tired, angry, or scared. Psychological effects can cause a change in the patient's present mental state (elated, anxious, more relaxed) on the basis of his or her past experiences and memory storage/retrieval by the limbic system.

The limbic system of the brain (particularly the hippocampus and amygdale) functions to determine the emotional state of mind. It is a principal player in memory storage, recall, and emotional interpretation of events (54). The limbic system also modulates motivation and libido, controls appetite and sleep, and processes sense of smell. Behavior reinforcement pathways include hindbrain centers for taste and forebrain centers for cognitive interpretation.

The nucleus accumbens is at the crossroads of the systems in that it interprets the signals of taste from the prefrontal cortex (olfaction) and communicates with the motor system for action and the globus pallidus and hypothalamus for appetite and motivation. The neurotransmitters involved include NE, 5-HT, and DA. NE *stimulates* feeding by activating alpha 2 NA receptors and *inhibits* via alpha 1 receptors. 5-HT suppresses food intake by inhibiting alpha 2 NA in the midhypothalamus. DA positively reinforces a behavior/action by generating appetite/want/motivation and, then, reward/pleasure. It also promotes escape from aversive stimulus (i.e., being hungry/lack of pleasure) (53). Genetic defects in the DA receptors have been implicated in the development of obesity (55–58) resulting in a "Reward Deficiency Syndrome," whereby the patient is at risk for using more and more of the substance (e.g., sugar) to get the same satisfied feeling (59,60). Another hypothesis of some studies that overstimulation of receptors and then withdrawal of the substance (e.g., sugar) creates a relative "depletion" of the dopamine signal (61) and processes/behaviors similar to addiction (62) Also, along with hormonal factors such as leptin and insulin resistance (63), this process has been postulated as an evolutionary advantage, in that the obese patient becomes a thrifty storer of energy as a survival mechanisms, but it now becomes a negative in the environment of abundant food (energy input) and less physical activity required to survive (energy output) (64,65).

Every being behaves in certain ways and may or may not always know why. The antecedent thought, anticipation of a specific behavior or behavioral outcome, for example, may produce neurochemicals that reinforce the behavior. Behavior may be modified by tracing those thoughts and actions that lead to the behavior (back-chaining) and then substituting new, healthier (or at least not self-defeating) behaviors (e.g., reading, playing a game, or engaging in some other pleasurable activity as opposed to doing work [laundry]) that give a reward/feeling or neurochemical response in the limbic system of the brain. Insert a new behavior closest to the desired outcome (or extinguish the old behavior closest to the undesired outcome). Then work backward by changing each action step and linking it to the new one changed before it. It takes many repetitions of practice to change an imprinted behavior pattern. For example, if you always overeat a certain trigger food at a holiday event, think why (e.g., your relative is a "food pusher" or you did not eat before being presented with the trigger). Then, learn to decline the food (e.g.," No, thank you." "No, I'm good."). You could plan ahead to have a small portion and eat plenty of healthy satisfying food beforehand. You could bring a nontriggering, acceptable substitution. You could choose to show up at the event after dinner is over or you could decline to attend altogether. Even bad habits are sometimes more comfortable than new habits, and attempting to change the action will cause anxiety (remember NE) or, especially in the beginning, not give you the same pleasure (dopamine). Anticipating and planning ahead for what action you will take, as well as training/repetition, ensures more likelihood of success. Some common stress-reduction techniques include relaxation training through biofeedback, listening to pleasing music, and deep breathing exercises. Hypnosis also has some success in reframing/retraining thoughts or feelings surrounding food choices. As in our previous example, if it makes you anxious or nervous to decline a relative's famous dish, you could opt to say, "It looks very tasty but I am so full. Could I please have the recipe?" You can also take a relaxing breath and repeat your answer, "No, thank you." Or excuse yourself to go talk to another relative away from the food table (avoidance) (1,66).

Assisting the patient in discovering the *why* (the thoughts and emotions surrounding and preceding the action/behavior) and *how* to change or override the neurotransmitter feedback may be the future key to long-term success (15). Well-trained medical bariatricians are in the best position to know, listen to, and advise obese patients on how to apply the most recent research findings on behavioral change strategies. Thus, they are also the best resource to help the obese patient achieve long-term, healthy weight maintenance and an improved quality of life (67).

REFERENCES

1. Kennedy M. Intermediate Bariatrics Course. Long-term Weight Management. Costa Mesa, CA: American Society of Bariatric Physicians, 2009.
2. Koop CE. A quest for the healing roots of medicine. The Chronicle of Higher Education. July 1, 1992:A5.
3. The American Board of Family Medicine Practice Guidelines, 2002.
4. Adding Magic to Medicine: Using Techniques From the Behavioral Sciences to Treat Obesity. Denver, CO: American Society of Bariatric Physicians, 2002.
5. Stuart R. Behavioral control of overeating. Behav Res Ther 1967; 5:357.
6. Jackson DN. Personality Research Form. 6th ed. Research Psychologists Press Inc, 1997. London, Ontario, Canada.
7. Jackson DH, Hoffman H. Common dimensions of psychopathology from the MMPI and Basic Personality Inventory. J Clin Psychol 1987; 43(6):661–669.
8. www.Pearsonsassessments.com. (Accessed February 2010).
9. Williamson DA, Perrin LA. Behavioral therapy for obesity. Endocrinol Metab Clin North Am 1996; 25:943–955.
10. Bray GA, Bouchard C. Handbook of Obesity. New York, NY: Marcel and Dekker, Inc, 2004.
11. Black DR, Cameron R. Self-administered interventions: a health strategy for improving population health. Health Educ Res 1997; 12(4):531–545.
12. American Medical Association. http://www.ama-asn.org. (Accessed February 2010).
13. Brownell KD, Wadden TA. The Learn Program for Weight Control. Dallas, TX: American Health Publishing Co, 1998.
14. Van Dorsten B. Behavioral modification in the treatment of obesity. In: Barnett AH, Kumar S, eds. London, England: Obesity and Diabetes, 2004.
15. Ludwig DS, Mjzaub JA, Al-Zahrani A. High glycemic foods, overeating, and obesity. Pediatrics 1999; 103(3):E26.

16. Keebler C. Board Review Course. Behavioral Modification. Nashville, TN: American Board of Bariatric Medicine, 2007.
17. Wansink B. Mindless Eating: Why We Eat More Than We Think. New York, NY: Bantam Dell, 2007.
18. Prochaska JO, DiClemente CC. Toward a comprehensive model change. In: Miller WR, ed. Treating Addictive Behaviors. New York, NY: Plenum, 1986:3–27.
19. Prochaska JO. Systems of Psychotherapy: A Transtheoretical Analysis. Homewood, IL: Dorsey Press, 1979.
20. Prochaska JO, DiClemente CC, Norcross JC. In search of how people change. Application to addictive behaviors. Am Psychol 1992; 47(9):1102–1114.
21. Biener L, Abrams DA. The contemplation ladder: validation of a measure of readiness to consider smoking cessation. Health Psychol 1991; 10:360–365.
22. Wing R, Hall J. The National Weight Control Registry. http://www.nwcr.ws. (Accessed February 2010).
23. Jeffrey RW, Folsom AR, Luepker RV, et al. Prevalence of overweight and weight loss behavior in a metropolitan adult population: the Minnesota Heart Survey experience. Am J Public Health 1984; 74;349–357.
24. Van Dorsten B. Obesity Course. Maintaining Patient Motivation in Long-term Weight Management: Combining Creativity with Genius. Atlanta, GA: American Society of Bariatric Physicians, 2005.
25. Wing RR, Jeffrey RW. Benefits of recruiting participants with friends and increasing social support for weight loss and maintenance. J Consult Clin Psychol 1999; 67(1):132–138.
26. Meyers A, Graves TJ, Whelan JP, et al. An evaluation of a television-delivered behavioral weight loss program: are the ratings acceptable? J Consult Clin Psychol 1996; 64:172–178.
27. Harvey B. Changing health behavior via telecomm technology. Behav Ther 1998; 29:505–59.
28. Webber KH, Tate DF, Quintiliani LM. Motivational interviewing in internet groups: a pilot study for weight loss. J Am Diet Assoc 2008; 108(6):1029–1032.
29. Hung SH, Hwang SL, Su MJ, et al. An evaluation of weight loss programs incorporating E-learning for obese junior high school students. Telemed J E Health 2008; 14(8):783–792.
30. Byrne SM. Psychological aspects of weight maintenance and relapse in obesity [review]. J Psychosom Res 2002; 53(5):1029–1036.
31. Jeffrey RW, Levy RL, Langer SL, et al. A comparison of maintenance-tailored therapy & standard behavioral therapy for treatment of obesity [published online ahead of print August 18, 2009]. Prev Med 2009; 49(5):384–389.
32. DiMarco ID, Klein DA, Clark VL, et al. The use of motivational interviewing techniques to enhance the efficacy of guided self-help behavioral weight loss treatment. Eat Behav 2009; 10(2):134–136.
33. Temple JL, Bulkley AM, Badawy RL, et al. Differential effects of daily snack food intake on the reinforcing value of food in obese and nonobese. Am J Clin Nutr 2009; 90(2):304–313.
34. Rollnick S. Behavior change in practice; targeting individuals. Int J Obes Relat Metab Disord 1996; 20:S22–S26.
35. Pollak KI, Østbye T, Alexander SC, et al. Empathy goes a long way in weight loss discussions. J Fam Pract 2007; 56(12):1031–1036.
36. West DS, DiLillo V, Bursac Z, et al. Motivational interviewing improves weight loss in women with type 2 diabetes. Diabetes Care 2007; 30(5):1081–1087.
37. Carels RA, Darby L, Cacciapaglia HM, et al. Using motivational interviewing as a supplement to obesity treatment: a stepped-care approach. Health Psychol 2007; 26(3):369–377.
38. Miller WR, Rollnick S. Motivational Interviewing: Preparing People for Change. Guilford Press, New York, NY 2002.
39. Sim MB, Wain T, Khong E.. Influencing behavior change in general practice—Part 1-brief intervention and motivational interviewing. Aust Fam Physician 2009; 38(11):885–888.
40. Ruback S, Sandbaek A, Lauritzen T, et al. Motivational interviewing: a systematic review and meta-analysis. Br J Gen Pract 2005; 55(513):305–312.
41. Houng V. Putting prevention into practice: counseling patients to prevent and decrease obesity. J Okla State Med Assoc 2005; 98(6):252–254.
42. Burke BL, Arkowitz H, Menchola M. The efficacy of motivational interviewing: a meta-analysis of controlled clinical trials. J Consult Clin Psychol 2003; 71(5):843–861.
43. Roberts RE, Deleger S, Strawbridge WJ, et al. Prospective association between obesity and depression evidence from the Alameda County Study. Int J Obes Relat Metab Disord 2003; 27(4):514–521.
44. Perri, MG, Corsica JA. Improving the maintenance of weight lost in behavioral treatment of obesity. In: Wadden T, Stunkard A, eds. Handbook of Obesity Treatment. New York, NY: Guilford Press, 2002.
45. Goldberg JH, Klernan M. Innovative techniques to address retention in a behavioral weight-loss trial. Health Educ Res 2005; 20(4):439–447.

46. Davis JF, Tracy AL. Exposure to elevated levels of dietary fat attenuates psychostimulant reward and mesolimbic dopamine turnover in rats. Behav Neurosci 2008; 122(6):1257–1263.
47. Tsujino N, Sakurai T. Orexin/hypocretin: a neuropeptide at the interface of sleep, energy homeostasis and reward system. Pharmacol Rev 2009; 61(2):162–176.
48. Zheng H, Lenard NR, Shin AC, et al. Appetite control and energy balance regulation in the modern world: reward-driven brain overrides repletion signals. Int J Obes 2009; 33(2):8–13.
49. Stoeckel LE, Kim J, Weller RE, et al. Effective connectivity of a reward network in obese women [published online ahead of print May 23, 2009]. Brain Res Bull 2009; 79(6):388–395.
50. Adam TC, Epel ES. Stress, eating and the reward system [published online ahead of print April 14, 1007]. Physiol Behav 2007; 91(4):449–458.
51. Shin AC, Zheng H, Berthoud HR. An expanded view of energy homeostasis: neural integration of metabolic, cognitive, and emotional drives to eat [published online ahead of print February 12, 2009]. Physiol Behav 2009; 97(5):572–580.
52. Jay K. Food addiction and the weight-loss surgery patient. Obesity Action Coalitions News 2007; 15–17.
53. Wang GJ, Volkow ND, Fowler JS. The role of dopamine in motivation for food in humans: implications for obesity. Expert Opin Ther Targets 2002; 6(5):601–609.
54. Suyama S, Takano E, Iwasaki Y, et al. Roles and functional interplay of the gut, brain stem, hypothalamus and limbic system in regulation of feeding [in Japanese]. Nippon Rinsho 2009; 67(2):277–286.
55. Thanos PK, Michaelides M, Ho CW, et al. The effects of two highly selective dopamine D3 receptor antagonists (SB-277011 A and NGB-2904) on food self administration in a rodent model of obesity. Pharmacol Biochem Behav 2008; 89(4):499–507.
56. Hajnai A, Margas WM, Covasa M. Altered dopamine D2 receptor function and binding to obese OTETF rat. Brain Res Bull 2008; 75(1):70–76.
57. Hajnai A, De Jonghe BC, Covasa M. Dopamine D2 receptors contribute to increased avidity for sucrose in obese rats lacking CCK-1 receptors. Neuroscience 2007; 148(2):584–592.
58. Hajnai A, Acharya NK, Grigson PS, et al. Obese OLETF rats exhibit increased operant performance for palatable sucrose solutions and differential sensitivity to D2 receptor antagonism. Am J Physiol Regul Integr Comp Physiol 2007; 293(5):R1846–R1854.
59. Comings DE, Blum K. Reward deficiency syndrome: genetic aspects of behavioral disorders. Prod Brain Res 200; 126:325–341.
60. Geiger BM, Haburcak M, Avena NM, et al. Deficits of mesolimbic dopamine neurotransmission in rat dietary obesity. Neuroscience 2009; 159(4):1193–1199.
61. Reinholz J, Skopp O, Breitenstein C, et al. Compensatory weight gain due to dopaminergic hypofunction: new evidence. Nutr Metab (Lon) 2008; 5:35.
62. Avena NM, Rada P, Hoebel BG. Evidence for sugar addiction: behavioral and neurochemical effects of intermittent excessive sugar intake. Neurosci Biobehav Rev 2008; 32(1):20–39.
63. Bello NT, Hajnai A. Alterations in blood glucose levels under hyperinsulinema affect accumbens dopamine. Physiol Behav 2006; 88(1–2):138–145.
64. Berthoud HR. Interactions between the "cognitive" and "metabolic" brain in the control of food intake. Physiol Behav 2007; 91(5):486–498.
65. Lenard NR, Berthoud HR. Central and peripheral regulation of food intake and physical activity: pathways and genes. Obesity (Silver Spring) 2008; 16(3):11–22.
66. Epstein LH, Leddy JJ, Temple JL, et al. Food reinforcement and eating: a multilevel analysis. Psychol Bull 2007; 133(5):88.
67. American Society of Bariatric Physicians. http://www.asbp.org; and American Board of Bariatric Medicine. http://www.abbmcertification.org. (Accessed February 2010).

8 Pharmacotherapy

Ed J. Hendricks

INTRODUCTION

This chapter is intended to be a practical guide to clinically useful prescription weight management medications in current use. There are only a handful of FDA approved drugs available for treating obesity. The newer drugs, sibutramine and orlistat, which are approved for long-term use, are recommended by many standard texts simply because FDA sanctioned long-term trials of a year or more have been conducted and published. The older drugs, phentermine, diethylpropion, and phendimetrazine are ignored or considered inappropriate by some experts because these are not approved for long-term use (long-term trials were not in vogue when the FDA approved them 50 years ago) and because they are amphetamine congeners. Although long-term trials tailored to current FDA specifications have not been conducted, the older drugs have been tested practically through long usage. In the opinion of experienced practicing bariatric physicians, the older drugs are more effective than the newer drugs, they share very few characteristics with amphetamine, they are considerably less expensive, and they are just as safe as the new drugs, if not safer. When patients who pay for their own medications are allowed to try any of the anti-obesity drugs, they invariably end choosing one of the older drugs, most often phentermine.

This chapter discusses the evidence supporting these opinions that are held by a majority of experienced bariatric physicians. The lack of evidence supporting the conjectures in the FDA labeling of the older drugs is discussed. This chapter is not meant to be an academic review of all pharmaceutical agents used in weight management in the past, present, or in the future. Only a few new drugs that have yet to be approved by the FDA are discussed. The remainder of experimental unapproved drugs for weight loss and the over-the-counter vitamins and supplements said to be helpful in weight loss are not discussed. Drugs that have been found most useful in practice are discussed in detail; less effective drugs are briefly discussed but not elaborated upon.

Pharmacotherapy is a mainstay in obesity treatment, but it should always be used within the context of a comprehensive approach to treating the illness. Pharmacotherapy should never be used alone but in combination with caloric restriction for weight loss or dietary control for maintenance, and behavior modification. An increase in exercise frequency and intensity are important behavior modifications for nearly all patients. For optimum effectiveness, pharmacotherapy should be long-term; patient and physician should mutually agree that medications selected should be used for as long as the drug is effective, provided undesirable side effects are absent or, if present, manageable.

CAUTIONS FOR PRESCRIBING PHYSICIANS

Although experienced bariatric physicians have found the drugs discussed here to be both effective and safe, many nonbariatric physicians believe them to be inherently dangerous—more dangerous than the obesity for which they are prescribed, at least until the patient is egregiously overweight. One reason for this opinion is that weight management drugs in general, and anorectics in particular, have had a history of unexpected adverse effects (1). Although there is little evidence in the medical literature the dangers enumerated in the product labeling for the older drugs have actually occurred, neither is there much documentation of long-term safety and efficacy for the older weight management drugs. As a result, unproven conjectures based on chemical structural similarities to amphetamine regarding the sympathomimetic amine drugs, phentermine, diethylpropion, and phendimetrazine, persist and the potential benefits of effective obesity pharmacotherapy with these older drugs have been greatly restricted.

In 2008, the American Society of Bariatric Physicians (ASBP) conducted a national survey examining how bariatric physicians employ pharmacotherapy in obesity treatment (2). The survey revealed a striking discrepancy between how bariatric medicine physicians actually prescribe pharmacologic agents in treating obesity and academic obesity treatment guidelines. The obesity treatment guidelines promulgated by many academic medical societies follow closely the recommendations of the National Institutes of Health's clinical guidelines for the diagnosis and treatment of obesity issued in September 1998 (3). The expert committee, in formulating the NIH guideline, decided that diagnosis and, therefore, treatment decisions should be predicted entirely upon body mass index (BMI) thresholds. This decision, controversial because it was based on opinion and not evidence, and because it restricted treatment—especially obesity pharmacotherapy, was opposed by some clinicians at the time the NIH guidelines were adopted and published (4). Currently, the only obesity treatment guide that places emphasis on diagnostic thresholds other than the BMI is the guideline of the ASBP (5). This national society of physicians practicing obesity treatment developed practice standards and obesity treatment guidelines long before obesity was officially recognized as a disease and long before the use of the BMI came into vogue. BMI, originally an epidemiology tool, which correlates best with obesity mortality, is known to be an insensitive indicator of abdominal adiposity (6–8) and of the typical morbidities associated with obesity (9). In particular, BMI is an insensitive indicator for cardiovascular risk (10,11).

It is the opinion of the author that patients should be selected and treated by following the guidelines of the ASBP. The recommendations in this chapter, therefore, in some cases, may deviate from what is uniformly recommended in the product labeling, the Physicians Desk Reference (PDR) or the NIH guidelines. However, physicians who treat obesity should be cognizant that some state medical boards insist physicians adhere strictly to the NIH guidelines. We are aware of cases in some states where physicians have been disciplined by their boards for prescribing obesity drugs off-label. Physicians who treat obesity should make themselves aware of the stance of their own state medical board on these issues before deciding how to use these drugs.

Selection of patients for whom controlled substance anorectic medications can be prescribed has become increasingly controversial since FDA approval of dexfenfluramine in 1996 and the subsequent Phentermine/Fenfluramine crisis (12). The ASBP first formalized and published their Anorectic Usage Guidelines in 1990 following the 1985 NIH Consensus Conference, which first defined Obesity by BMI thresholds: BMI $\geq$ 27.2 in women or $\geq$ 27.8 in men. The ASBP guidance emphasized that pharmacotherapy for the chronic progressive illness called obesity in any individual patient should be based on the physician's judgment and not on arbitrary thresholds. Subsequently, in 1995, an expert committee of the World Health Organization opined that obesity should be defined as a BMI $\geq$ 30, whereupon the FDA mandated BMI restrictions in clinical trials for anti-obesity drugs, and added BMI threshold restrictions to dexfenfluramine as it was approved in 1996. Subsequently, the FDA added the same BMI restrictions to sibutramine upon its approval in 1999 and, at the same time, extended BMI restrictions to the older drugs, including phentermine. After 40 years of safe use, the older drugs suddenly were declared unsafe by government fiat; physicians who prescribed the drugs in patients who did not fit the government decreed thresholds were suddenly prescribing "off-schedule." In 1998, the NIH published "Clinical guidelines on the identification, evaluation, and treatment of overweight and obesity in adults—the evidence report." These guidelines have also been adopted by a variety of medical associations including the Obesity Society (formerly NAASO, now TOS) (3), the AMA (13), the American College of Physicians (14), and by numerous other organizations (15). These all define obesity by BMI threshold and offer guidance to restrict treatment with anti-obesity drugs to patients with BMI $\geq$ 30 or with BMI $\geq$ 27 if the patient has diabetes, hypertension, or hyperlipidemia. Although these were offered only as treatment guides, not intended to override clinicians' judgment, it is the view of many government agencies and state medical boards that the official guidelines are *the standard of practice*. It appears that only the ASBP obesity treatment guidelines recommend treatment using criteria other than the BMI.

Be forewarned that, although the author believes the recommendations given here are sound and are in the best interests of your patients, not all physicians, medical boards, and insurance companies will agree. Each physician will have to decide which of the guidelines to use in their own practice and how far they can stray "off-schedule." Although the physician may believe it not in a patient's best interests, the safest course for the physician to follow in protecting his right to practice medicine is to prescribe controlled substance weight management medications strictly in accordance with product labeling.

WHY USE PHARMACOTHERAPY?

One might ask why pharmacotherapy is a treatment mainstay; why use pharmacotherapy at all if it is so controversial? There have been numerous clinical trials in the past of all the weight management drugs and these have been reviewed in several extensive meta-analyses, all of which agree that pharmacotherapy is an effective addition to obesity treatment (16–20).

Several more recent studies have shown that patients in weight loss programs who are placed on a weight management drug lose more weight than those on the same program without the drug, in both short-term trials and year-long trials. Patients given sibutramine, in a study by Wadden et al. (21), lost 12% of their original weight at 52 weeks while those on the same program with no drug lost 6%. In an unpublished study from the author's clinic, patients on phentermine lost 15% of their original weight in 12 weeks while those on the same program on no drug lost 10% in the same time period (22). Haddock has reported that, compared with published long-term studies, both better 52-week weight loss and better patient retention occurred when phentermine was combined with caloric restriction in a private practice setting (23).

Bariatric physicians who employ pharmacotherapy are generally in agreement with Haddock's assertion that the rate of patient retention is higher in patients placed on weight management medications than in those on no medication. Obesity is a chronic illness; obviously, the longer patients stay in therapy the higher the likelihood of both short-term weight loss and long-term successful weight maintenance.

Pharmacotherapy can also produce beneficial effects other than weight loss and metabolic improvements produced by weight loss. There is evidence that quality of life (QOL) improves with weight loss (24), and that pharmacotherapy producing greater weight loss enhances QOL improvement (25).

MEDICATIONS USEFUL IN TREATING OBESITY

Agents for Weight Loss and Maintenance

Phentermine

Phentermine is safe and effective for nearly every patient; if an anorectic is to be used phentermine should always be the first choice unless there is some reason to avoid it. Phentermine is the most widely used weight management agent in current use. The ASBP survey revealed that 97% of the responding bariatric physicians used pharmacotherapy in treating obesity and 98% of them used phentermine in an average of 50% of their patients (2) (Table 1).

Phentermine, a sympathomimetic amine derived from β-phenylethylamine, is thought to produce an anorectic effect by releasing norepinephrine that acts through α_1-adrenergic receptors in the paraventricular nucleus in the central nervous system to reduce food intake. The β-phenylethylamine skeleton is also the framework for the neurotransmitters epinephrine, norepinephrine, and dopamine. In clinical use, phentermine has two distinctly different therapeutic effects in all patients. The first and most obvious is short-term appetite suppression. The second, more subtle but long-term effect, is improved or stronger eating restraint. Appetite

Table 1 Percentage of Bariatric Medicine Specialists Prescribing Specific Drugs for Weight Management (2008 ASBP Survey of Bariatric Physicians Prescribing Practices)

Drug prescribed	% Physicians
Phentermine	98
Diethylpropion	58
Phendimetrazine	56
Sibutramine	46
Topiramate	45
Orlistat	44
Zonisamide	8

suppression tends to fade with time but eating restraint persists and is still present after the patient has been taking phentermine for years. Patients experience less hunger or even no hunger when started on phentermine, and this effect diminishes with time on any given dose. If the dose is increased, the patient may again experience less hunger but this effect diminishes even more rapidly. Typically, if the drug is discontinued, as the labeling advises, hunger reappears and the patient begins to gain weight even while still attempting to diet. On the other hand, if the drug is continued even though the patient does not think it is effective, the patient will often continue to lose weight or maintain their weight loss without regain or with minimal regain. Patients who have taken phentermine long-term to assist with maintenance say that they take it every day and notice no effect whatsoever. However, if they stop taking the phentermine they soon notice increased hunger and that their food servings are larger. They also notice a diminution of restraint and weight gain often soon ensues. This second long-term effect of phentermine has long been ignored but is clearly the basis for better success with long-term maintenance when phentermine is included in a maintenance regimen (23).

Some, but not all, patients also notice another long-term clinical effect—a diminution of carbohydrate cravings. Such cravings typically disappear quickly in the early stages of a weight management program, especially if the caloric restriction component also restricts carbohydrate intake. Very low-carbohydrate diets with daily carbohydrate restricted to 20 g or less work best in this regard. Carbohydrate cravings disappear promptly on such diets when no weight management medications are employed and it is impossible to tell if phentermine helps much in allaying cravings after the first three days on such a diet. Patients having carbohydrate intakes greater than 20 g daily and no phentermine will sometimes still complain of carbohydrate cravings, and it is in these patients that the addition of phentermine will sometimes produce diminution of cravings. If later in the course of weight loss or during maintenance carbohydrate cravings become a problem, the addition of phentermine or an upward adjustment of phentermine dose may alleviate cravings. The addition of 5-hydroxytryptophan combined with carbidopa added to the phentermine, discussed later, may be helpful in patients with carbohydrate cravings.

Duration of action—Phentermine is long acting with a biological half-life of 18 to 24 hours.

Clinical usefulness—Phentermine is the most useful weight management agent of all.

Absolute contraindications—The three conditions that are absolute contraindications to prescribing phentermine are pregnancy, nursing an infant, and previous severe allergic reaction to phentermine. Although pregnancy is an absolute contraindication now, phentermine and other anorectics were widely used to prevent excessive weight gain during pregnancy from 1959 until 1979 without any adverse effects on either the gestation or the fetus. After the FDA introduced Pharmaceutical Pregnancy Categories in 1979, and gave phentermine a category C rating, obstetricians stopped prescribing phentermine during pregnancy. There are no known teratogenetic effects ascribed to phentermine. Patients can be advised to continue taking it while trying to get pregnant and then discontinue it once pregnancy is diagnosed.

Nursing mothers should not have phentermine prescribed since the drug will find its way into her milk producing an anorectic effect in the infant. Phentermine given to someone who has had a prior severe allergic reaction may induce anaphylaxis.

Ages—Although phentermine labeling states that the drug should not be used in patients aged 16 years and younger, the drug has been used in children as young as age 3 without ill effects (26,27). Typically, guidelines for treating obesity in children and adolescents either omit mentioning the sympathomimetic amine anorectics or condemn their use (28). The 2008 ASBP survey revealed that 56% of practicing bariatric physicians prescribed anorectics for adolescents (the question did not specify an adolescent age range). Some caution is advisable here since pediatricians seem to be uniformly opposed to using the older anorectics. It is indeed incongruous that the very same pediatricians who will willingly employ schedule II controlled substance amphetamines to treat attention deficit hyperactivity disorder (ADHD) in their patients refuse to consider far less dangerous schedule IV controlled substances such as phentermine and diethylpropion for treating obesity. Informed consent should be obtained from the parents before prescribing phentermine for an adolescent and the parents should be forewarned that the patient's pediatrician would likely be opposed to the use of phentermine. There is no upper age limit for phentermine.

Dose—The normal starting dose for adults is 18.75 mg (1/2 of a 37.5 mg tablet) once or twice daily with the second dose before 3 PM, if a second dose is needed. Although the drug has a biological half-life of 18 to 24 hours and once daily dosing should be efficacious, some patients benefit from twice daily dosing. Phentermine has stimulant effects that typically are mild and fade quickly. In patients who have a history of over-reacting to stimulants, or have panic or anxiety, a lower starting dose of 15 mg may be advisable. An even lower starting dose could be achieved by breaking the 37.5 mg tablet into quarters to achieve a dose approximating 9 mg. Eight milligram tablets, available before the Phen/Fen crisis in 1997, are no longer manufactured. The starting dose for younger adolescents should be either ~ 9 or 15 mg/day. Later in the course doses may be adjusted as discussed in the following section. One early study reported that patients given phentermine on an alternating month schedule had the same weight loss as patients given phentermine continuously (29). This practice is not recommended since it interrupts weight loss, sometimes with significant weight gain. Patients who have been taken off phentermine often begin to gain weight in the first month, become discouraged and disillusioned with their treatment, and are lost to follow-up.

Dose ranging—Although some early clinical trials used dose-to-effect titration of phentermine doses (30), there are only a few modern papers reporting phentermine doses exceeding 37.5 mg per day for treating obesity. There are no modern, double-blind, randomized, placebo-controlled, prospective phentermine dose ranging clinical trials in the medical literature. There are, however, several reports suggesting that dose-to-effect titration has been in use for phentermine for many years. In the study reported by Haddock the authors state, "In cases of excessive hunger, the initial starting dosage was doubled for Phentermine-HCL" (23). Their starting dose was either 30 or 37.5 mg/day, so evidently some patients were started on either 60 or 75 mg/day. Another report from a private obesity treatment clinic reports starting compounded doses of 40 mg phentermine with 5-HTP (5-hydroxytryptophan)/carbidopa per day that are often then titrated to phentermine 55 mg per day within the first month (31). The 2008 ASBP Prescribing Practices Survey asked the question "... what are the lowest and highest doses you prescribed [of phentermine] ..." and although the *average* high dose was reported as 56 mg/day, significant numbers of physicians prescribed more than the average high dose. Responses to the survey were anonymous to encourage honesty and to protect respondents from trial lawyers, governmental agencies, and malpractice insurers. The raw data from the survey revealed that while 5% of respondent physicians prescribed 56 mg/day as their highest dose, 11% prescribed 60 mg/day, 19% prescribed 75 mg/day, 3% prescribed 90 mg/day, 4% 112 mg/day, 1% prescribed 150 mg/day, and 1% prescribed 180 mg/day as their highest dose (2). The responses indicate that 44% of the physicians surveyed have titrated phentermine doses beyond the PDR recommended highest dose. This practice, dose-to-effect titration of phentermine, although never before reported in the peer-reviewed medical literature, is therefore very commonly employed in bariatric medicine.

In phentermine dose-to-effect titration, the dose, which may have been set low initially to avoid undesirable stimulant side effects, is adjusted upward if the patient complains of hunger or if weight loss is less than expected. Early in the course of phentermine therapy, as tachyphylaxis occurs, dose adjustments are made focusing on phentermine short-term anorectic effect. Later dose adjustments are made focusing on the long-term eating restraint effect or on the long-term anti-carbohydrate craving effect. Doses may be adjusted up or down at any time during the course of the treatment depending on the patient's weight response, on their perception of either hunger or their ability to exercise eating restraint, or on the anti-carbohydrate craving effect. Some patients may comfortably stay at their starting dose for years, while others may need higher doses soon after starting, and still others may benefit from an adjustment up or down after many months. Anytime a patient reaches a plateau in weight loss in spite of good compliance, dose adjustment upward should be considered. Anytime the patient notes weakening of eating restraint or recurrence of carbohydrate cravings, dose adjustments should be considered. Conversely, if side effects appear at any dose, dose reduction should be considered, if side effects cannot be managed otherwise. If at any time the patient believes he/she no longer needs the drug or that phentermine is no longer effective, it should be discontinued. Often in such cases, after phentermine is discontinued, the patient finds that it was more helpful than he/she realized. In such cases the drug can always be restarted.

Dose-to-effect titration is a common practice in medicine that is employed with a wide variety of pharmacologic agents. Dose-to-effect titration of amphetamine drugs is the standard of practice in treating ADHD where physicians employ three approaches:

1. Prescribe a low dose, then judge effectiveness
2. Gradually titrate to higher doses until behavior improves
3. Ramp up until side effects appear, then reduce dose to the level before they appeared (32).

A wide range of amphetamine doses are used in ADHD patients; clearly some patients tolerate higher doses than the recommended starting doses. The 2008 ASBP survey did not specifically ask about dose-to-effect titration but the ranges of starting doses and highest doses reported suggest that the physicians who adjust phentermine doses higher use an analogous approach. Although there is not an extensive literature on dose-to-effect phentermine titration, this approach has clearly been long employed in practice without reports of problems, suggesting this is a safe and effective strategy. There are also anecdotal reports that adult obese patients with ADHD require (and tolerate) higher doses of phentermine, which might be expected in view of the range of effective amphetamine doses observed in ADHD patients. Dose-to-effect titration for the older anorectics has been presented and discussed numerous times in scientific sessions at the meetings of the ASBP and at the Annual Review Course of the American Board of Bariatric Physicians (33–46).

Dose-to-effect titration seems to be safe and effective for the patient, but this approach can jeopardize the physician's license or his malpractice insurance in states where medical boards insist on strict adherence to FDA drug labeling.

Other beneficial effects—Obviously the most important beneficial effect of phentermine therapy is additional weight loss but there are others. Low energy is a frequent complaint of obese patients at initial evaluation. Weight reduction therapy in general improves energy level in these patients, but the addition of phentermine to their therapy often provides an added improvement. In some cases, patients on phentermine report an aroused interest in their daily activities and improvements in mood. This may be seen both in patients with previously undiagnosed depression and in patients already on anti-depressant medication. Generally patients with attention deficit disorder (ADD) or ADHD experience some improvement in their ADHD or ADD on phentermine. This is true for most patients on no medication but may also be true for patients already on a stimulant medication for ADD or ADHD. Occasionally some patients experience anticholinergic effects that are beneficial. Since phentermine can produce decreased gastrointestinal motility, some patients with chronic diarrhea or who suffer from rapid gastrointestinal transit time notice improvement on phentermine. Women with stress incontinence may note symptomatic improvement.

Adverse side effects—Since phentermine works by increasing norepinephrine release, which then acts through β-adrenergic receptors pervasive throughout the entire nervous system, it should not be surprising that the drug can produce a diverse variety of side effects. Some side effects may be beneficial, as noted earlier, while others limit the effectiveness of the drug. The adverse side effects discussed in the following paragraphs are those that have actually been observed in practice. Potential adverse effects, of theoretical interest, which have not been, or have rarely been observed, are discussed in the following section. Where possible, estimates of the rate of occurrence of each reaction described are included. The incidence rates apply if the patient is taking the medication as directed. Incidences of adverse reactions may go up if the patient is taking more than advised.

Phentermine is a mild stimulant; patient's reactions to the stimulant effects of phentermine vary widely. Some patients notice "feeling speedy" with initial doses of phentermine, but most patients do not notice or complain of this. Other patients report being pleasantly energized. Rarely, a patient becomes so stimulated they cannot be persuaded to ever take phentermine again. Generally, stimulant effects occur early, are mild, and disappear with continued exposure to the drug. Perhaps 20% of patients experience some stimulant effect, and perhaps, 1 in 100 has such severe stimulation, and in that case, the drug must be discontinued. If stimulation is a problem, a useful antidote is to give such a patient a β-blocker such as pindolol 5 mg once or twice daily; this will mitigate the stimulation without interfering with the anorectic effect.

In some patients undesirable mood altering effects occur. There are patients who will stop phentermine because they experience mood changes and do not like the way they feel. In some cases, increased irritability appears while on the drug. Irritability in some patients can be controlled with pindolol; if not, discontinuation of phentermine may be advisable.

Insomnia, another stimulant effect, is pretty common in the population of patients presenting for obesity treatment. Insomnia is frequent in the general population and may have already been a problem before phentermine was started. The clinician should always question patients about their sleep patterns before the initiation of phentermine. Insomnia, where the patient cannot go to sleep, occurs early on in phentermine therapy. This is a stimulant effect that, if it occurs at all, is generally mild and disappears if the patient continues the drug. Sleep deprivation symptoms are rare. The incidence of insomnia is perhaps 3% one month after initiation of phentermine therapy. There is a second form of insomnia that can occur after the patient has been on phentermine for months or years in which the patient goes to sleep easily but awakens after a few hours and cannot go back to sleep. Sleep deprivation symptoms can become problematic with this form of insomnia. The incidence of late-appearing insomnia is generally less than 1 in 1000 patients. Early onset insomnia typically responds to pindolol at bedtime. Late onset insomnia will sometimes respond to melatonin; if not, then pindolol or trazadone should be tried rather than a benzodiazapine. If all remedies fail, discontinuation of the phentermine may be required for resolution of the insomnia.

Undesirable anticholinergic effects include dry mouth, constipation, light-headedness, and difficulty with urination. Many patients complain of mild dry mouth—generally so mild that it only serves to remind them to drink the 64 ounces of water daily we recommend. A rare patient will have such severe dry mouth that mucosal erosions may occur—the incidence of such severe dry mouth is found in less than 1 in 1000 patients. If constipation appears, it is usually due to the change in fiber intake with caloric restriction, or it may be due in part to the phentermine. Constipation usually responds to strategies to increase fiber intake. Light-headedness or dizziness occurs in about 2% of patients, but in bariatric patients these are more often due to transient hypoglycemia invoked by caloric restriction or postural hypotension due to inadequate sodium intake when on a ketogenic diet rather than being due to phentermine. Other, more serious anticholinergic effects, such as increased intraocular pressure, confusion, disorientation, and symptoms associated with delirium, have not been observed in practice.

Phentermine-induced mild bladder outlet sphincter contraction can be counteracted with tamsulosin 0.4 mg daily or twice daily. Headache, occurring in about 1% of patients, is usually of the tension type and responds favorably to therapy. Patients with migraine, in whom stimulant medications provoke attacks, may experience a migraine headache upon initiation of phentermine, but most patients with migraine tolerate phentermine initiation without headache.

Uncommon side effects include allergic reactions, impotence, and intensification of pre-existing tremors. Allergic reaction to phentermine, most often manifest as urticaria, is uncommon but does occur in less than 1 in 1000 patients. Intensification of pre-existing tremor does sometimes occur, as can happen with any stimulant in this condition.

Potential/theoretical adverse effects—Phentermine adverse effects that typically occur in practice are enumerated in the paragraph above. In addition to these, phentermine labeling includes a long list of potential side effects. With rare exceptions, none of the other potential side effects listed in phentermine labeling have actually been observed in practice. Most of these are *theoretical conjectures* and are not based on fact but rather upon the supposition that since the phentermine molecule is very similar to amphetamine then phentermine should have adverse effects identical to or very similar to those of amphetamine. Phentermine has been in use for 50 years. If these potential problems have not appeared as yet, the potential risk of these theoretical adverse effects must be either vanishingly low or do not exist. Phentermine effects and adverse effects *are not identical* to those of amphetamine or methamphetamine.

Phentermine labeling lists nine contraindications including advanced arteriosclerosis, cardiovascular disease, hypertension, moderate to severe, hyperthyroidism, hypersensitivity or idiosyncrasy to sympathomimetic amines, glaucoma, agitated states, and history of drug abuse. Phentermine labeling also includes warnings concerning, use in combination with other weight loss drugs, use in combination with selective serotonon reuptake inhibitors, primary pulmonary hypertension, valvular heart disease, tolerance, and impairment in ability to drive or operate machinery. Finally, phentermine labeling includes a paragraph on drug abuse and dependence that discusses six issues implying that all of these are hazards of phentermine therapy including: abuse, intense psychological dependence, severe social dysfunction, addiction, chronic intoxication, and psychosis. While some of these are well-known problems associated with amphetamine, or more often, with methamphetamine, none have ever been observed with phentermine. Every one of these is theoretical and is based solely on the conjecture that phentermine adverse effects *must* be identical to amphetamine and methamphetamine effects. A literature search on PubMed will reveal that there are a few rare exceptions to these last two statements, but closer investigation of the exceptions reveals that most of them do not withstand careful scrutiny (42).

Space constraints prohibit detailed examination of each and every one of these accusations against phentermine, but a few of them should be rebutted. The most fearsome of these are valvular heart disease, hypertension, pulmonary hypertension, and abuse or addiction. It is now clear that phentermine does not and never has produced valvular heart disease (47–49). Amphetamine may elevate blood pressure and there is a widespread assumption that the same is true of phentermine. Evidence in the medical literature of phentermine blood pressure effects is scant but, aside from a few anecdotal cases to the contrary (30), the evidence from clinical trials (50), and from retrospective reports (22,23,31), suggests that blood pressure decreases in phentermine-treated patients in weight loss programs. Phentermine, in the dose ranges discussed here, does not appear to induce sustained elevations of blood pressure. The author, in an ongoing study of phentermine and blood pressure in a weight management program, has observed transient increases in blood pressure at one week after initiation of phentermine therapy in less than 1% of patients, and more rarely, transient increases in blood pressure at one week after phentermine dose increases (22). When a patient in a weight management program is found to have a blood pressure ≥140 systolic or ≥90 diastolic, a prudent course of action would be to withhold phentermine until blood pressure is in control. If the patient is not on antihypertensive medications, either daily hydrochlorothiazide 50 mg or a daily dose of the combination of 25 mg of hydrochlorothiazide and 25 mg of spironolactone will often bring blood pressure in control quickly. Once blood pressure is in control, phentermine may be initiated or resumed.

The incidence of primary pulmonary hypertension in patients on phentermine is lower than the incidence in the general population; phentermine has not and does not induce primary pulmonary hypertension (51). The hallmark of substance addiction is intense craving for the substance (52). This is present both during chronic substance use and upon substance cessation. Neither patients on long-term phentermine nor patients who abruptly cease phentermine exhibit phentermine cravings, nor do such patients manifest amphetamine-like withdrawal (53). There is not a single literature report of abuse, addiction, or withdrawal with phentermine. Clearly phentermine is not an addicting substance; abuse or addiction, as defined in the Diagnostic and Statistical Manual of Mental Disorders, fourth edition, does not occur in the context of phentermine pharmacotherapy.

Combinations—Although some on-line chemical databases (54) list a variety of drug interactions, the listings are for drug interactions for amphetamine and not for phentermine. Phentermine can be used in combination with any drug—there are neither known drug interactions nor known contraindications to combining phentermine with any other drug. Several combinations of phentermine with other drugs with effects on weight have been found useful and will be discussed in section "Useful Combinations."

Diethylpropion

Diethylpropion is a safe and effective weight management drug that is widely used. The 2008 ASBP medication survey revealed that 58% of bariatric physicians utilize it in an average of 15% of their patients (Table 1), making diethylpropion the second most frequently prescribed drug for weight management.

Diethylpropion is another sympathomimetic amine derived from β-phenylethylamine and the molecular structure also resembles that of amphetamine. The FDA has long presumed that all the sympathomimetic amines, including this one, have effects and adverse effects very similar to, if not identical with, amphetamine. As a result, the product labeling for diethylpropion includes all the same conjectures discussed earlier under phentermine. The mechanism of action is thought to be very similar to that of phentermine.

Diethylpropion has therapeutic effects similar to those of phentermine. Patients on diethylpropion notice suppression of appetite at first. When this fades, they notice better eating restraint and sometimes suppression of carbohydrate cravings.

Duration of action—Diethylpropion has a biological half-life of four to six hours. The clinical duration of action is about four hours.

Clinical usefulness—Diethylpropion is a very useful weight management agent. It should be the second choice considered in any patient if phentermine is ineffective or poorly tolerated. Patients in whom phentermine produces insomnia are candidates for diethylpropion. Some patients can tolerate a low dose of phentermine in the morning may benefit from a morning dose of phentermine and an afternoon dose of diethylpropion.

Absolute contraindications—Absolute contraindications to diethylpropion are identical to those of phentermine—pregnancy, nursing an infant, and prior allergic reactions to diethylpropion. The drug was frequently prescribed for prevention of excessive weight gain during pregnancy with no known problems for 20 years after diethylpropion was approved in 1959 until 1979 when the FDA Pharmaceutical Pregnancy Categories were introduced. Since there have been no controlled clinical trials of diethylpropion during pregnancy the drug was assigned a C category and obstetricians abruptly stopped prescribing the drug.

Ages—Diethylpropion labeling admonishes that the drug not be used in children younger than 16 years of age. The situation is analogous to the situation with phentermine; pediatricians once used diethylpropion for children, but then stopped for reasons unrelated to the diethylpropion itself. There is no upper age limit.

Dose—The drug is available as 25 mg immediate-release tablets and 75 mg controlled-release tablets. The usual dose with either is 75 mg daily. Some patients do well with 25 or 50 mg daily. Thirty percent of the bariatric physicians responding to the 2008 ASBP survey indicated that they sometimes used higher doses of 100 to 150 mg daily.

Adverse side effects—Diethylpropion has adverse effects similar to those of phentermine. In general, adverse effects due to diethylpropion are less frequent and of lower intensity than are those due to phentermine.

Potentialtheoretical adverse effects—Here again the FDA presumes, without evidence, that the adverse effects of diethylpropion are identical to those of amphetamine and methamphetamine. Diethylpropion labeling includes all of the same theoretical objections listed in phentermine labeling.

Combinations—Although various databases list drug interactions with diethylpropion, the interaction are amphetamine interactions. These have not been observed with diethylpropion. Diethylpropion is very safe and may be used in patients taking any other drug including other weight management drugs.

Phendimetrazine

Clinical usefulness—Fifty-six percent of bariatric physicians have found phendimetrazine to be a useful drug; those who utilize it do so in 18% of their patients. Phendimetrazine is another sympathomimetic amine derived from β-phenylethylamine and the molecular structure also resembles that of amphetamine. The FDA has long presumed that all the sympathomimetic amines, including this one, have effects and adverse effects very similar to, if not identical with, amphetamine. As a result, the product labeling for phendimetrazine includes all the same conjectures discussed earlier under phentermine. The mechanism of action is thought to be very similar to that of phentermine.

Phendimetrazine has therapeutic effects similar to those of phentermine. Patients on phendimetrazine first notice suppression of appetite, then when this fades, they notice better eating restraint and sometimes suppression of carbohydrate cravings.

Absolute contraindications—These are the same as for phentermine.

Mechanism of action—In the body, phendimetrazine is converted to phenmetrazine, which is the active metabolite. Phenmetrazine is a sympathomimetic with anorectic properties.

Dose—The typical dose is 35 mg three times daily. The maximum dose listed in package labeling and PDR is 70 mg three times daily.

Dose ranging—Some patients tolerate more than the typical dose. The 2008 ASBP survey found that only 51% of bariatric physicians prescribed phendimetrazine at the recommended daily dose of 105 mg. Of the remainder, 16% prescribed 140 mg/day, 5% prescribed 175 mg/day, 26% prescribed 210 mg/day, and 1% each prescribed 280 mg and 315 mg as their highest dose.

Beneficial effects, adverse side effects, and potential or relative contraindications are all very similar to those of phentermine. Phendimetrazine can be used in combination with the same drugs as is used with phentermine.

Orlistat

Clinical usefulness—Orlistat has not proven to be useful in clinical practice because few patients tolerate the gastrointestinal side effects. Although 44% of medical bariatric specialists prescribe Orlistat, these physicians only use it in about 8% of their patients. Orlistat is a very safe, but only modestly effective, weight loss drug. It is an intestinal lipase inhibitor that will prevent absorption of some of the fat a patient consumes for a few hours after taking the drug. Its effectiveness is limited by its unpopularity with the vast majority of patients. Some patients find it useful for maintenance. It is available as a prescription 120 mg capsule marketed as Xenical and also as an over-the-counter 60 mg capsule (Alli).

Dosages–Either 60 mg or 120 mg three times daily.

Adverse reactions/side effects—The most common side effects of Orlistat are abdominal discomfort, oily stools, oily diarrhea, and increased flatus. Other side effects are listed in the PDR.

Management of adverse reactions/side effects—Severe adverse reactions are virtually unheard of, but the gastrointestinal side effects are all too common. Most patients learn to skip the drug if they plan to eat a fatty meal. Side effects are lessened by lowering the amount of fat ingested during the meal.

Sibutramine

Clinical usefulness—Although this drug is favored by academic centers because the FDA has approved it for long-term use, sibutramine has not proven to be very useful in clinical practice. Forty-eight percent of bariatric medicine specialists prescribe sibutramine in an average of just 3% of their patients. Sibutramine is a safe weight loss drug. Most patients have found it disappointing and, given the opportunity, will switch to phentermine, which most find more effective. Sibutramine is a category IV controlled substance, although there is no evidence whatsoever of any addiction potential, and no cases of addiction have ever been reported. One report suggests that sibutramine should be considered in olanzapine-associated weight gain (55). Long-term sibutramine therapy can be effective in long-term maintenance of weight loss (56,57), possibly because it increases metabolic rate (58).

Topiramate

Shortly after this sulfamate-substituted monosaccharide was introduced as an antiepileptic, topiramate was noted to produce weight loss in treated subjects. Clinical trials demonstrated weight loss comparable with the other anti-obesity drugs (59,60), and currently 45% bariatric medicine specialists prescribe topiramate for weight loss in their patients. Once a very expensive drug, the patent for topiramate has lapsed, and the drug is now available as a generic.

Clinical usefulness—Topiramate has been found to be very useful in treating Binge Eating Disorder (61,62) and in treating drug-induced weight gain produced by anti-depressants and some other psychiatric drugs (63). Topiramate can be used as a single agent and, since it is not a controlled substance, it can be used as an alternative to the older drugs.

Absolute contraindications—Known sensitivity to sulfamates is an absolute contraindication.

Dose—Effective doses for weight management range from 25 to 200 mg/day. The typical starting dose for weight management is 25 mg at bedtime. If this dose does not produce the desired effect, the dose can be slowly titrated up in 25 mg increments. By increasing the dose once every two weeks or at monthly intervals one can often avoid annoying side effects. Most patients do not need more than 100 mg/day in the first year or two of treatment. Some patients eventually require 200 mg/day.

Beneficial effects—Patients with binge eating often experience diminution in frequency and intensity of binge eating. Patients with iatrogenic drug-induced weight gain either lose weight or stop gaining weight. Other patients note a decrease in hunger or eating or both.

Adverse side effects—Topiramate is a weak carbonic anhydrase inhibitor and can produce symptoms suggestive of peripheral neuropathy. These usually disappear if the drug is continued. Memory loss for recent events, psychomotor slowing, difficulty with concentration, depression, speech or language problems, and paresthesia are common at doses used for epilepsy but unusual at doses for weight management.

Patients started on topiramate should be watched carefully for eye symptoms. Patients continued on topiramate should have intraocular pressures checked periodically, at least quarterly. Always discontinue topiramate immediately if the patient complains of eye pain or any change in visual acuity. Patients who present with eye symptoms should be immediately referred to an ophthalmologist, since untreated secondary angle glaucoma can result in blindness. The practitioner should speak directly to the patient's ophthalmologist stressing the acuteness of the situation and ask for an urgent consultation. If an ophthalmologist cannot be reached, then the practitioner should call the closest hospital emergency room and speak directly to the physician in charge. If for any reason the practitioner thinks there will be a delay in having the patient seen by an ophthalmologist, then the practitioner should prescribe furosemide 40 mg to be taken immediately and twice daily. Patients should be cautioned to watch for hypotension and should be seen in follow-up within 24 to 48 hours.

Neurological reactions can often be alleviated with dose reductions.

Combinations—In December 2009, Vivus Pharmaceuticals applied for FDA approval for Qnexa, a combination of topiramate and phentermine. Data from clinical trials conducted by Vivus suggest that phentermine and topiramate are an effective combination (64).

Zonisamide

Zonisamide is another antiepileptic drug that can induce weight loss. A clinical trial with zonisamide as monotherapy indicated a respectable weight loss (65) and other clinical trials have shown that it useful in binge eating (66,67). Another clinical trial has shown good results with a combination of bupropion and zonisamide (68), and yet another suggests zonisamide is useful in preventing olanzapine-associated weight gain (69). Probably as a result of these reports, 8% of bariatric physicians now use zonisamide in a few of their patients (2). However, at the present time, zonisamide is not often used alone for obesity treatment.

ADD-ON AGENTS

Certain drugs are useful as adjuncts in obesity pharmacotherapy. Generally, these have not proven to be effective in producing weight loss when used alone.

Metformin is an agent useful in treating diabetics or patients with insulin resistance. The addition of metformin in treating diabetes or insulin resistance can prevent or diminish the weight gain attendant to other drugs used in treating these conditions, and will occasionally produce a modest weight loss. More often there is either minimal or no weight loss. Metformin offers no benefit to a patient with a normal fasting glucose and insulin levels.

Bupropion is dopamine and norepinephrine reuptake inhibitor. Used as monotherapy it can produce a modest weight loss that plateaus within a few months (70). Bupropion should be considered when obese patients require an anti-depressant. This drug should also be considered when a patient is gaining weight on another anti-depressant. The 2008 ASBP Prescribing Practices Survey indicated that 25% of bariatric physicians were using bupropion in 7% of their patients.

Weight loss is more impressive when naltrexone is combined with bupropion (71).

Glucagon-like peptide-1 receptor agonists (GLP-1 agonist), including exenatide and liraglutide, enhance insulin secretion, suppress glucagon, and slow gastric emptying. Clinical trials in patients with type 2 diabetes have demonstrated weight loss in the range of 1 to 3 kg over 26 to 52 weeks (72). Till the time of writing this chapter, liragltide (Victoza) is available only in Europe but Novo Nordisk anticipates FDA approval soon. Exenatide (Byetta) is currently available in the United States. These agents are intended as add-on drug for use in diabetics with poor glucose control and are not intended for monotherapy either for diabetes control or for weight loss.

OTHER AGENTS TO CONSIDER

Spironolactone will, in some women, inhibit premenstrual chocolate, sugar, and other carbohydrate cravings. Spironolactone 25 mg daily for a few days prior to menses often reduces or eliminates cravings. The combination of hydrochlorothiazide and spironolactone, 25 mg of each, is equally effective and is less expensive.

5-HTP/carbodopa—5-HTP is the immediate precursor of serotonin (5-hyydroxytryptamine). 5-HTP has long been known to have anorectic properties and to have the effect of relieving carbohydrate cravings (73). The 5-HTP is converted to serotonin in the brain and activates the leptin-melanocortin anorexigenic signaling pathway (74). 5-HTP works because it crosses the blood–brain barrier and is then converted to serotonin in the brain. However, because of rapid decarboxylation of 5-HTP and conversion to serotonin in the gut, liver, and bloodstream, high oral doses of 5-HTP are required to produce even small increases in brain serotonin. If 5-HTP is given alone, high doses of up to 900 mg per day produce the best results. Many patients have nausea and other gastrointestinal side effects at such a high doses limiting the effectiveness of 5-HTP alone. A few patients do well with 150 to 300 mg 5-HTP per day but for most patients low doses are not effective.

Carbidopa is a peripheral inhibitor of L-aromatic amino acid decarboxylation and inhibits premature decarboxylation of 5-HTP to serotonin before the 5-HTP can cross the blood–brain barrier. Carbidopa, at a 5 mg dose, has no other pharmacologic effect. L-dopa/carbidopa combinations are used in treating Parkinson's disease. The carbidopa inhibits decarboxylation of the L-dopa, increasing its effectiveness. Combining carbidopa with 5-HTP increases the effectiveness of the 5-HTP dramatically. 5-HTP/carbidopa in combination has been used extensively in Europe as a treatment for depression, generally at higher doses of 5-HTP than needed for anorectic use (75).

Patients can be started on a dose of 5 mg 5-HTP with 5 mg carbidopa, taken three times daily with food. If the patient has a good response and no side effects, then the dose may be gradually increased, first to 10 mg, then 15 mg, and eventually up to 20 mg or 25 mg 5-HTP, always with 5 mg carbidopa (2,31). Occasional patients benefit from a fourth, nighttime dose. 5-HTP can cause gastrointestinal side effects in higher doses. Carbidopa is not used alone therapeutically and has no known side effects. Side effects for carbidopa reported in the medical literature are those of the L-dopa with which the carbidopa is compounded. The only significant adverse side effects are gastric irritation or nausea when the 5-HTP/carbidopa medication is taken with an empty stomach. Neither serotonin syndrome nor cardiac valvulopathy has ever been reported in patients on 5-HTP at any dose level (76).

5-HTP/carbidopa can be thought of as safe replacement for the fenfluramines and like the fenfluramines is best used in combination with phentermine. Patients treated with 5-HTP/carbidopa alone generally neither experience a significant weight loss nor notice a diminution of sugar or other carbohydrate cravings.

USEFUL COMBINATIONS

Phentermine and 5-HTP/carbidopa is a useful combination with a mechanism of action similar to Phen/Fen but with no risk of cardiac pathology. The 5-HTP tends to modulate the stimulant effect of the phentermine so that patients tolerate the phentermine with fewer side effects. Weight loss with the combination when both phentermine and 5-HTP/carbidopa are started in a new patient is similar to that seen with Phen/Fen (31). Some physicians prefer to start the patient on phentermine and add the 5-HTP/carbidopa at a later time. One report suggests a 16% weight loss at six months with phentermine, and an optimum protein restricted carbohydrate diet at which point the 5-HTP/carbidopa is added resulting in a 17% weight loss at one year (2).

Phentermine and *topiramate* is the combination used in Vivus Pharmaceutical's new drug Qnexa discussed later. However, both drugs are currently available as generics and can be prescribed or dispensed by bariatric physicians. The only clinical trials that have been conducted are those with Qnexa. The best weight loss in those trials occurred at the maximum doses tested—15 mg phentermine combined with 92 mg topiramate daily. The phentermine dose is below the usual and customary dose for this drug and the topiramate dose is higher than the initial dose recommended, but well below the maximum dose recommended. By prescribing these drugs in combination, one could avoid the disadvantages of a fixed dose combination with the possible benefit of producing greater weight loss. The 2008 ASBP survey found that 18% of the physicians who used combinations of anti-obesity drugs used phentermine and topiramate.

Phentermine and *diethylpropion* is a combination useful for patients who benefit from phentermine but can only tolerate low early morning doses and experience return of hunger and appetite in the late afternoon or evening. The addition of one or two doses of diethylpropion after 12 noon may be of benefit. Diethylpropion used in this way seldom provokes insomnia or overstimulation because of its short duration of action.

Phentermine and *fluoxetine*, thought to be an effective combination by some (77), has not been found useful by most bariatric specialists. The 2008 ASBP survey found that 3% of physicians using combinations used phentermine and fluoxetine in combination.

Bupropion and *naltrexone* is the combination of drugs in the new drug contrave discussed later. Both individual drugs have been approved for other indications, so one could prescribe the combination prior to FDA approval for contrave but naltrexone is prohibitively expensive, limiting its use.

Bupropion and *zonisamide* is a combination with which Orexigen believes has some promise. Patients in an initial 12-week trial with this combination reportedly achieved an 8.5% weight loss (68). Orexigen has completed one phase II trial but had not reported their results at the time this is written. Both drugs have been approved, so some bariatric physicians are using the combination.

NEW DRUGS

Three companies, Vivus, Arena, and Orexigen, have new drugs awaiting FDA approval. These companies have reported their results for their completed phase III clinical trials. Table 2 is a summary of results in completers in these very large trials (64,78,79) compared with an observational study on phentermine monotherapy and with a small clinical trial with topiramate. Of the three new drugs, Qnexa ostensibly produces the greater weight loss, which is not surprising, since we know both drugs used in monotherapy do produce significant weight loss, and combinations of effective drugs are often more effective than single drugs. Note that results comparable with Qnexa at 12 months were obtained when either drug was used as monotherapy. Of course, the explanation is probably that the number of subjects in latter studies was a small fraction of the numbers in the phase III clinical trials. However, the speculation remains that Qnexa would be more effective if the phentermine dose were higher.

In December 2009, Arena and Vivus applied for FDA approvals for Lorcaserin and Qnexa respectively, and Orexigen filed for approval of Contrave in March 2010. All three drugs are approvable, based on the FDA's recommended criteria, but FDA approval is not guaranteed.

Qnexa, under consideration for FDA approval, is a combination of phentermine and topiramate. It is anticipated that Vivus will apply for approval of the highest dose tested that

Table 2 Effectiveness of New Drugs Compared with Phentermine and Topiramate Monotherapy

Drug	Dose mg/day	Categorical weight loss 5%	Categorical weight loss 10%	Categorical weight loss 15%	Completers at 12 months (%)	Weight loss at 12 months (%)
Lorcaserin	20	63%	35%	NA	59	8
Qnexa	Phent. 15 Top. 96	84%	60%	43%	59	15
Contrave		56%	33%	15%	52	8
Phentermine compared (23)	30	84%	61%	NA	24	13–14
Topiramate (59)	96	96%	78%	49%	31	17

Data, rounded to whole numbers, are from company reports of clinical trials. Data selected are best case when several trials were conducted. Weight loss at 12 months is observed weight loss in completers without placebo subtraction. Haddock's (23) data are from a 12-month retrospective study in a fee-for-service private practice, not from a clinical trial.

produced a 14.7% weight loss at one year in obese patients without comorbidities and a 13.2% weight loss in obese patients with comorbidities at one year (64). Reductions in blood pressure, total and low density lipoprotein (LDL) cholesterol, triglycerides, inflammatory markers, glucose, and insulin were seen, as would be expected with this magnitude of weight loss. Eighteen percent of patients on the highest dose dropped out because of side effects. The most common adverse side effects that differed significantly from those observed in patients on placebo were dry mouth, tingling, constipation, altered taste, insomnia, and headache.

Lorcaserin, a new drug under consideration for FDA approval, is a novel 5-HT_{2C} receptor agonist that has no effect on the 5-HT_{2B} receptors implicated in drug-induced valvulopathy. Arena has reported that the drug produces an 8% weight loss at one year and that 66% of patients lost 5% and 36% lost 10% of their initial weight (78). Side effects occurred early, generally disappeared after a few weeks, and were limited to nausea and headaches. The possible occurrence of drug-induced cardiac valvulopathy was monitored carefully and was not observed. Lorcaserin was engineered to be a safe replacement for the fenfluramines. Many patients and physicians will want to try lorcaserin in combination with phentermine; the possibility that this combination will be used off-schedule could influence the FDA and the drug advisory committee in considering approval.

Contrave, now being considered for FDA approval, is a combination of bupropion and naltrexone. Orexigen has reported that contrave has produced an 8.2% weight loss at 52 weeks with 56% of patients achieving a 5% weight loss and 33% achieving a 10% weight loss (79).

MEDICATIONS KNOWN TO CAUSE WEIGHT GAIN

The list of drugs, both prescription and over-the-counter, that are known to induce weight gain in some patients is long and continues to grow. In some cases, the patient is conscious of the culprit drug, but more often the patient is unaware that a drug is inducing weight gain. The classes of drugs with central nervous system effects most often involved include antidepressants, antipsychotics, anticonvulsants, mood stabilizers, and migraine preventatives. Drugs without a CNS action that can induce weight gain include β-blockers, calcium channel blockers, anti-diabetics, steroids, clonidine, clofibrate, antihistamines, antiretrovirals, and some chemotherapy agents. A recent excellent review provides more detail (80).

RECOMMENDED PRESCRIBING PRACTICES

Practical Considerations

Pharmacotherapy is one mainstay of obesity treatment; dietary treatment, motivation, behavior modification, and exercise are the others. A combination of all these can produce greater weight loss and promote lasting success for compliant patients than can any single component. *A danger to carefully avoid, not previously mentioned in this chapter, in including anti-obesity drugs is that of reducing hunger or appetite so much that the patient eats insufficient protein.* Patients who lose weight on protein-deficient diets lose muscle mass. In the author's opinion, patients on any anti-obesity drug should have prescribed protein intake quotas and continuously questioned about their protein intake to assure such patients consume enough protein to avoid net muscle protein loss. *Patients who cannot or will not eat the required protein should have their anti-obesity drug dose reduced or discontinued.*

The amount of daily protein intake suggested by the Recommended Dietary Allowance is inadequate and fails to recognize that dietary protein need is inversely proportional to energy intake (81). As a result of this failure, both the food pyramid diet and any diet that stipulates caloric restriction combined with setting protein intake to a percentage of caloric intake are *protein-deficient diets* (82). Such diets for weight loss should be avoided. Recent studies suggest that a minimum threshold protein dose of 30 g is required for the initiation of muscle protein synthesis (83), leading to the recommendation that adults should consume this threshold dose three times daily and eat a minimum of 120 g protein daily (82).

In recognition of these recent developments in protein research, some bariatric physicians now prescribe a start-up restricted carbohydrate diet with a minimum of 120 g protein (more for women taller than 70 in. or men taller than 72 in.), combined with 20 g of low glycemic carbohydrates, and 25 g of fat. The same protein intake is maintained when carbohydrate intake is liberalized to a low-calorie diet or to maintenance. The danger of inducing insufficient protein intake with an anorectic is considerably lessened if such a diet is prescribed. One must still continue to ascertain that the patient is eating enough protein despite the anorectic.

After three days on such a diet, hunger and carbohydrate cravings typically disappear (84) and the patient may discover that an anorectic medication is superfluous. Even so, many patients are more comfortable continuing their medication.

Primary drug choice—Phentermine should be the first drug considered at start-up. If phentermine cannot be used, diethylpropion is a logical second choice. A third choice should fall between phendimetrazine and topiramate. Sibutramine and orlistat as the primary drug should be the last choices. This order of preference will be subject to revision if, and when, the new drugs discussed earlier are approved. Topiramate for patients with Binge Eating Disorder or drug-induced weight gain should be started as soon as the diagnosis is established.

Add-on choices—If a carbohydrate-reduced diet is utilized for weight loss, the medications for carbohydrate cravings such as 5-HTP/carbidopa and spironolactone usually are not necessary until the patient starts eating more than 20 g of carbohydrates daily. In some patients, carnitine will suppress carbohydrate cravings; it may be best to verify the patient is taking or has tried carnitine before prescribing either 5-HTP/carbidopa or spironolactone. Obviously, if the patient is diabetic and is not already taking metformin, it should be added. Metformin may be given in combination with any anti-obesity drug.

Eventually, when the patient begins eating more carbohydrates, an anorectic medication becomes more important. Many patients eventually experience a decrease of their weight loss or reach a plateau. It is at this point that the addition of 5-HTP/carbidopa, or spironolactone or both should be considered.

One reason successful maintenance is difficult because patients enter a "weight reduced" metabolic state characterized by decreased metabolic rate, decreased sympathetic tone, and low circulating leptin, thyroxin, and tri-iodothyronine levels (85). Continued phentermine, or phentermine and 5-HTP/carbidopa, usually enables the patient to comfortably eat less. Free T3 and free T4 levels should be assayed and, if either one is low, consideration should be given to treatment to return the levels to normal. Leibel and associates have shown that low-dose leptin reverses the syndrome. One day perhaps we will have leptin for our maintenance patients.

Cautions—Bariatric physicians who are treating their patients according to this chapter are using the medications "off-schedule." Physicians who prescribe rather than dispense these medications expose themselves to the risk that a zealous pharmacist will report the physician to the state medical board for "overprescribing" a controlled substance. Some medical boards (including the California Medical Board) will accuse the physician of "indiscriminately prescribing controlled substances" that may be considered grounds for suspending the offending physician's license to practice.

Physicians who dispense controlled substances in their offices should make themselves aware of Drug Enforcement Administration (DEA) regulations and follow them scrupulously. The DEA requires that every pill that come into and goes out of a physician's office be accounted for. Dispensing logs, patient records, and patient accounts must be kept in exact correspondence. The DEA also expects a precise inventory that must be in exact agreement with invoices of drugs received and with the dispensing logs. The DEA can levy a $5000 fine for each and every discrepancy their agents can find. If the DEA agents suspect that a physician is deliberately deviating from their rules or is not cooperative, they have the authority to shutter the physician's office, seize every asset, and take the physician away in handcuffs. On the other hand, physicians who follow the rules, keep meticulous records, and are cooperative have nothing to fear if DEA agents arrive unexpectedly.

The state medical boards vary in their regulation of office dispensing practices; practitioners who wish to dispense medications should be aware of local requirements. Nearly every state board requires a good faith examination of a patient before any medication is prescribed or dispensed. Patients on maintenance on any of the controlled medications should be seen at least once every three months.

WEIGHT MAINTENANCE

Most patients will have better long-term success with weight maintenance if anti-obesity drugs are continued indefinitely after weight loss. Pharmacotherapy should always be offered to patients who lost weight without it anytime they begin to gain weight after weight loss. This is particularly true after bariatric surgery. Bariatric surgery patients typically lose weight for perhaps a year after surgery, and then reach a weight plateau. Typically then, after a variable interval, these patients begin to gain weight—sometimes reaching or exceeding their preoperative weight. The addition of weight management drugs at this point may prevent further weight gain and is preferable to allowing the patient to regain. Little has been published on this strategy, and surgeons seldom think of prescribing anti-obesity drugs.

REFERENCES

1. Colman E. Anorectics on trial: A half century of federal regulation of prescription appetite suppressants. Ann Intern Med 2005; 143:380–385.
2. Hendricks EJ, Rothman RB, Greenway FL. How physician obesity specialists use drugs to treat obesity. Obesity (Silver Spring) 2009; 17:1730–1735.
3. NIH. Clinical guidelines on the identification, evaluation, and treatment of overweight and obesity in adults—The evidence report. National Institutes of Health. Obes Res 1998; 6(suppl 2):51S–209S.
4. Atkinson RL, Hubbard VS. Report on the NIH workshop on pharmacologic treatment of obesity. Am J clin Nutr 1994; 60:153–156.
5. ASBP. Overweight and Obesity Evaluation and Treatment. Aurora, CO: American Society of Bariatric Physicians, 2009. http://www.asbp.org. Accessed May 10, 2010.
6. Zhang C, Rexrode KM, van Dam RM, et al. Abdominal obesity and the risk of all-cause, cardiovascular, and cancer mortality: Sixteen years of follow-up in us women. Circulation 2008; 117:1624–1626.
7. Pischon T, Boeing H, Hoffmann K, et al. General and abdominal adiposity and risk of death in Europe. N Engl J Med 2008; 359:2105–2120.
8. Fox CS, Massaro JM, Hoffmann U, et al. Abdominal visceral and subcutaneous adipose tissue compartments: Association with metabolic risk factors in the Framingham heart study. Circulation 2007; 116:39–48.
9. Bays HE, Gonzalez-Campoy JM, Bray GA, et al. Pathogenic potential of adipose tissue and metabolic consequences of adipocyte hypertrophy and increased visceral adiposity. Expert Rev Cardiovasc Ther 2008; 6:343–368.
10. Romero-Corral A, Somers VK, Sierra-Johnson J, et al. Diagnostic performance of body mass index to detect obesity in patients with coronary artery disease. Eur Heart J 2007; 28:2087–2093.
11. Romero-Corral A, Somers VK, Sierra-Johnson J, et al. Normal weight obesity: A risk factor for cardiometabolic dysregulation and cardiovascular mortality. Eur Heart J 2010; 31(6):737–746.
12. Connolly HM, Crary JL, McGoon MD, et al. Valvular heart disease associated with fenfluramine-phentermine. N Engl J Med 1997; 337:581–588.
13. Kushner RF. Roadmaps for Clinical Practice: Case Studies in Disease Prevention and Health Promotion—Assessment and Management of Adult Obesity: A Primer for Physicians. Chicago: American Medical Association, 2003.
14. Snow V, Barry P, Fitterman N, et al. Pharmacologic and surgical management of obesity in primary care: A clinical practice guideline from the American College of Physicians. Ann Intern Med 2005; 142:525–531.
15. NGC. National Guideline Clearinghouse. http://www.guideline.gov/. Updated 2010. Accessed May 10, 2010.
16. Glazer G. Long-term pharmacotherapy of obesity 2000: A review of efficacy and safety. Arch Intern Med 2001; 161:1814–1824.
17. Haddock CK, Poston WS, Dill PL, et al. Pharmacotherapy for obesity: A quantitative analysis of four decades of published randomized clinical trials. Intern J Obes Relat Metab Disord 2002; 26:262–273.
18. Li Z, Maglione M, Tu W, et al. Meta-analysis: Pharmacologic treatment of obesity. Ann Intern Med 2005; 142:532–546.
19. Padwal R, Li SK, Lau DC. Long-term pharmacotherapy for overweight and obesity: A systematic review and meta-analysis of randomized controlled trials. Int J Obes Relat Metab Disord 2003; 27:1437–1446.
20. Shekelle PG, Morton SC, Maglione MA, et al. Pharmacological and surgical treatment of obesity.. Evidence Report/Technology Assessment No. 103. Rockville, MD: U.S. Department of Health and Human Services, 2004:1–172.
21. Wadden TA, Berkowitz RI, Womble LG, et al. Randomized trial of lifestyle modification and pharmacotherapy for obesity. N Engl J Med 2005; 353:2111–2120.

22. Hendricks EJ, Westman EC. Phentermine therapy in obesity treatment: Effect on blood pressure 582P. Obesity 2008; 16(suppl 1):S216.
23. Haddock CK, Poston WS, Foreyt JP, et al. Effectiveness of medifast supplements combined with obesity pharmacotherapy: A clinical program evaluation. Eat Weight Disord 2008; 13:95–101.
24. Fullerton G, Tyler C, Johnston CA, et al. Quality of life in Mexican-American children following a weight management program. Obesity (Silver Spring) 2007; 15:2553–2556.
25. Gadde KM, Kolotkin RL, Peterson CA, et al. Changes in weight and quality of life in obese patients treated with topiramate plus phentermine 272P. Obesity 2007; 15:A85.
26. Lorber J. Obesity in childhood. A controlled trial of anorectic drugs. Arch Dis Child 1966; 41:309–312.
27. Rothman RB. Treatment of a 4-year-old boy with ADHD with the dopamine releaser phentermine. J Clin Psychiatry 1996; 57:308–309.
28. Spear BA, Barlow SE, Ervin C, et al. Recommendations for treatment of child and adolescent overweight and obesity. Pediatrics 2007; 120:S254–S288.
29. Munro JF, MacCuish AC, Wilson EM, et al. Comparison of continuous and intermittent anorectic therapy in obesity. Br Med J 1968; 1:352–354.
30. Douglas A, Douglas JG, Robertson CE, et al. Plasma phentermine levels, weight loss and side-effects. Int J Obes 1983; 7:591–595.
31. Rothman RB. Treatment of obesity with "combination" pharmacotherapy [published online ahead of print April 19, 2009]. Am J Ther doi: 10.1097/MJT.1090b1013e31818e31830 da.
32. Manos MJ. Pharmacologic treatment of ADHD: Road conditions in driving patients to successful outcomes. Medscape J Med 2008; 10:5.
33. Bruner DE, Richardson L, Steelman GM. Use of Anorectic Medications. Eastern Regional Obesity Course. Louisville, KY: American Society of Bariatric Physicians, 2006.
34. Hendricks EJ. Pharmacotherapy of Obesity. Annual Review Course. Atlanta, GA: American Board Bariatric Medicine, 2001.
35. Hendricks EJ. Pharmacotherapy of Obesity. Annual Review Course. Denver, CO: American Board Bariatric Medicine, 2002.
36. Hendricks EJ. Pharmacotherapy of Obesity. Annual Review Course. Las Vegas, NV: American Board Bariatric Medicine, 2003.
37. Hendricks EJ. Pathophysiology of Obesity. Annual Review Course. Scottsdale, AZ: American Board of Bariatric Medicine, 2004.
38. Hendricks EJ. Pharmacotherapy of Obesity. Annual Review Course. Scottsdale, AZ: American Board of Bariatric Medicine, 2004.
39. Hendricks EJ. Pharmacotherapy of Obesity. Annual Review Course. Atlanta, GA: American Board of Bariatric Medicine, 2005.
40. Hendricks EJ. Pharmacotherapy of Obesity. Annual Review Course. Lexington, KY: American Board of Bariatric Medicine, 2006.
41. Hendricks EJ. Pharmacotherapy of Obesity. Annual Review Course. Nashville, TN: American Board of Bariatric Medicine, 2007.
42. Hendricks EJ. Adverse reactions to phentermine. Evidence versus conjecture. In: 58th Annual Obesity & Associated Conditions Symposium. Tampa, FL: American Society of Bariatric Physicians, 2008.
43. Hendricks EJ. Is phentermine addicting? In: 59th Annual Obesity & Associated Conditions Symposium; October 10, 2009. Costa Mesa: American Society of Bariatric Physicians, 2009.
44. Steelman GM. Controversies in the Use of Anti-Obesity (Anorectic) Medications. Western Regional Obesity Course; May 13. Portland, OR: American Society of Bariatric Physicians, 2000.
45. Steelman GM. The Art of Tailoring Drug Therapy to Your Patients. In: 51st Annual Obesity and Associated Conditions Symposium; October 27. San Diego, CA: American Society of Bariatric Physicians, 2001.
46. Steelman GM. Difficult Decisions with Anorectic Use. Western Regional Obesity Course; May 17. Denver, CO: American Society of Bariatric Physicians, 2002.
47. Bonow RO, Carabello BA, Chatterjee K, et al. 2008 focused update incorporated into the ACC/AHA 2006 guidelines for the management of patients with valvular heart disease: A report of the American College of Cardiology/American Heart Association Task Force on Practice Guidelines. Circulation 2008; 118:e523–661.
48. Roth BL. Drugs and valvular heart disease. N Engl J Med 2007; 356:6–9.
49. Rothman RB, Baumann MH. Serotonergic drugs and valvular heart disease. Expert Opin Drug Saf 2009; 8:317–329.
50. Kim KK, Cho HJ, Kang HC, et al. Effects on weight reduction and safety of short-term phentermine administration in Korean obese people. Yonsei Med J 2006; 47:614–625.
51. Rich S, Rubin L, Walker AM, et al. Anorexigens and pulmonary hypertension in the United States: Results from the surveillance of North American pulmonary hypertension. Chest 2000; 117:870–874.

52. Heinz AJ, Epstein DH, Schroeder JR, et al. Heroin and cocaine craving and use during treatment: Measurement validation and potential relationships. J Subst Abuse Treat 2006; 31:355–364.
53. Hendricks EJ, Greenway FL. A study of abrupt phentermine cessation in patients in a weight management program. Am J Ther 2009; in Press, Manuscript AJT-20082603.
54. INCHEM. Phentermine. International Programme on Chemical Safety. 2009. http://www.inchem.org/documents/pims/pharm/pim415.htm. Updated August 1997. Accessed May 10, 2010.
55. Henderson DC, Copeland PM, Daley TB, et al. A double-blind, placebo-controlled trial of sibutramine for olanzapine-associated weight gain. Am J Psychiatry 2005; 162:954–962.
56. Mathus-Vliegen EM. Long-term maintenance of weight loss with sibutramine in a GP setting following a specialist guided very-low-calorie diet: A double-blind, placebo-controlled, parallel group study. Eur J Clin Nutr 2005; 59(suppl 1):S31–S38; discussion S39.
57. James WP, Astrup A, Finer N. Effect of Sibutramine on weight maintenance after weight loss: A randomized trial. STORM Study Group. Sibutramine Trial of Obesity Reduction and Maintenance. Lancet 2000; 356:2119–2125.
58. Astrup A. Thermogenic drugs as a strategy for treatment of obesity. Endocrine 2000; 13:207–212.
59. Astrup A, Caterson I, Zelissen P, et al. Topiramate: Long-term maintenance of weight loss induced by a low-calorie diet in obese subjects. Obes Res 2004; 12:1658–1669.
60. Bray GA, Hollander P, Klein S, et al. A 6-month randomized, placebo-controlled, dose-ranging trial of topiramate for weight loss in obesity. Obes Res 2003; 11:722–733.
61. Appolinario JC, McElroy SL. Pharmacological approaches in the treatment of binge eating disorder. Curr Drug Targets 2004; 5:301–307.
62. Guerdjikova AI, Kotwal R, McElroy SL. Response of recurrent binge eating and weight gain to topiramate in patients with binge eating disorder after bariatric surgery. Obes Surg 2005; 15:273–277.
63. Khazaal Y, Chatton A, Rusca M, et al. Long-term topiramate treatment of psychotropic drug-induced weight gain: A retrospective chart review. Gen Hosp Psychiatry 2007; 29:446–449.
64. Vivus. Equip and Conquer Study Results, September 9, 2009. http://www.vivus.com/newsroom/publications/qnexa982009.pdf. Updated September 8, 2009. Accessed May 10, 2010.
65. Gadde KM, Franciscy DM, Wagner HR II, et al. Zonisamide for weight loss in obese adults: A randomized controlled trial. JAMA 2003; 289:1820–1825.
66. McElroy SL, Kotwal R, Guerdjikova AI, et al. Zonisamide in the treatment of binge eating disorder with obesity: A randomized controlled trial. J Clin Psychiatry 2006; 67:1897–1906.
67. McElroy SL, Kotwal R, Hudson JI, et al. Zonisamide in the treatment of binge-eating disorder: An open-label, prospective trial. J Clin Psychiatry 2004; 65:50–56.
68. Gadde KM, Yonish GM, Foust MS, et al. Combination therapy of zonisamide and bupropion for weight reduction in obese women: A preliminary, randomized, open-label study. J Clin Psychiatry 2007; 68:1226–1229.
69. Wallingford NM, Sinnayah P, Bymaster FP, et al. Zonisamide prevents olanzapine-associated hyperphagia, weight gain, and elevated blood glucose in rats. Neuropsychopharmacology 2008; 33:2922–2933.
70. Anderson JW, Greenway FL, Fujioka K, et al. Bupropion SR enhances weight loss: A 48-week double-blind, placebo-controlled trial. Obes Res 2002; 10:633–641.
71. Greenway FL, Whitehouse MJ, Guttadauria M, et al. Rational design of a combination medication for the treatment of obesity. Obesity (Silver Spring) 2009; 17:30–39.
72. White J. Efficacy and safety of incretin based therapies: Clinical trial data. J Am Pharm Assoc (2003) 2009; 49(suppl 1):S30–S40.
73. Garfield AS, Heisler LK. Pharmacological targeting of the serotonergic system for the treatment of obesity. J Physiol 2009; 587:49–60.
74. Heisler LK, Jobst EE, Sutton GM, et al. Serotonin reciprocally regulates melanocortin neurons to modulate food intake. Neuron 2006; 51:239–249.
75. Turner EH, Loftis JM, Blackwell AD. Serotonin a la carte: Supplementation with the serotonin precursor 5-hydroxytryptophan. Pharmacol Ther 2006; 109:325–338.
76. Rothman RB, Baumann MH. Appetite suppressants, cardiac valve disease and combination pharmacotherapy. Am J Ther 2009; 16:354–364.
77. Whigham LD, Dhurandhar NV, Rahko PS, et al. Comparison of combinations of drugs for treatment of obesity: Body weight and echocardiographic status. Int J Obes (Lond) 2007; 31:850–857.
78. Arena. Blossom trial results presentation. 2009. http://files.shareholder.com/downloads/ARNA/719082264x0x320104/d78a7f2d-2294-42a1-8225-f4147e4848af/BLOSSOMResults.pdf. Updated September 18, 2009. Accessed May 10, 2010.
79. Orexigen. Phase 3 clinical trial results. http://ir.orexigen.com/phoenix.zhtml?c=207034&p=irol-newsArticle&ID=1308920&highlight=/. Updated July 20, 2009. Accessed May 10, 2010.

80. Davtyan C, Ma M. Drug-induced weight gain. In: Proceedings of UCLA Healthcare; September 10, 2008; Los Angeles, CA, 12:1.
81. Millward DJ. Macronutrient intakes as determinants of dietary protein and amino acid adequacy. J Nutr 2004; 134:1588S–1596S.
82. Layman D. Dietary guidelines should reflect new understandings about adult protein needs. Nutr Metab 2009; 6:12.
83. Symons TB, Sheffield-Moore M, Wolfe RR, et al. A moderate serving of high-quality protein maximally stimulates skeletal muscle protein synthesis in young and elderly subjects. J Am Diet Assoc 2009; 109:1582–1586.
84. Martin CK, O'Neil PM, Pawlow L. Changes in food cravings during low-calorie and very-low-calorie diets. Obes Res 2006; 14:115–121.
85. Rosenbaum M, Goldsmith R, Bloomfield D, et al. Low-dose leptin reverses skeletal muscle, autonomic, and neuroendocrine adaptations to maintenance of reduced weight. J Clin Invest 2005; 115:3579–3586.

9 Maintenance of weight loss

Scott Rigden

INTRODUCTION

Losing weight and keeping it off is a very difficult accomplishment in our society. Wadden's research team reported (1) that only 5% of patients maintained their full weight loss five years after treatment, while 62% had regained all of their approximately 15 kg loss. A review of the weight loss maintenance literature shows that weight regain is a problem regardless of the treatment used. Obese individuals in commercial weight loss programs do not seem to perform any better than those in research studies. A survey conducted by Consumer Reports (2) found that participants typically regained 30 to 40% of their weight loss one year after treatment; one quarter regained all of it.

Weight maintenance studies are rare compared with the prolific number of weight loss studies. The commercialization of weight loss hardly ever includes a catchy announcement or advertisement regarding long-term maintenance. My experience has been that even bariatricians, who should be especially sensitive to maintenance of weight loss issues, prefer to discuss, almost exclusively, exceptional cases of weight loss. Perhaps the lack of excitement and emphasis on weight loss maintenance is a symptom of our society, which is oriented to fast, instant, and quick resolutions of problems. My experience as a veteran bariatrician is that very few new obese patients come in to the office with any thought of weight loss maintenance. All would agree that maintenance is not nearly as much fun and exciting as the initial weight loss with its associated positive feelings and physiological changes.

DEFINITION OF MAINTENANCE

One common definition of long-term weight loss that has been used in medical research is the intentional weight loss of at least 10% or more of the original weight and maintaining this weight loss for one year. The National Heart, Lung, and Blood Institute (NHLBI) definition of success is at least 10% weight loss from baseline, <3-kg weight regain at two years, and sustained reduction in waist circumference of at least 1.6 in. (3). Many bariatricians seem to agree with the criteria used by the National Weight Control Registry, whose definition of "successful losers" is a minimum of 30 lb of weight loss maintained for a minimum of one year (4). No matter what criteria that would be favored by bariatricians, it is clear that overweight patients have very unrealistic goals for weight loss that may lead to disappointment and, ultimately, undermine their zeal to continue working intensely on their weight. Foster's study (5) of weight loss goals and expectations revealed most considered a hypothetical 17% reduction disappointing; a 33% weight loss was a typical goal weight. Fortunately, maintaining a weight loss as little as 5% to 10% of the original weight can have very significant medical results (1).

REVIEW OF THE MEDICAL LITERATURE ON MAINTENANCE

Maintenance and Nutritional Approaches

Toubro and Astrup (6) reviewed one year of maintenance among 43 subjects. One group of subjects was put on an ad-lib low fat, high carbohydrate diet; another group was put on a fixed calorie, exchange list diet. The mean weight loss of the participants was 12.6 kg prior to the maintenance period. During maintenance, the subjects attended sessions two to three times per month. At one-year follow-up, 65% of the ad-lib low fat group and 40% of the fixed calorie group had maintained a weight loss of 5 kg or more.

At the conclusion of a 12-month maintenance program, Perri et al. (7) concluded that one-on-one contact was superior to peer-group support or "no contact" conditions. They recommended multifaceted maintenance programs including ongoing professional contact, skills training, social support, and exercise.

After completing a very low calorie diet (VLCD), 210 subjects were followed for 15 months by Agras et al. (8). They found that use of prepackaged foods did not enhance successful maintenance. In fact, this strategy correlated with worse compliance and attendance in the maintenance condition.

Hartman et al. (9) conducted a long-term weight loss maintenance program after weight loss with supplemental fasting. One hundred and two subjects were evaluated for two to three years following treatment in a combined behavior therapy and VLCD program. Average weight loss was 27.2 kg; at follow-up the mean weight loss was 11.3 kg. Fifty-six subjects participated in the optional maintenance program; 46 did not. Factors associated with long-term success were high levels of exercise and participating in the maintenance program for more than eight months. The maintenance program consisted of regular group visits, occasional physician visits, review of nutrition and exercise topics, and visits to restaurants and grocery stores.

Walsh and Flynn reported a 54-month evaluation of weight maintenance after a popular VLCD program (10). After initial weight loss for males of 27.2 kg and 19.3 kg for females, the average maintained loss 54 months after program entry was 5.1 kg. Twenty-six of 145 patients maintained a medically significant weight loss of 20% of their entry weight. Because longer program attendance and continued exercise were the main correlates with successful maintenance, Walsh recommended at least two years of a maintenance program after reaching goal weight.

What happens in a prospective study of weight maintenance in obese subjects reduced to normal body weight without an associated weight loss training program? Hensrud et al. (11) directed 24 obese dieting women to diet until they lost 10 kg. They were not taught any weight management skills and then were followed until they attained their initial weight. At one year, they regained 42% of their weight loss and at four years they had regained 87% of the weight previously lost.

Maintenance and Anorectic Agents

Goldstein (12) looked at long-term weight loss and the effect of pharmacologic agents. He reviewed 20 weight reduction studies on the effect of at least six months of pharmacologic therapy on weight loss maintenance. The agents investigated included phentermine, mazindol, fenfluramine, dexfenfluramine, and fluoxetine. Ten of the clinical trials investigated the effect of therapy used intermittently or continuously for six months; nine investigated the effects for more than one year. The conclusion of the article was that the long-range benefits of medication as an aid to weight loss maintenance exceeded the risks.

Weintraub's (13) important publication on long-term weight control was a meticulous 210-week study. The treatment plan was multimodal with a combination of behavior therapy, nutrition counseling, exercise, and anorectic agents. His data clearly showed that, whenever the drug treatment was discontinued, patients rapidly regained their lost weight despite adjunctive counseling.

A national task force on the prevention and treatment of obesity published its findings in 1996 (14). The two key points were: (*i*) pharmacotherapy for obesity, when combined with appropriate behavioral approaches to change diet and physical activity, helps some obese patients lose and maintain weight loss for at least one year, (*ii*) pharmacotherapy for weight loss maintenance is not recommended for routine use in obese individuals, although it may be helpful in carefully selected patients.

Based on years of clinical experience and the experience of many other bariatricians, the author and the American Society of Bariatric Physicians (ASBP) believed that pharmacotherapy can be a very effective tool in carefully selected patients, when professionally monitored according to the ASBP guidelines (15).

Maintenance and the Internet

An example of the use of the Internet for weight maintenance can be seen in an article by Svetkey et al. (16), which compared three strategies for sustaining weight loss. One thousand and thirty-two subjects were followed for 30 months after a six-month weight loss phase. The average weight loss was 8.5 kg. Then the subjects were divided into three maintenance groups: (*i*) a monthly personal contact group, (*ii*) a group with unlimited access to an interactive technology-based intervention, (*iii*) self-directed control group. The results showed that all three maintenance groups regained weight, but the personal contact group regained less weight (4 kg) than the self-directed and technology group (5.5 kg). Interestingly, the interactive technology-based intervention provided early but transient benefit. Apparently, the subjects were likely to "burn out" on using the Internet for their maintenance intervention.

Maintenance Physiology

There have been a number of articles that identify compensatory physiological changes the body makes after weight loss. These changes, such as the stability of the number of fat cells, improved insulin sensitivity, decreased energy expenditure, and increased lipoprotein lipase activity, are used to justify a pessimistic view that permanent weight loss is unlikely (17). Recently, however, Voelker, in "Losers Can Win at Weight Maintenance," refutes the popular assumption that the overweight body is always destined to return to its set-point weight (18). He discusses many studies that have not found an inappropriate decrease in resting metabolic rate for the reduced body size. My experience in bariatric practice certainly supports Volker's assertion. Table 1 shows four typical case studies of successful long-term maintenance from our practice; obviously, weight maintenance efforts were not overridden by some inevitable physiological set-point in these cases.

CLINICAL TRIALS OF INTENSIVE BEHAVIORAL PROGRAMS

The NIH-sponsored Diabetes Prevention Program (DPP) and Action for Health in Diabetes (Look AHEAD) studies were two recent landmark multiyear, multicenter research investigations (19,20). They compared the relative effectiveness of intensive behavioral and pharmacological approaches while treating body weight, diabetes status, and cardiovascular risk factors in adults with prediabetes and type 2 diabetes mellitus.

Table 1 Four Examples of Successful Long-Term Maintenance

Date	Weight
Case study #1: 40-year-old female	
2/2001	159.4 lb
8/2001	141 lb
2/2002	137.6 lb
5/2005	132.6 lb
9/2005	126.8 lb
7/2007	135.8 lb
Case study #2: 42-year-old native American male	
1/2007	474 lb
7/2007	412.4 lb
1/2008	398.6 lb
6/2008	377.8 lb
Case study #3: 48-year-old female	
6/2000	185 lb
3/2001	184.2 lb
4/2002	148.6 lb
3/2003	151.8 lb
3/2004	150.2 lb
3/2006	155.4 lb
3/2007	163.2 lb
2/2008	149.6 lb
Case study #4: 32-year-old female	
1/2002	266.8 lb
6/2003	150.2 lb
6/2004	177.8 lb
6/2006	213.4 lb
12/2007	155.8 lb
6/2008	160 lb

The DPP study interventions were intensive lifestyle, medication (metformin), and placebo. Each group had almost 1100 participants. The lifestyle intervention group featured an intensive program with the following specific goals: (*i*) >7% total body weight loss and maintenance of weight loss, (*ii*) <25% of calories from fat, (*iii*) a calorie goal of 1200 to 1800 kcal/day, (*iv*) >150 minutes of physical activity per week. The lifestyle intervention structure included a 16-session core curriculum over 24 weeks, a long-term maintenance program, supervision of each individual by a case manager, and access to a lifestyle support staff including a dietitian, behavior counselor, and exercise specialist. Education and training in diet and exercise in addition to behavior modification skills were featured in the 16-session course conducted over 24 weeks. There was special emphasis on self-monitoring techniques, problem solving, individualizing programs, self-esteem, empowerment, and social support. There was frequent contact with the case manager and staff. After the core program, self-monitoring and other behavioral strategies were emphasized during monthly visits. Supervised exercise sessions were offered along with periodic group classes and motivational campaigns. The subjects were provided exercise videotapes and pedometers and were encouraged to enroll in a health club and/or cooking class. The retention and participation of the subjects in the intervention group was excellent, with an average follow-up of 2.8 years (range of 1.8–4.5 years). The study conclusively showed the results in the lifestyle intervention group to be superior to the metformin and placebo groups in increasing physical activity, losing weight, reducing the incidence of diabetes, and improving fasting glucose and hemoglobin A1 C values. Seventy-four percent of the intensive lifestyle arm subjects achieved the study goal of >150 minutes of activity per week at 24 weeks. This group also had a more significant mean weight loss of 9.9 lb at three years. The researchers in the DPP study summarized that intensive lifestyle intervention reduced development of diabetes by 58% compared with metformin reducing the development of diabetes by 31% ($P < 0.001$). They also confirmed that modest weight loss improves health, modest increases in physical activity can be sustained, and long-term adherence to lifestyle interventions is possible. The study clearly shows that people really will make lasting lifestyle changes with good maintenance strategies.

The Look AHEAD study is now in progress and also employing lifestyle intervention to improve diabetes mellitus and show health benefits such as decreased rates of cardiovascular death, nonfatal myocardial infarction, and nonfatal stroke. Using similar education and support sessions developed in the DPP protocol, the preliminary results after one year (19) are very exciting. At one year, the Look AHEAD intensive intervention resulted in a clinically significant weight loss of 8.6%, with the control group only losing 0.7%.

COHORT STUDIES OF SELF-REPORTED WEIGHT LOSS AND MAINTENANCE

The National Weight Control Registry (NWCR) is an observational cohort study of self-reported, long-term successful weight loss maintenance (4,21). Started in 1994, the NWCR is tracking over 5000 individuals who have lost at least 30 lb and kept it off for at least one year. Registry members have lost an average of 66 lb and kept it off for 5.5 years. The weight losses have ranged from 30 to 300 lb; the duration of successful weight loss has ranged from 1 to 66 years. Some individuals lost the weight rapidly, while others lost weight very slowly, over as many as 14 years. The demographics show 80% of persons in the NWCR are female, 20% male. The average woman is 45 years of age and currently weighs 145 lb, while the average man is 49 years of age and currently weighs 190 lb. About half of the participants lost the weight on their own and the other half lost weight with the help of some type of program. Most of the registry participants had childhood onset obesity. Forty-six percent report being overweight by 11 years of age, 28.3% report being overweight by 12 to 18 years of age, and 28.3% report being overweight by 18 years of age. Forty-six percent report one parent was overweight, while 26.8% report both parents were overweight. Ninety-eight percent of these participants report they modified their food intake in some way to lose weight; 94% increased their physical activity, with the most frequently reported form of activity being walking.

Successful Weight Loss in the NWCR

By far, the highest single predictor of success in this group seems to be high levels of activity (22). Ninety percent exercise, on average, about one hour per day. The average energy expenditure

Table 2 Successful Weight Maintenance Strategies by NWCR Members

1. Low-fat diet
2. Low-carbohydrate diet
3. Low-calorie diet
4. High daily levels of physical activity, minimize watching television
5. Regularly eat breakfast, eat several times daily, avoid eating out
6. Frequent self-monitoring

per week is staggering, at almost 2700 kcal. In addition to aerobic activities, 24% of the males and 19.5% of the females included weight lifting in their regimen. Sixty-four percent watch less than 10 hours of television per week.

The current eating habits of registry participants show a low average caloric intake of 1380 calories; the macronutrient balance of their diet averages 24% fat, 19% protein, and 56% carbohydrate. The successful maintainers tend to eat five times daily; very few eat less than twice a day. Seventy-eight percent eat breakfast every day and they eat out three times a week on the average. Interestingly, only 0.9% of subjects reported eating a diet less than 24% carbohydrate. Self-monitoring is used by a majority of the NWCR members. Seventy-five percent (75%) weigh more than once a week; 44% weigh once a day; 50% still count calories and/or fat grams. Table 2 summarizes the successful weight maintenance strategies used by NWCR participants.

ENHANCING SUCCESSFUL WEIGHT MAINTENANCE

Behavioral Aspects

Dr. John Foreyt, a faculty member of the Psychology Department at Baylor Medical School, has contributed much to the understanding of the psychology of weight maintenance (23,24). He has found that consistent behaviors that correlate with successful maintenance include regular physical activity, self-monitoring, and continued contact with health professionals. He reports that successful programs stress the importance of maintenance from the start of the weight loss program. Realistic goals need to be discussed with the patient from the initial appointment. The patients need to identify intrinsic health reasons why they want to have a healthier weight (e.g., improved energy and feel better about themselves). Extrinsic reasons such as losing weight for a class reunion seldom sustain motivation. Structured eating patterns with regular breakfast and several feedings a day are important. Health professionals need to be a resource to help provide social support and help the patient solve problems. Weight regain is more likely to occur with inconsistent and restrictive dieting, elevated life stress, negative coping styles, and emotional or binge eating patterns.

Dr. Brian Wansink, Department of Psychology at Cornell University, has many helpful insights into long-term successful eating behaviors (25,26). Based on his behavioral research, Wansink reports that people make well over 200 decisions about food very day. Unfortunately, these decisions are usually unconscious, robotic, and automatic. Therefore, much of our inappropriate eating is due to a variety of environmental stimuli and unconscious cues that could be improved with the development of new behaviors. For example, he has shown that overeaters will often consume smaller amounts of food, and feel just as full, if they use smaller plates and dishes.

Medication-Related Weight Gain

An often overlooked problem in long-term weight loss maintenance is the frequent prescription of medications that cause weight gain as a common side effect (27). Since there are often alternative agents that do not cause such problems, it is hoped that prescribing professionals and patients will become more aware of this issue. As shown in Table 3, many different types of medications can lead to weight gain, including insulin, oral hypoglycemics, corticosteroids, antipsychotics, and antidepressants.

Table 3 Medications That Can Lead to Weight Gain

1. Anticonvulsants: valproic acid, carbamazepine
2. Antidepressants: tricyclic antidepressants, including Elavil (Amitriptylene), monoamine oxidase (MAO) inhibitors like Nardil, serotonin reuptake inhibitors (SSRIs) including Paxil and Zoloft; Remeron
3. Anticancer agents: e.g., Arimidex
4. Corticosteroids: e.g., Prednisone
5. Insulin: up to 17 lb weight gain can occur in an intensive three-month treatment course
6. Lithium: gains can be 22 lb or more in 6–10 years
7. Oral contraceptives: e.g., ethinylestradiol (6, 100, 200 mcg) leads to dose-dependent increases in body fat
8. Oral hypoglycemic agents (sulfonylureas): usual weight gain is more than 11 lb during 3–12 months of therapy
9. Antipsychotics: Haloperidol, Loxipine, Olanzapine, and Clozapine are the most likely culprits

Obstructive Sleep Apnea

In multiple recent studies, body mass index has been shown to increase with sleep durations significantly less than eight hours per night (28). Epidemiological studies have demonstrated a relationship between short sleep duration and increased risk of diabetes (28). Experimental studies have shown a strong relationship between acute sleep restriction and the development of abnormalities in glucose and insulin levels, serum cortisol, thyroid stimulation hormone, leptin, ghrelin, and sympathovagal balance (28). These physiological disturbances all contribute to weight gain. Bariatricians highly suspect obstructive sleep apnea when evaluating obese patients with central obesity, a neck circumference greater than 16 in., and an association with metabolic syndrome. Fortunately, these metabolic dysfunctions can be improved by treating obstructive sleep apnea with CPAP or similar technology. It is logical to include this important area for investigation and treatment to facilitate the probability of long-term successful weight loss maintenance. Table 4 contains some simple questions that can help the practitioner decide whether a sleep study evaluation is needed.

PUTTING IT ALL TOGETHER

In my personal clinical experience, it is imperative to stress to the patient at his first appointment that we conceive of a weight problem as requiring two strategies: phase A, the weight loss phase, and phase B, weight maintenance. We inform the patient they will see the physician and staff at least once a month for 12 to 18 months after reaching goal weight, planting the seeds of a maintenance strategy from the start. We reiterate frequently that our program is "a marathon, not a sprint." Although they may sound trite and corny, our patients hear often and respond to "you are the little engine that could," "you are the tortoise that beats the hare," and "don't forget 'LSD,' long slow distance!" Throughout the weight loss phase, the key to long-term professional contact is personal bonding to the office and staff and physician; we try to promote that bond by making visits enjoyable, frequently using laughter, humor, and awards to make the appointments a positive experience. All of our patients, while in the weight loss phase, receive a psychological and behavioral curriculum that goes beyond nutrition education and implementation of an exercise program. These include modules on stress management, self-esteem, understanding eating triggers, self-nurturing, dealing with slumps, positive attitude, and mindful eating. It is important for patients to master the art of eating out and learn how to deal with holidays and special occasions. All patients are exposed to the ideas of relaxation

Table 4 Sleep History Questions

1. Do you snore?
2. Has anyone seen you stop breathing while you were asleep?
3. Has anyone observed long irregular pauses between breaths while you are sleeping?
4. Are you often too sleepy during the day?

breathing, stretching exercises, and pet therapy. To provide a manual for our patients, we put this information together in a book (27).

In summary, the art and science of successful weight maintenance is still in its infancy. Most people underestimate the effort it takes to assist people in losing weight. Many breakthroughs are needed and expected in the next decade. At present, when all is said and done, persistence by the patient and physician seems to be the key. The importance of persistence was best stated by former president Calvin Coolidge: "Nothing in this world can take the place of persistence. Talent will not; nothing is more common that unsuccessful men with talent. Genius will not; unrewarded genius is almost a proverb. Education will not; the world is full of educated derelicts. Persistence and determination alone are omnipotent. The slogan 'press on' has solved and always will solve the problems of the human race."

REFERENCES

1. Wadden TA, Steen SN. Improving the maintenance of weight loss: The ten per cent solution. In: Angel A, Anderson H, Bouchard D, et Al, eds. Progress in Obesity Research. London: John Libbey, 1996:745–749.
2. Losing weight: What works. What doesn't. Consumer Reports June 1993; 58:347–353.
3. Wing RR, Hill JO. Successful weight loss maintenance. Annu Rev Nutr 2001; 21:323–341.
4. Klem ML, Wing RR, McGuire MT, et al. A descriptive study of individuals successful at long-term maintenance of substantial weight loss. Am J Clin Nutr 1997; 66:239–246.
5. Foster GD, Wadden TA, Kendall PC, et al. Psychological effects of weight loss and regain: A prospective evaluation. J Consult Clin Psychol 1996; 64(4):752–757.
6. Toubro S, Astrup A. Randomised comparison of diets for maintaining obese subjects' weight after major weight loss: Ad lib, low fat, high carbohydrate diet v fixed energy intake. BMJ 1997; 314(7073): 29–34.
7. Perri MG, Sears SF Jr, Clark JE. Strategies for improving maintenance of weight loss. Toward a continuous care model of obesity management. Diabetes Care 1993; 16:200–209.
8. Agras WS, Berkowitz RI, Arnow BA, et al. Maintenance following a very-low-calorie diet. J Consult Clin Psychol 1996; 64(3):610–613.
9. Hartman WM, Stroud M, Sweet DM, et al. Long-term maintenance of weight loss following supplemented fasting. Int J Eat Disord 1993; 14:87–93.
10. Walsh MF, Flynn TJ. A 54-month evaluation of a popular very low calorie diet progam. J Fam Pract 1995; 41:231–236.
11. Hensrud DD, Weinsier RL, Darnell BE, et al. A prospective study of weight maintenance in obese subjects reduced to normal body weight without weight-loss training. Am J Clin Nutr 1994; 60:688–694.
12. Goldstein DJ, Potvin JH. Long-term weight loss: The effect of pharmacologic agents. Am J Clin Nutr 1994; 60:6747–6657.
13. Weintraub M. Long-term weight control: The national heart, lung and blood institute funded multimodal intervention study. Clin Pharmacol Ther 1992; 51:581–646.
14. National task force on the prevention and treatment of obesity. Long-term pharmacotherapy in the management of obesity. JAMA 1996; 276(23):1907–1915.
15. American Society of Bariatric Physicians. www.asbp.org. Updated May 2010.
16. Svetkey LP, Stevens VJ, Brantley PJ, et al. Comparison of strategies for sustaining weight loss: The weight loss maintenance randomized controlled trial. JAMA 2008; 299(10):1139–1148.
17. Leibel RL, Rosenbaum M, Hirsch J. Changes in energy expenditure resulting from altered body weight. N Engl J Med 1995; 332(10):621–628.
18. Voelker R. Losers can win at weight maintenance. JAMA 2007; 298(3):272–273.
19. Look AHEAD Research Group. Reduction in weight and cardiovascular disease risk factors in individuals with type 2 diabetes: One-year results of the look AHEAD trial. Diabetes Care 2007; 30:1374–1383.
20. Diabetes Prevention Program Research Group. Reduction in the incidence of Type 2 diabetes with lifestyle intervention or metformin. N Engl J Med 2002; 346:393–403.
21. Shick SM, Wing RR, Klem ML, et al. Persons successful at long-term weight loss and maintenance continue to consume a low-energy, low-fat diet. J Am Diet Assoc 1998; 98:408–413.
22. Phelan S, Wyatt H, Nassery S, et al. Three-year weight change in successful weight losers who lost weight on a low-carbohydrate diet. Obesity 2007; 15:2470–2477.
23. Foreyt JP, Goodrick G. Attributes of successful approaches to weight loss and control. Appl Prev Psychol 1994; 3:209–215.
24. Foreyt JP, Goodrick GK. Evidence for success of behavior modification in weight loss and control. Ann Intern Med 1993; 119:698–701.

25. Wansink B. Environmental factors that increase the food intake and consumption volume of unknowing consumers. Annu Rev Nutr 2004; 24:455–479.
26. Wansink B, Sobal J. Mindless eating: The 200 daily food decisions we overlook. Environ Behav 2007; 39(1):106–123.
27. Rigden S. Chapter 7: Weight gain with chronic illness and impaired liver detoxification. In: The Ultimate Metabolism Diet. Eat right for your metabolic type. Alameda, California: Hunter House, 2008:185–188.
28. Tatman J. Impaired Sleep and Obesity. Obesity Course. Phoenix, AZ: American Society of Bariatric Physicians, 2008:176–190.

10 Surgical treatment of the obese individual

John B. Cleek

INTRODUCTION

A discussion of the current treatment of obesity is not complete without a review of the surgical options. "Bariatric surgery" is the term used for the surgical treatment of obesity. The number of bariatric surgery operations has climbed steadily over the last 10 years to represent 121,055 cases in 2004. In his recent review, Buchwald outlines the research that demonstrates the reduction in obesity-related morbidity and mortality with the use of bariatric surgery (1–3). The bariatric surgery literature gives the best-published view of how health can improve with weight loss. For example, hypertension is reduced or eliminated in 78.5% of patients, hyperlipidemia in 70%, and obstructive sleep apnea improved in 83.6%. Analyses have now been published that show a reduction in mortality when compared with usual care treatments. When compared with control groups that do not achieve substantial weight loss, there is a reduction in mortality in those who had bariatric surgery. In a retrospective study of 7900 patients with an average follow-up of 7.1 years, the mortality reduction at 7.1 years was 40% including a 56% reduction in death from coronary artery disease, a 92% reduction in death from diabetes mellitus, and a 60% reduction in deaths from cancer. The overall reduction in mortality over a 10.9-year period was 29% (4,5).

WHO SHOULD HAVE BARIATRIC SURGERY?

With such dramatic outcomes, the question is which patients qualify for surgery? Current recommendations state that those patients with a body mass index (BMI) greater than 40 may be considered candidates for bariatric surgery (6–9). Patients may be considered also if the BMI is greater than 35 with other medical comorbidities such as hypertension, diabetes mellitus, and obstructive sleep apnea. The patient should have had a complete medical and psychological evaluation to rule out an endocrinologic, psychiatric, or metabolic cause of obesity. Other qualifiers for candidacy include prior attempts at weight loss with no long-term success, commitment to regular health care follow-up as well as long-term diet and exercise programs. Patients must be able to understand the surgical risks as well as their long-term commitment.

Contraindications to bariatric surgery are specific as well. Female patients who may wish to become pregnant in the 18 months postoperatively should not be considered for surgery. Patients with major psychiatric disorder, such as uncontrolled depression, suicidal ideation, and personality disorder, are not candidates for bariatric intervention. Active substance abuse is also an absolute contraindication to surgery.

Preoperative Evaluation

The preoperative evaluations ensure that the patients meet the required criteria for surgery and help insure patient safety. A thorough history and physical examination is necessary to optimize patient care, including identification of preoperative risk factors. Laboratory testing helps identify additional risk factors for surgical complications. The preoperative evaluations include psychological evaluation and often exercise evaluation as well.

A comprehensive history should include weight history and nutrition history. Prior weight loss attempts should be recorded including method employed, results, and length of success. Barriers to success need to be reviewed for correction preoperatively or postoperatively. Further history should address perioperative risks. For example, increased perioperative risk is associated with a history of thromboembolic events, smoking, sleep apnea, and unstable angina.

The physical examination should screen for causes of obesity as well as complications of obesity. Vital signs including blood pressure, heart rate, height, and weight should be documented. Skin should be inspected for striae suggestive of Cushing's syndrome. The oropharynx is evaluated for airway size and possible risk for sleep apnea. Pulmonary examination checks for pulmonary edema suggestive of uncompensated heart failure. Cardiac examination evaluates

Table 1 Possible Postoperative Complications for Bariatric Surgery Patients

Possible complications during hospitalization
Intraluminal hemorrhage
Intraperitoneal hemorrhage
Anastomotic leak
Wound complications (ventral hernias, infection, and fascial dehiscence)
Deep venous thrombophlebitis (DVT)
Pulmonary embolism
Pneumonia
Possible posthospital discharge complications
Protein malnutrition
Vitamin deficiencies: vitamin A, vitamin B1 (thiamine), vitamin B12, vitamin D, vitamin K, folate
Micronutrient deficiencies: iron, magnesium, zinc, calcium, copper, selenium
Steatorrhea
Dumping syndrome
Anastomotic stricture or ulceration
Internal and ventral hernias
Bowel obstruction
Fistulas
Cholelithiasis
Islet cell hypertrophy
Insufficient weight loss

for murmurs and possible structural heart defects. Abdominal examination evaluates for hepatosplenomegaly associated with fatty liver disease. All other systems should also be checked for changes suggestive of unrecognized disease.

Laboratory testing should be comprehensive as well. Complete blood cell count, fasting blood sugar, comprehensive metabolic panel, and thyroid stimulating hormone are drawn at a minimum. Many centers routinely screen for Helicobacter Pylori, but this practice is not universal among bariatric surgery programs. Other laboratory testing should be based on the clinical situation of the individual patient.

No specific recommendations have been adopted for nutritional laboratory screening. In a series of patients reported by Flancbaum et al., vitamin D deficiency was found in 68% preoperatively (10). Additionally, iron deficiency was found in 43.9% and thiamine deficiency in 29% of the preoperative patients. Replacement of deficiencies needs to be undertaken prior to surgery, as replacement is problematic in the postoperative state.

Exercise evaluation is generally recommended preoperatively. While the exact best testing modality is not known, the four-minute walk test is commonly employed. Patients with poor physical conditioning have twice the risk of serious postoperative complications compared with those with higher exercise tolerance (11). Patients with poor exercise tolerance may benefit from cardiology screening such as a dobuatmine stress echocardiographic testing. Screening allows preoperative intervention to increase the operative safety.

Electrocardiograms are generally advised in men older than 45 years or women older than 55 years and any patients with known or suspected heart disease. Patients with multiple risk factors such as hypertension, diabetes mellitus, dyslipidemia should have an electrocardiogram taken, as should patients on diuretic therapy, due to the subsequent risk for electrolyte abnormalities.

Table 2 Suggested Routine Vitamin and Mineral Supplementation After Bariatric Surgery

Complete multivitamin with iron daily (chewable form in the early postoperative)
Calcium citrate 1200–1800 mg daily with vitamin D3 800–1000 IU daily
Ferrous sulfate 325 mg 2–3 times daily as needed
Oral vitamin B12 1000 μg daily
Folic acid 1 mg daily as needed
Zinc sulfate 100 mg as needed

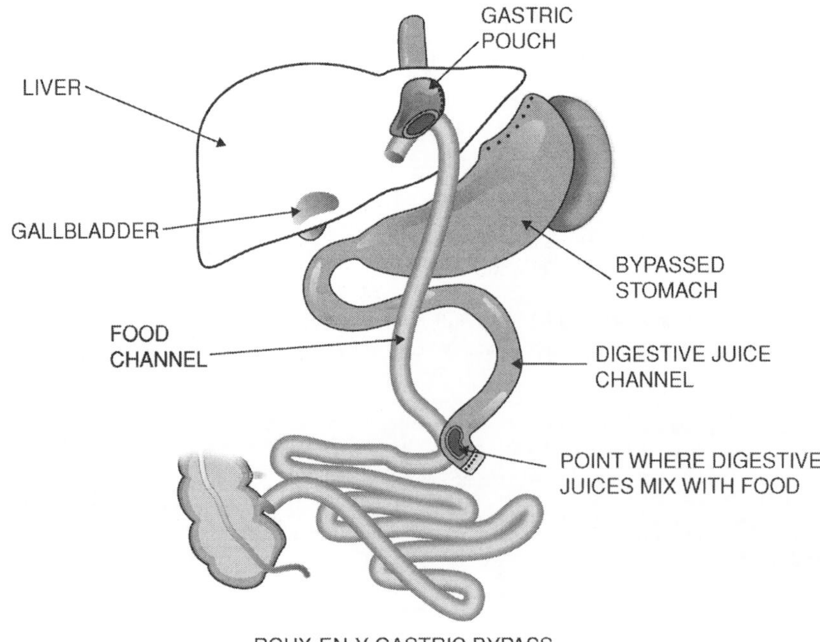

Figure 1 Gastric bypass using Roux-en-Y.

Diagnostic chest radiographs should be obtained for patients with known pulmonary disease, history of congestive heart failure, or who are older than 60 years. Many centers routinely screen every patient for sleep apnea as well.

A psychological evaluation is recommended for each patient. No standardized guidelines exist for this evaluation; however, most bariatric surgery centers use self-administered tests such as the Beck Depression Inventory, Minnesota Multiphasic Personality Inventory, or Millon Behavioral Medicine Diagnostic among other potential instruments. These instruments, in collaboration with the interview, are used to identify eating disorders, major depressive disorders, suicidality, personality disorders, and substance abuse disorders, in particular. In a 2004 review by Herpertz et al., 27% to 41% of preoperative patients have an Axis I diagnosis while 22% to 24% have an Axis II disorder (12). In a review by Sarwer et al., 62.2% of preoperative patients received a psychological diagnosis. Thirty-one percent of patients were referred for further evaluation and therapy prior to surgery (13). Mood disorders were the most common diagnosis, occurring in 19% to 60% of preoperative patients. Historically, 5% to 20% of patients are excluded from surgery based on their psychological evaluation.

A more controversial area of behavioral issues in the surgical candidate is the role of eating disorders, primarily binge eating disorder and nocturnal eating disorder, and subsequent outcome. Ten to fifty percent of patients presenting for bariatric surgery have binge eating disorder (14). Initially this disorder was felt to be potential for poor weight loss results after surgery and therefore patients were felt to be poor candidates. More recently, Fujioka et al., showed the excess weight loss is no different from controls at 12 and 24 months postoperatively (15). No change in perioperative complications is seen in this same period. Bocchieri-Ricciardi et al. also demonstrate no difference between binge eaters and nonbinge eaters at 18 months in terms of weight loss (16). Eating disorders, especially binge eating, does not appear to be a contraindication for surgery at this time.

Up to 40% of patients presenting to a weight loss center have night eating syndrome (14). Night eating syndrome is characterized by anorexia in the morning, evening hyperphagia, nocturnal awakenings, and eating during the awakenings. Generally, more than one-half of consumed calories in the day are after 5 PM. There is a lack of literature available relative to any role this disorder has in the approach to the surgical patient.

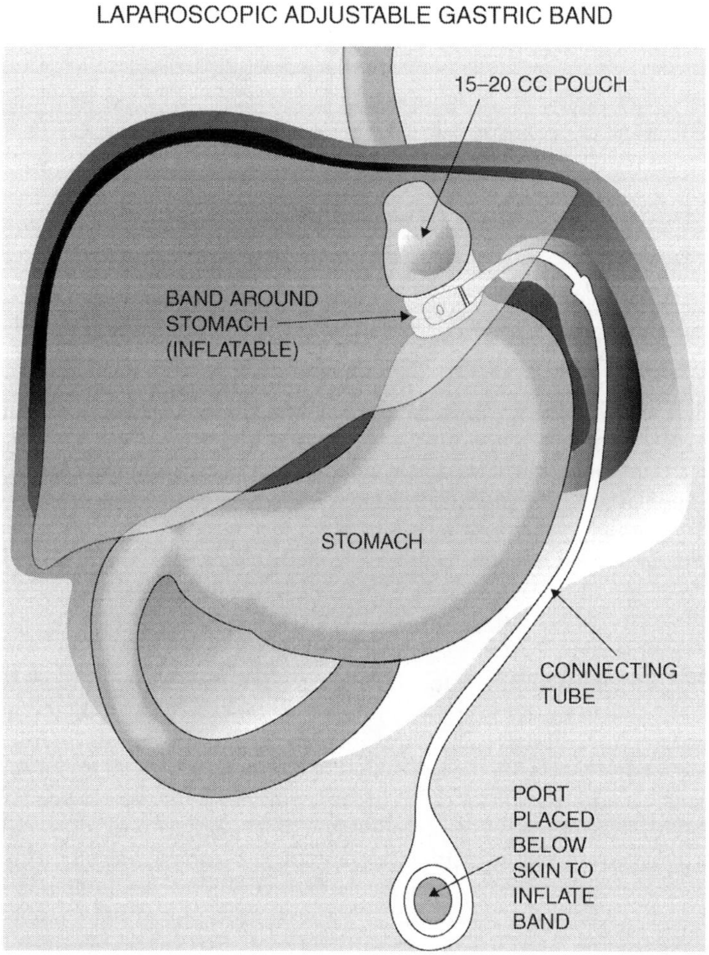

Figure 2 Example of gastric banding.

Perioperative Complications

Overall, the major risk factors for perioperative complications appear to include male sex, age older than 45 years, hypertension, diabetes, obstructive sleep apnea, unstable angina, congestive heart failure, and asthma. Risk factors for cirrhosis and pulmonary embolism increase perioperative complications. The super obese with a BMI greater than 50 have a significantly higher risk for perioperative complications, as well. Patients with limited exercise capacity (e.g., the inability to walk four blocks or two flights of stairs) have twice the risk of serious postoperative complications as compared with those with unlimited exercise capacity.

Preoperative Treatment

A preoperative program may be required by the bariatric surgery center or by the patient's insurance provider, though there are no studies to support the use of these programs. Typically varying in duration from 3 to 12 months, these programs may include patient education regarding exercise, nutrition, and lifestyle change. Compliance to the multiple visits of a preoperative program is thought to give a demonstration of the ability of the patient to comply with postoperative recommendations. Future research is needed to examine the importance of this type of program.

Preoperative weight loss is beneficial for improvement of operative complications (17–19). The more obese the patient is, the greater the risk of death or major perioperative complication

Vertical Banded Gastroplasty

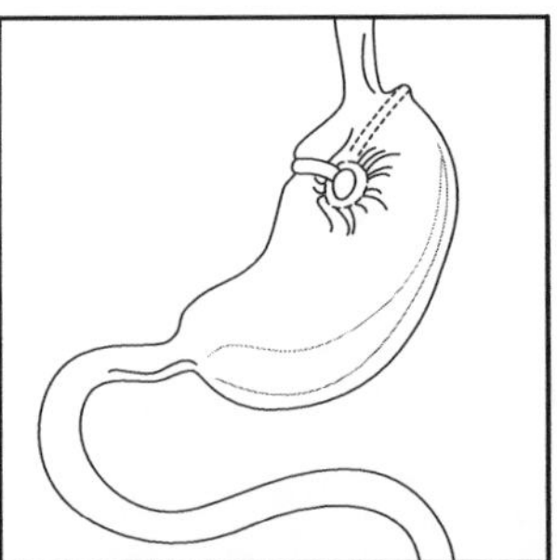

Roux-en-Y Gastric Bypass

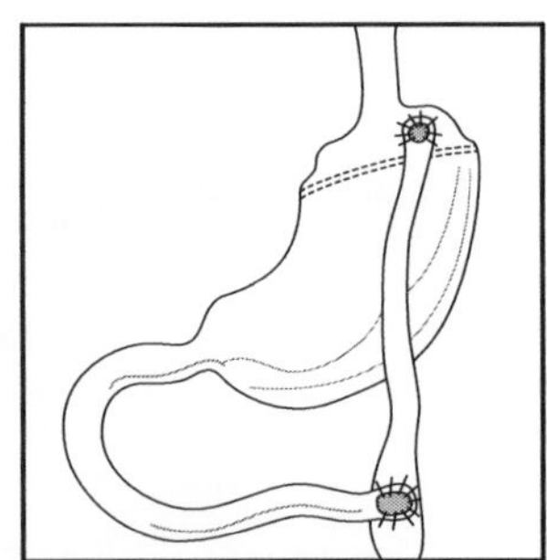

when undergoing certain operative bariatric procedures. For medical comorbidities, as little as 10% total body weight loss improves multiple conditions, including obstructive sleep apnea, cardiovascular risk, thromboembolic risk, and elevated blood glucose. Because increased abdominal adiposity and enlarged liver are major factors in having to convert from a laparoscopic to an open procedure, reducing adipose tissue in the abdomen and liver fat before the surgery reduces the technical difficulty of the surgery. Preoperative weight loss is also associated with less intraoperative blood loss.

Types of Bariatric Surgery

Although bariatric surgery started in the 1960s, a recent increase in surgeries has occurred because of the increased recognition of obesity as a serious medical problem, the use of minimally invasive surgery and laparoscopy, and increased reimbursement by insurance companies. Surgeries are generally classified on the basis of the mechanism of action. According to the Society of American Gastrointestinal and Endoscopic Surgeons, the type of bariatric surgery can be categorized into (*i*) mostly restrictive, (*ii*) mostly malabsorptive, and (*iii*) purely restrictive.

Purely restrictive procedures include horizontal gastroplasty, silastic ring gastroplasty, vertical banded gastroplasty, and adjustable gastric band (20). Vertical banded gastroplasty (see above sketch) consists of creating a fixed gastric pouch in the proximal stomach with a fixed band. The adjustable gastric band has been approved in the United States since June 2001 (21). The device has an inflatable cuff inside a silicone ring. A reservoir is attached to the inflatable cuff allowing for the adjustment of the band circumference through saline injection into the reservoir. The reservoir is placed in a subcutaneous location, allowing for improved access. Anatomically the reservoir or port is placed superior and left of the umbilicus. The band is placed around the gastric cardia, creating a 15 to 30 mL pouch. The wall of the stomach may be sutured over the top of the band to hold it in place. The band, therefore, creates a purely restrictive element to the gastrointestinal tract. The degree of restriction can be varied by the amount of saline placed in the reservoir and, hence, the cuff.

Currently, the most commonly performed bariatric surgery is a "mostly restrictive" procedure called the Roux-en-Y gastric bypass (RYGB), or simply gastric bypass (see above and Figure 1 on page 110). In this procedure, the stomach is transected into two pieces. One piece is a pouch of 15 to 30 mL size created from the cardia of the stomach. The second part of the stomach is larger and sealed at the site of the transection and otherwise remains intact. The jejunum is divided approximately 3 ft from the gastric outlet. The end of the jejunum originating from the stomach, or Y limb, is reanastomosed to the jejunum 100 to 150 cm from the newly created end of the jejunum. This section is attached to the gastric pouch and is called the Roux limb. A standard Roux limb is 75 to 150 cm in length, while a "long-limb" procedure creates a Roux limb of 150 to 200 cm. The Roux limb carries incompletely digested food from the stomach pouch, while the Y limb carries digestive enzymes from the stomach and pancreas. The digestion proceeds in the common channel of the unchanged small intestine.

"Mostly malabsorptive" procedures include long limb gastric bypass and biliopancreatic diversion with or without duodenal switch. In a long-limb gastric bypass, the Roux limb is lengthened to 200 cm or longer. The increase in length of the Roux creates a greater malabsorption. In the biliopancreatic diversion procedure, a partial gastrectomy is performed with a sleeve of lesser gastric fundus remaining intact, creating 100 to 150 mL gastric pouch. The small intestine is transected in the first part of the duodenum. A new anastomosis is created with the new limb of the small intestine and the remaining intact duodenum. The common channel is created 50 cm from the ileocecal valve. In a biliopancreatic diversion with duodenal switch, the common channel is lengthened to 100 cm. These procedures are reserved for patients with a BMI greater than 50 because of the complications of the severe malabsorption.

Surgical Mortality

The mortality rate is directly influenced by surgeon and hospital facility expertise. Published inpatient death rates range from 0.19% to 0.3%. High volume bariatric centers performing more than 100 cases annually had 0.3% mortality rate compared with 1.2% mortality rate in those centers performing less than 50 cases annually. These same high volume centers had lower complication rate at 10.2% compared with 14.5% in low volume centers (22). The rationale for developing "centers of excellence" for bariatric surgery relate, in part, to the variability in these statistics.

Possible Complications During Hospitalization

Intraoperative complications include bleeding, injury to surrounding structures, and staple misfire. Bleeding complications occur from the staple line, anastomosis site, or mesenteric vessels, and occur in about 4% of patients (23). Bleeding may be in the intestinal or gastric lumen, or intraperitoneal. Signs suggesting bleeding problems include hematemesis, bloody drain output, or a drop in hemoglobin. Treatment includes fluid resuscitation, transfusion as needed, and correction of any coagulopathy. Esophagogastroduodenoscopy (EGD) is indicated for intraluminal evaluation but reoperation may be required for persistent intraperitoneal bleeding.

Anastomotic leak is an early postoperative complication of bariatric surgery. These leaks are reported in 0% to 3% of patients after gastric bypass. Anastomotic leaks are more common at the gastrojejunum anastomosis due to ischemia in the region thought to be due to tension in the sutures. Worsening abdominal pain, leukocytosis, fever, distress, oliguria, and tachycardia with a rate greater than 120 beats per minute suggest an intra-abdominal leak. Often the presentation of the patient is tachycardia without other symptoms. Rapid surgical exploration of the abdomen is required (22).

Wound complications include ventral hernias, infection, and fascial dehiscence. Infection is more common in the obese with a reported rate of 2.9% in laparoscopic gastric bypass. Ventral hernias or incisional hernias are reported in the same study as to occur in 0.45% of cases. Wound dehiscence happens in less than 1% of patients (24).

Obesity is linked to a higher risk of deep venous phlebitis and pulmonary embolism. The risk of venous thromboembolism increases with higher BMI, and the published rate is 0 to 3%. Pulmonary embolism accounts for 50% (23) of the early postoperative deaths. All patients should receive prophylaxis, including subcutaneous heparin. Strong consideration should be given to placement of a vena caval filter if the patient has multiple risk factors including prior deep vein thrombosis, hypercoagulable syndrome, and venous stasis. A patient with tachycardia, shortness of breath, and oxygen desaturation should be evaluated for pulmonary embolus.

Pneumonia can occur after laparoscopic procedures, related to increased intra-abdominal pressure reducing diaphragmatic excursion. This condition also predisposes to pulmonary effusion. Dyspnea, fever, leukocytosis suggests this possible problem. A chest radiograph can help confirm the diagnosis.

Possible Posthospital Discharge Complications

Long-term complications of surgery include anastomotic strictures, cholelithiasis, intestinal obstruction, internal and ventral hernias, and gastrointestinal bleeding. Unique to the adjustable gastric band procedure are band slippage, band erosion, and port problems. With respect to the duodenal switch with biliopancreatic diversion, steatorrhea is a common problem (23).

Anastomotic strictures develop in 2% to 16% of patients after gastric bypass. Strictures are more common when the stoma diameter is less than 1 cm (25). Presenting symptoms include dysphagia, nausea, and vomiting, or excessive weight loss. Most commonly, the stricture occurs at the gastojejunal junction. Diagnosis of the stricture is made by upper gastrointestinal series or by EGD. The majority of cases are managed by simple balloon dilatation at the time of endoscopy. Rarely, surgical revision is required.

Anastomotic ulceration occurs in up to 4% for anastomotic ulceration of patients after gastric bypass. Ulceration usually occurs within the first three months. Symptoms include abdominal pain, nausea, vomiting, bleeding, and, rarely, perforation with an acute abdomen presentation. Ulcers are treated with proton pump inhibitors, sucralfate, and rarely surgical revision. These ulcers represent the most common cause of gastrointestinal bleeding.

Bowel obstruction is a later complication of surgery. Intraluminal causes of obstruction include blood clot, edema of the bowel wall or stoma, or in the case of adjustable gastric band, a band that is overly restrictive. Postoperative adhesions, incisional or internal hernias can also cause late onset bowel obstruction. Presenting symptoms include abdominal pain, nausea, and vomiting. A plain radiograph such as KUB (kidney, ureter, and bladder) may aid in the diagnosis. Computerized tomography is more sensitive in diagnosis. Specifically, a swirl sign, in which the mesentery and perhaps intestine are visualized twisting through an internal mesenteric defect created during the surgery, is the most specific finding. Typically surgery will be required to definitively treat the problem.

Cholelithiasis is common with any rapid weight loss and weight loss following bariatric surgery is no exception. After bariatric surgery, 38% to 52% of patients develop cholelithiasis within one year (23). Patients with gallstones at the time of surgery may have elective cholecystectomy at the time of their bariatric procedure. This technique is controversial and generally performed only with symptomatic gallstones at the time of bariatric intervention. Cholecystectomy is performed in 15% to 28% of patients within three years of a gastric bypass (23).

Steatorrhea is a problem in those patients having a malabsorptive procedure such as long-limb gastric bypass or biliopancreatic diversion with duodenal switch. The steatorrhea is generally due to the short common jejunoileal channel. If the common channel is less than 100 cm, then the risk for increased malabsorption and subsequent steatorrhea is increased. The only therapy for severe steatorrhea in a patient with a common channel that is shorter than 100 cm is surgical repair to create a longer common channel.

Complications unique to the adjustable gastric band procedure relate to the device itself. The band may erode into the stomach and even cause perforation. The band may slip, causing intolerance of the band with dysphagia or vomiting. The band may become infected, often with redness and drainage at the site of the port. The port may migrate or flip making access difficult and causing a loss of the ability to adjust the band. The pouch may dilate, as well as the esophagus, if the patient continues to overfill the pouch. Generally, surgical removal will be required to solve these issues.

Postoperative care is specialized to the bariatric patient, in particular for the gastric bypass patient. Adjustable laparoscopic band procedures are performed on an outpatient basis. The band needs to be adjusted at the first postoperative visit, usually two weeks after the surgical procedure. On the other hand, the gastric bypass patient remains hospitalized for two to three days and more stringent care is needed. In order to lessen the likelihood of pouch obstruction in the immediate postoperative period, no sustained release medications are given. Close blood sugar monitoring is required, as medications need to be reduced rapidly. Most diabetics are discharged from the hospital no longer on diabetes medications.

Diet and hydration are monitored closely. Feeding may be started as soon as the nasogastric tube is removed. Continual sipping of clear liquids helps maintain hydration. The goal is to maintain 40 mL per hour of urine output after the first two postoperative hours. The diet for the first two days after surgery is clear liquids. On day 3, full liquids are initiated. During days 4 to 30, pureed foods with six small meals a day are included. A mechanical soft diet with five meals a day ($^1/_2$ cup of food at each meal) is recommended for days 31 to 60. Meals of $^1/_2$ to $^3/_4$ cup, four times a day, are utilized from day 61 to day 90. After day 90, regular food is consumed in 3 to 5 meals a day, with each meal containing 1 to 1.5 cups. Patients are encouraged to drink at least 1.5 L of fluid daily. Recommendations include 5 to 8 fruits and vegetables daily, no concentrated sweets, and 80 to 120 g of protein daily. Patients are asked not to drink fluids with meals, as the fluid may empty the pouch more quickly and reduce satiety. Small bites, chewed thoroughly, are encouraged, with each meal lasting at least 30 minutes. Common food intolerances after surgery include bread, rice, pasta, chicken, milk, dairy foods, and carbonated beverages.

Patients require lifetime vitamin support especially after the malabsorptive or partial malabsorptive procedures (26). A general multivitamin is recommended daily, one or two tablets. Supplementation of calcium with calcium citrate at 1200 to 2000 mg daily is recommended. Citrate is better absorbed in the low acid environment after any form of gastric resection. The dosage of vitamin D is not entirely agreed upon though 400 to 800 IU have been the standard. Folate at a dose of 1 mg daily should be taken. Elemental iron at 65 mg is recommended daily. Vitamin B12, 500 μg, is the minimum dose for daily supplementation.

Dumping syndrome generally occurs within six months of surgery. Seventy to seventy-six percent of patients will experience dumping syndrome on at least one occasion (from a lecture at Cleveland Clinic, December 3rd, 2005, by Dr. Jeffrey Mechanick). When high sugar foods are consumed, the patient may experience abdominal pain, nausea, vomiting, diarrhea, flushing, headache, weakness, dizziness, and syncope. Signs of dumping syndrome include tachycardia and hypotension. The etiology of dumping syndrome remains unclear, with some postulating an increase in glucagon-like peptide-1, resulting in beta cell hyperplasia and a reactive hypoglycemia (from a lecture at Cleveland Clinic, December 3rd, 2005, by Dr. Jeffrey Mechanick).

Nutritional deficiencies are common postoperatively, especially with the purely malabsorptive and partially malabsorptive surgeries. Purely restrictive surgery is less likely to cause nutritional deficits. The deficits arise because of reduction in the stomach size and the lower vitamin and mineral absorption due to malabsorption.

Fat-soluble vitamin deficiencies are more common after biliopancreatic diversion but may also be a complication of gastric bypass. Vitamin A deficiency is reported in 52% to 69% of patients after biliopancreatic diversion and in 10% of patients after gastric bypass (27). A case report of night blindness occurring 10 years after gastric bypass underscores the need for recognition (28). Oral replacement therapy is sufficient.

Vitamin K deficiency is reported in 51% to 68% of patients after biliopancreatic diversion with duodenal switch, and improved after vitamin K supplementation (27).

With respect to vitamin E, little evidence exists to support clinically significant changes in level. In study by Slater et al. (27), vitamin E levels did not change over a four-year period after biliopancreatic diversion. Preoperative evaluation of micronutrients reveals an incidence of about 2% of vitamin E deficiency, but the importance of this is unknown.

Vitamin D has been extensively studied in the last several years. Vitamin D deficiency, as stated earlier, is evidenced in up to 68% of patients seen preoperatively. Malabsorption creates a risk for new onset or worsening of the vitamin D deficiency. In postoperative patients, the concern for inadequate vitamin D has surrounded bone loss. Vitamin D deficiency leads to secondary hyperparathyroidism, which may cause bone loss. Dexa scans for detection of bone loss are recommended at baseline and one year postoperatively.

Vitamin B deficiencies are a common postoperative nutritional complication. Folate is generally low because of reduced intake. Zero to thirty-eight percent of patients after gastric bypass have folate deficiency. Folate deficiency may cause anemia and is of particular importance prenatally for reduction (29) in neural tube birth defects.

Thiamine (vitamin B1) is lowered because of food intake restrictions, reduction in acidity from creation of the pouch, and because of duodenal exclusion (highest area of absorption). Thiamine deficiency is seen as early as six weeks postoperatively from malabsorptive procedures, especially in patients with recurrent vomiting. Beriberi may be seen at this early postoperative time. Thiamine deficiency may result in confusion, ophthalmoplegia, ataxia, and nystagmus, as in Wernicke's encephalopathy. Recognition of Wernicke's encephalopathy is critical for treatment to prevent long-term sequelae. Symptoms of beriberi may develop, not only early, but several years after surgery with symptoms of peripheral neuropathy, including pain and weakness of the lower extremities.

Vitamin B12 deficiency is created by achlorhydria preventing nutrient release from food, by the low tolerance to milk and dairy, and by the reduced production of intrinsic factor. Deficiency of vitamin B12 may, most commonly, produce a megaloblastic anemia or peripheral neuropathy.

Micronutrient and mineral deficiencies are frequently observed postoperatively, especially after malabsorptive procedures. In particular magnesium, zinc, iron, selenium, calcium, and copper may need to be evaluated postoperatively.

Iron deficiency is caused by the limitation in food intake, reduced acid production, and duodenal exclusion. The greatest proportion of iron absorption occurs in the duodenum. Iron deficiency is reported to occur from 13% to 52% of patients after gastric bypass, two to four years after surgery, but up to 33% of patients may develop it by the first year postoperatively. An anemia is recognized in up to 50% of patients after gastric bypass with higher incidence in menstruating young women (30). Testing includes complete blood count, iron level, and ferritin. Ferritin is the most sensitive for detecting low iron.

Zinc absorption is impaired after malabsorptive procedures, since zinc is absorbed primarily in the duodenum and proximal jejunum. Zinc deficiency results in dermatitis of the nasolabial folds and hands, reduced wound healing, and altered taste perception. Up to 50% of patients after biliopancreatic diversion will have zinc deficiency (31).

Magnesium deficiency is reported in just fewer than 5% of patients preoperatively. Patients may experience a loss of magnesium with excessive diarrhea or steatorrhea. A recent study by Johansson et al. (32) reports a slight increase in magnesium levels at one year after gastric bypass. Magnesium should be checked in those patients with spasms or myalgias. No routine recommendation exists for checking levels in asymptomatic patients.

Calcium changes are common after malabsorptive surgeries. In a study by Newbury et al. (33), 25% of patients had hypocalcemia after biliopancreatic diversion. Attention should be given to calcium and ionized calcium levels in particular.

Copper deficiency can be seen after gastric bypass. Copper deficiency may cause a neuropathy that resembles vitamin B12 deficiency. Rarely copper can be an etiologic factor in anemia. Selenium deficiency is reported in up to 15% of patients after biliopancreatic diversion. Low selenium is reported in three percent of gastric bypass patients after one year. A case report by Boldery et al. reveals a cardiomyopathy related to selenium deficiency in a patient after gastric bypass (34). Evaluation of selenium has not been a routine recommendation.

From a macronutrient standpoint, protein malnutrition is a postoperative risk. With greater amount of malabsorption, the risk of protein-calorie malnutrition increases. Reduced intake due to gastric restriction and food intolerance contributes to inadequate protein level. Signs of protein malnutrition include edema, anasarca, hair loss, and muscle wasting. Prealbumin and albumin levels are markers of protein stores. Severe inadequacy is marked by total protein of less than 5 g per deciliter and albumin less than 2.5 g/dL. Lowest levels of albumin occur one to two years after a gastric bypass. Treatment consists of increased intake of high protein foods, protein supplements, and may require enteral or parenteral nutrition.

Hypoglycemia is increasingly reported as a complication to surgery, specifically after gastric bypass. Neuroglycopenia appears to be related to islet cell hypertrophy. The hypertrophy origin is a point of controversy. The hypertrophy may be in response to weight gain, which necessitated the surgery, or due to increase in incretin hormone glucagon-like peptide-1 response postoperatively. The common link is excessive insulin secretion in response to a meal, with resultant delayed hypoglycemia. A portion of these symptomatic patients will require partial pancreatectomy while most can be managed with diet and pharmacotherapy when needed.

The effects of surgery on gastrointestinal hormones are under intense scrutiny. The advantage of malabsorptive surgeries may rely on the changes in these hormones such as PYY, ghrelin, and glucagon-like peptide-1 in particular. The rapid resolution of diabetes mellitus following gastric bypass as compared with adjustable gastric band suggests factors beyond weight loss account for the difference in effect (see Figure 2 on page 111). The gastrointestinal hormones are hypothesized to account for that difference in diabetic resolution, as 80% to 100% of patients after gastric bypass have diabetes resolution compared with 30% to 70% of patients after gastric banding. In particular, patients after gastric bypass have an earlier rise in glucose after a meal compared with nonsurgical patients. This glucose rise precipitates a rise in postprandial insulin that is earlier and more pronounced than in nonsurgical patients. Glucagon-like peptide-1 (GLP-1) and PYY are enhanced postprandially in the surgical patient. The rise in PYY and GLP-1 may contribute to the satiety of the postoperative patient, as these hormones are known to be anorexigenic. These hormones, PYY and GLP-1, are not increased with gastric band procedures and seem to account for the improved satiety after gastric bypass in comparison with gastric band. Additionally, plasma ghrelin, orexigenic in nature, has a blunted response to weight loss in gastric bypass patients. This decrease in ghrelin contributes to the improved satiety after gastric bypass compared with gastric banding.

A long-term complication of surgery may be insufficient weight loss. Defined as a loss of less than 40% to 50% of excess weight, 15% to 17% of patients after gastric bypass and adjustable gastric band will fail to lose expected amount of weight. Reasons for insufficient weight loss include lack of dietary adherence, lack of exercise, psychological causes, and surgical technique complications. From surgical standpoint, a large or dilated pouch, short Roux limb, or gastrogastric fistula can create increased nutrient absorption. Surgical interventions may be the best treatment option in these cases.

Nonsurgical etiologies of insufficient weight loss are typically lifestyle related. In a study of 100 patients after gastric bypass, Elkins et al. report 37% patients eat snacks, 2% drink sodas, 11% fail to take vitamin supplements, and 41% do not exercise (35). A program combining aerobic activity and strength training is recommended. The program should be a gradually progressive program taking into account the patient's clinical status and physical ability. In a study by Evans et al., participation in 150 minutes per week of moderate or higher intensity activity yields higher weight loss at 6 and 12 months postoperatively after gastric bypass (36).

With respect to pregnancy, women are encouraged to wait one to two years after surgery before planning pregnancy. With proper nutritional evaluation and support, minimal adverse effects have been noted. Specifically, iron, vitamin B12, vitamin A, folate, calcium, and vitamin D need to be followed closely as these nutrients have a direct impact on fetal development. A study by Weintraub et al., in fact, shows that postsurgically treated women experience fewer diabetes and hypertension complications and have a reduced risk of neonatal macrosomia (37). A study by Sheiner et al. of 298 patients reveals no increase in pregnancy or perinatal complications in women after weight loss surgery (38). A literature review by Grundy et al. presents similar outcomes in terms of pregnancy morbidities (39).

Several other newer procedures are becoming increasingly used for weight reduction. Gastric sleeve surgery is the most common of these procedures. A gastric sleeve procedure is a restrictive procedure in which the stomach is resected along the greater curvature leaving a tubular stomach of 60 to 80 cm. The antrum and pylorus of the stomach are preserved. The procedure has been performed in patients with Crohn's disease, ulcerative colitis, cardiomyopathy with low ejection fraction, and renal transplant patients. A review by Iannelli et al. revealed weight loss of 83% at 12 months though a study by Almogy et al. revealed an excess weight loss of 45.1% at 12 months (40,41). Mortality rate in the reviewed studies by Iannelli et al. is 0.9% and morbidity 10.3% (40). This procedure is often used as part of a two-stage approach for the super-obese patient with second-stage duodenal switch. Till et al. report use of a gastric sleeve procedure as in four adolescent cases (42).

Future surgical therapies may include gastric stimulator, intragastric balloon, endoluminal sleeve, and gastric pouch revision. The intragastric balloon, gastric pouch revision, and endoluminal sleeve are endoscopic procedures. Intragastric balloons are used for short-term weight loss with 26% excess weight loss. The balloon promotes satiety. The potential complications include pressure ulcers, balloon rupture, and distal gastric obstruction.

Neuromodulation is a potential course of bariatric therapy. Variations include vagal pacemaker, sympathetic nerve stimulator, intragastric stimulator, implantable intestinal stimulator, and gastric implantable stimulator. By changing the nerve signals to the central nervous system, the hope is for significant reduction in intake and, hence, weight loss.

The endoluminal sleeve is endoscopically placed at the gastric outlet. The sleeve uncurls resulting in blockage of nutrient contact with the duodenum and proximal jejunum. Studies at this time do not extend beyond six months. The excess weight loss is 23.6%. Interestingly, four patients with diabetes had resolution of their diabetes (43).

In patients with gastric pouch dilatation, endoscopic revision has recently been undertaken. Revising from one type of surgery to another has been reported (such as from adjustable gastric band to gastric bypass). A variety of methods and procedures to improve the outcome from surgical intervention will continue to evolve.

Compared with other weight loss approaches at this time, surgery has demonstrated the greatest excess weight loss, the greatest reductions in comorbidities, and the first demonstration of reduced mortality compared with those receiving usual care. The safety of the procedures has been significantly improved and the result is a large increase in bariatric surgical procedures over the last 5 to 10 years. The immediate future will show an increase in surgical interventions until prevention or other pharmacotherapy makes significant improvements. The care of the postoperative patient requires careful attention to nutritional status but can be rewarding in view of the excellent results as described. It is important to note that there has never been a randomized trial of bariatric surgery versus effective pharmacologic or lifestyle modification treatment. This kind of study is needed to truly evaluate comparative effectiveness of these different therapies.

REFERENCES

1. Buchwald H, Avidor Y, Braunwald E, et al. Bariatric surgery: A systematic review and meta-analysis. JAMA 2004; 292(14):1724–1737.
2. Buchwald H, Estok R, Fahrbach K, et al. Weight and type 2 diabetes after bariatric surgery: Systematic review and meta-analysis. Am J Med 2009; 122(3):248–256.
3. Colquitt JL, Picot J, Loveman E, et al. Surgery for obesity. Cochrane Database Syst Rev 2009; 15(2):CD003641.
4. Adams TD, Gress RE, Smith SC, et al. Long-term mortality after gastric bypass surgery. N Engl J Med 2007; 357(8):753-761.
5. Sjöström L, Narbro K, Sjöström CD, et al. Effects of bariatric surgery on mortality in Swedish obese subjects. Swedish Obese Subjects Study. N Engl J Med 2007; 357(8):741–752.
6. National Institutes of Health, National Heart, Lung, and Blood Institute. The Practical Guide. Identification, Evaluation, and Treatment of Overweight and Obesity in Adults. Washington, DC: NIH, 2000.
7. Apovian CM, Cummings S, Anderson W, et al. Best practice updates for multidisciplinary care in weight loss surgery. Obesity (Silver Spring) 2009; 17(5):871–879.
8. Kelly JJ, Shikora S, Jones DB, et al. Best practice updates for surgical care in weight loss surgery. Obesity (Silver Spring) 2009; 17(5):863–870.
9. Mechanick JI, Kushner RF, Sugerman HJ, et al. American Association of Clinical Endocrinologists; Obesity Society; American Society for Metabolic & Bariatric Surgery. American Association of Clinical Endocrinologists, The Obesity Society, and American Society for Metabolic & Bariatric Surgery medical guidelines for clinical practice for the perioperative nutritional, metabolic, and nonsurgical support of the bariatric surgery patient. Obesity (Silver Spring) 2009; 17(suppl 1):S1–S70.
10. Flancbaum L, Belsley S, Drake V, et al. Preoperative nutritional status of patients undergoing Roux-en-Y gastric bypass for morbid obesity. J Gastrointest Surg 2006; 10(7):1033–1037.
11. Reilly DF, McNeely MJ, Doerner D, et al. Self-reported exercise tolerance and the risk of serious perioperative complications. Arch Intl Med 1999; 159:2185–2192.
12. Herpertz S, Kielmann R, Wolf AM, et al. Do psychosocial variables predict weight loss or mental health after obesity surgery? A systematic review. Obes Res 2004; 12(10):1554–1569.
13. Sarwer DB, Wadden TA, Fabricatore AN. Psychosocial and behavioral aspects of bariatric surgery. Obes Res 2005; 13(4):639–648.
14. Sarwer DB, Wadden TA, Fabricatore AN. Psychosocial and behavioral aspects of bariatric surgery. Obes Res 2005; 13(4):639–648.
15. Fujioka K, Yan E, Wang HJ, et al. Evaluating preoperative weight loss, binge eating disorder, and sexual abuse history on Roux-en-Y gastric bypass outcome. Surg Obes Relat Dis 2008; 4(2):137–143.
16. Bocchieri-Ricciardi LE, Chen EY, Munoz D, et al. Pre-surgery binge eating status: Effect on eating behavior and weight outcome after gastric bypass. Obes Surg 2006; 16(9):1198–1204.
17. Still CD, Benotti P, Wood GC, et al. Outcomes of preoperative weight loss in high risk patients undergoing gastric bypass surgery. Arch Surg 2007; 142(10):994–998.
18. Liu RC, Sabnis AA, Forsyth C, et al. The effect of acute preoperative weight loss on laparoscopic Roux-en-Y gastric bypass. Obes Surg 2005; 15(10):1396.
19. Alger-Meyer S. Preoperative weight loss as a predictor of long term success following Roux-n-Y gastric bypass. Obes Surg 2008; 18:772–775.
20. Folope V, Hellot MF, Kuhn JM, et al. Weight loss and quality of life after bariatric surgery: A study of 200 patients after vertical gastroplasty or adjustable gastric banding. Eur J Clin Nutr 2008; 62(8):1022–1030.

21. Nadler EP, Reddy S, Isenalumhe A, et al. Laparoscopic adjustable gastric banding for morbidly obese adolescents affects android fat loss, resolution of comorbidities, and improved metabolic status. J Am Coll Surg 2009; 209(5):638–644.
22. Nyugen NT, Paya M, Stevens CM, et al. The relationship between hospital volume and outcome in bariatric surgery at academic medical centers. Ann Surg 2004; 240:586–593.
23. Brethauer SA, Chand B, Schauer PR. Risks and benefits of bariatric surgery: Current evidence. Cleve Clin J Med 2006; 75(11):993–1007.
24. McGlinch BP, Que FG, Nelson JL, et al. Perioperative care of patients undergoing bariatric surgery. Mayo Clin Proc 2006; 81(10, suppl):S25–S33.
25. Podnos YD, Jimenez JC, Wilson SE, et al. Complications after laparoscopic gastric bypass: A review of 3464 cases. Arch Surg 2003; 138:957–961.
26. Malone M. Recommended nutritional supplements for bariatric surgery patients. Ann Pharmacother 2008; 42:1851–1858.
27. Slater GH, Ren CJ, Siegel N, et al. Serum fat-soluble vitamin deficiency and abnormal calcium metabolism after malabsorptive bariatric surgery. J Gastrointest Surg 2004; 8(1):48–55.
28. Lee WB, Hamilton SM, Schwab IR. Ocular complications of hypovitaminosis A after bariatric surgery. Ophthalmology 2005; 112(6):1031–1034.
29. Xanthakos SA, Inge TH. Nutritional consequences of bariatric surgery. Curr Opin Clin Nutr Metab Care 2006; 9(4):489–496.
30. McMahon MM, Sarr MG, Clark MM, et al. Clinical management after bariatric surgery: Value of a multidisciplinary approach. Mayo Clin Proc 2006; 81(10, suppl):S34–S45.
31. Slater GH, Ren CJ, Siegel N, et al. Serum fat-soluble vitamin deficiency and abnormal calcium metabolism after malabsorptive bariatric surgery. J Gastrointest Surg 2004; 6(1):48–55.
32. Johansson HE, Zethelius B, Ohrvall M, et al. Serum magnesium status after gastric bypass surgery in obesity. Obes Surg 2009; 19(9):1250–1255.
33. Newbury L, Dolan K, Hatzifotis M, et al. Calcium and vitamin D depletion and elevated parathyroid hormone following biliopancreatic diversion. Obes Surg 2003; 13(6):893–895.
34. Boldery R, Fielding G, Rafter T, et al. Nutritional deficiency of selenium secondary to weight loss surgery associated with life-threatening cardiomyopathy. Heart Lung Circ 2007; 16(2):123–126.
35. Elkins G, Whitfield P, Marcus J, et al. Noncompliance with behavioral recommendations following bariatric surgery. Obes Surg 2005; 15(4):546–551.
36. Evans RK, Bond DS, Wolfe LG, et al. Participation in 150 min/wk of moderate or higher intensity physical activity yields greater weight loss after gastric bypass surgery. Surg Obes Relat Dis 2007; 3(5):526–530.
37. Weintraub AY, Levy A, Levi I, et al. Effect of bariatric surgery on pregnancy outcome. Int J Gynaecol Obstet 2008; 103(3):246–251.
38. Sheiner E, Balaban E, Dreiher J, et al. Pregnancy outcome in patients following different types of bariatric surgeries. Obes Surg 2009; 19(9):1286–1292.
39. Grundy MA, Woodcock S, Attwood SE. The surgical management of obesity in young women: Consideration of the mother's and baby's health before, during, and after pregnancy. Surg Endosc 2008; 22(10):2107–2116.
40. Iannelli A, Schneck AS, Ragot E, et al. Laparoscopic sleeve gastrectomy as revisional procedure for failed gastric banding and vertical banded gastroplasty. Obes Surg 2009; 19(9):1216–1220.
41. Almogy G, Crookes PF, Anthone GJ. Longitudinal gastrectomy as a treatment for the high-risk super-obese patient. Obes Surg 2004; 14(4):492–497.
42. Till H, Blüher S, Hirsch W, Kiess W. Efficacy of laparoscopic sleeve gastrectomy (LSG) as a stand-alone technique for children with morbid obesity. Obes Surg 2008; 18(8):1047–1049.
43. Rodriguez-Grunert L, Galvao Neto MP, Alamo M, et al. First human experience with endoscopically delivered and retrieved duodenal-jejunal bypass sleeve. Surg Obes Relat Dis 2008; 4(1):55–59.

11 Medical treatment of pediatric obesity

Mary C. Vernon and Eric C. Westman

Treatment of overweight and obesity in children, and prevention of these conditions, is imperative. This is the first generation of children who may die before their parents because of the comorbidities of excess adiposity (1). The treatment of children is particularly complicated because they are particularly susceptible to advertising and peer pressure, both at home and at school. While the environment of a child may be difficult to control, the root cause of obesity is the same for children as it is for adults: hyperinsulinemia. The hormonal impact of insulin as a growth factor leads to macrosomia. Hyperinsulinemic children are not only obese, but they are also large for their age. This can be seen in the infants of diabetic mothers (IDM) who become hyperinsulinemic in the intrauterine environment due to maternal hyperglycemia.

Children have exposure both in school and via television and other electronic media, which define much of the social milieu today. It can be very difficult to control the source of food for children (Fig. 1). This has led to the ingestion of large amounts of sugar, much of it as fructose. Advice on "healthy diets" has often been interpreted as license to eat primarily sugars and starches under the label of fruits and vegetables. (Until recently, ketchup was considered a "vegetable" in school lunch programs.) Especially troublesome is the reality that sugar-sweetened beverages are part of the social interaction of adolescents, and even infants are given juice and colas from the time they take a bottle rather than the breast. This sugar consumption leads to hyperinsulinemia, which is the cause of the epidemic of type 2 diabetes and metabolic syndrome seen in children in the United States and now in other developed nations.

The role of parents in treatment of childhood obesity depends on the stage of the child's development. In children younger than pubertal age, parental support and engagement in lifestyle change are critical to the child's success. Pubertal and older teens often need to establish control over their bodies as evidence of individuation. In this case, helping the patient to strategize control over their food may need to be done with parental support but not parental responsibility. Only the clinician's judgment and relationship with the family can individualize such an approach.

DEFINITION OF OBESITY

Obesity in children is more difficult to define than in adults because of the changing height and normal growth of children. So, pediatric obesity is defined as excess adiposity relative to optimal growth parameters. Because of the relationship of weight gain to growth in children, body mass index (BMI), although the standard for defining obesity in adults, is not accepted universally for use among children. The Centers for Disease Control and Prevention (CDC) suggests two levels of concern for children on the basis of the BMI-for-age charts (2).

1. At the 85th percentile and above, children are "at risk for overweight";
2. At the 95th percentile or above, they are "overweight."

Some experts consider those children with a BMI-for-age above the 95th percentile to be "obese," corresponding to a BMI of 30 (considered obese in adults) (3) (Table 1). The use of percentage of body weight, which is fat mass, is also a good marker of obesity. Using the body fat percentage, boys >25% fat and girls >32% fat are considered obese. Body fat percentage can be measured in the office, and bariatricians often have access to equipment that can provide such a measurement.

GOAL OF TREATMENT

The goal of treatment of pediatric obesity depends, in part, on the physiologic age of the child. Although the reduction of excess adiposity in a safe, tolerable and sustainable way is still the treatment goal, the clinician must assess the child's growth to develop the treatment plan.

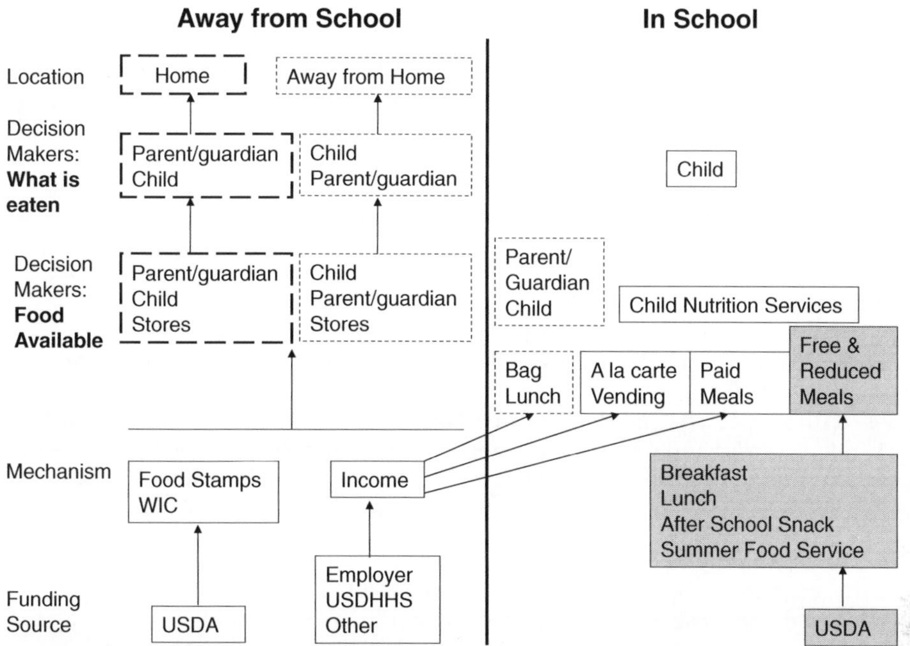

Figure 1 Factors influencing what a child eats. *Abbreviations*: USDA, United States Department of Agriculture; USDHHS, United States Department of Health and Human Services; WIC, USDA Women, Infants and Children Program.

Because children reach a point in their growth and development where linear growth ceases due to epiphyseal closure, the urgency and intensity of treatment may be impacted by how close the child is to cessation of linear growth. If the child is within a year or so of epiphyseal closure as noted by bone age and a BMI-for-age above the 90th percentile, then aggressive treatment options including carbohydrate and caloric restriction and adjunctive anorectic medications may be appropriate. Certainly, with any child for whom a surgical option is being discussed, a trial of vigorous medical therapy is indicated.

WHAT IS HEALTHY NUTRITION DURING WEIGHT LOSS?

Dietary protein is critical for appropriate growth, including bone and muscle development. The protein requirement for children is age dependent, and the values are based on extrapolations rather than on large population measurements (4). It appears that the protein concentration of breast milk (~150 mg protein/kg/day) is adequate for the first six months of life. After that, approximately 120 mg/kg/day appears sufficient by most standards until adult weight range is reached. This is assuming that the protein is of high biologic value (animal protein). If daily protein needs are fulfilled by lower biologic value proteins, then the daily requirement may be larger. The need for water and minerals parallels adult humans. Carbohydrates, fats and proteins are used to supply the energy needed for growth and development.

Table 1 BMI Categorization for Children

BMI category	Traditional terminology	Newer terminology
<5th percentile	Underweight	Underweight
5th–84th percentile	Healthy weight	Healthy weight
85th–94th percentile	At risk of overweight	Overweight
≥95th percentile	Overweight or obesity	Obesity

DIETARY TREATMENT

The use of diets that induce nutritional ketosis in children is historically supported, both by populations eating primarily meat and fat (Inuit) and by the use of the Ketogenic Diet to treat seizures. Children tolerate these diets well and are able to maintain appropriate growth and development. Therefore, in cases where ketogenic diets are needed to generate lipolysis of adipose stores, they have a history of safe use in children, with appropriate monitoring, of course. Children with less urgent or intense need for lipolysis may be able to "grow out of" their excess adiposity if sugary beverages and other forms of "empty" calories, primarily refined carbohydrates, are removed from the diet and replaced by adequate protein, leafy green vegetables, and limited consumption of complex carbohydrates (those with lower glycemic indices). If ketogenic or carbohydrate-restricted dietary approaches are used, then neither the amount nor the type of dietary fat is restricted. (Trans-fats limitation is considered appropriate.) Calories are also unrestricted in this approach. If a balanced deficit diet approach is used, without carbohydrate restriction, then fat calories may be restricted as part of the calculated caloric deficit. If a balanced deficit diet approach is used, then careful attention is needed to ensure adequate protein intake. Although dietary vitamins and minerals are required in small amounts and are found in food naturally, during any dietary approach to weight loss, a "multivitamin" is recommended as a "safety net."

CLINICAL ASSESSMENT

The bariatrician caring for a child typically obtains an initial measurement of lipids, chemistry profile, and fasting glucose and insulin levels. A two-hour postprandial glucose and insulin level is appropriate if any concern exists about the possibility of type 2 diabetes mellitus, as well as to assess the post-glucose challenge insulin response. An elevated c-peptide can also provide evidence of chronic hyperinsulinemia. Teenagers can easily tolerate a three-hour glucose tolerance test with insulin levels. Of course, topical anesthetic agents such as lidocaine/prilocaine (EMLA) cream can be employed, if desired, to decrease pain and anxiety. Abnormal laboratory values would be repeated at intervals—about three months is often adequate time for these abnormalities to correct. In addition, in all prepubertal patients, a bone age x-ray should be considered. If the bone age is more than one year ahead of the chronologic age, then the urgency of treatment increases, especially as the child approaches puberty. Therefore, the Tanner rating scale is used to assess the developmental progress toward puberty (5,6). A Tanner 3 with advanced bone age may need intense treatment and close follow-up to avoid premature epiphyseal closure.

Children are measured for height and weight at every visit and then these measurements are plotted on the BMI-for-age graph. It is not uncommon to see a linear growth spurt occur with weight loss, presumably because of improvement in chronic hyperinsulinemia. Measurement of percent body fat is also helpful, if available. Clothing sizes, belt, and waist measurement can also help document progress. Medical approaches to treat pediatric obesity include dietary and medication approaches (Table 2).

PHARMACOLOGICAL TREATMENT

Anorectic agents or insulin sensitizers are not labeled for use in children, but some research has been done in this area (7,8). However, children routinely receive medications for treatment of ADD/ADHD (attention deficit disorder/attention deficit hyperactivity disorder, which have chemical similarity to those used for appetite suppression. As mentioned above, it seems reasonable that any child or adolescent considering a surgical procedure for treatment of obesity should be given a trial period of intense medical management, which may include anorectic medication(s), if this is considered appropriate by the experienced treating physician.

Table 2 Medical Approaches to Treat Pediatric Obesity

- Carbohydrate-restricted diet
- Calorie-restricted diet
- Very low calorie diet
- Combined medication and dietary therapy

The monitoring interval may be more frequent than the usual monthly visit, as determined by the clinician. All appropriate risk/benefit discussions are documented and consent forms signed. Of course, anorectic medications must be prescribed within the regulatory confines of the state agencies supervising these medications.

DIETARY TREATMENT

Carbohydrate Restriction

Dietary carbohydrate is the primary insulin secretagogue. Because pancreatic insulin secretion is stimulated by the glucose/amino acid ratio in the portal vein and in response to the rate of increase in blood glucose, a powerful way to lower insulin levels is to reduce dietary carbohydrate. When the dietary intake of carbohydrate is reduced to less than 50 g/day, most individuals excrete ketones in the urine, leading to the descriptive name of "ketogenic diet." Several popular diets have used the recommendation of very low levels of carbohydrate (<20 g/day) in the early stages of the diet to enhance lipolysis (9–13). The presence of urinary ketones is an indicator of an increase in fat oxidation. Several research groups have referred to this approach as a "very low carbohydrate ketogenic diet" (VLCKD) or "low-carbohydrate ketogenic diet" (LCKD). When dietary carbohydrate is low (20 g/day), insulin secretion remains low—close to basal levels—and fat "burning" (lipolysis) and protein "burning" (gluconeogenesis) occur as glucagon levels rise. A "low-carbohydrate diet" is one that contains 50 to 150 g/day and is not typically associated with nutritional ketosis. When dietary carbohydrate is present in sufficient amounts for stimulating insulin secretion, fat storage will occur. This may even be true in situations where total energy intake is limited, resulting in fat storage and lean tissue breakdown. The dietary carbohydrate stimulates the hormonal signal for fat deposition, whereas the need for gluconeogenesis in energy-limited diets results in lean tissue utilization. In general, the low-carbohydrate diet will raise HDL-cholesterol, lower triglycerides, and have little effect on LDL-cholesterol. The average weight loss over 6 to 12 months in clinical trials ranged from 5.1 to 12.2 kg, although in private clinical settings larger amounts of weight loss have been reported. Examples of popular carbohydrate-restricted programs include the Atkins Diet, South Beach Diet, and Protein Power Plan.

Several studies have been published that support the safety and effectiveness of carbohydrate restricted diets in children. A randomized trial of 30 adolescents compared a low-carbohydrate diet with a low-fat diet over a 12-week period (14). The low-carbohydrate group was instructed to consume less than 20 g of carbohydrate per day for two weeks, and then less than 40 grams of carbohydrate per day for 10 weeks. The low-carbohydrate group lost more weight (mean 9.9 kg vs. 4.1 kg; $P < 0.05$) and had improvements in non–HDL-cholesterol levels ($P < 0.05$). The authors concluded that the low-carbohydrate diet was effective for short-term weight loss and that the diet did not harm the lipid profile.

In another study, 37 obese elementary school–aged children from a Pediatric Endocrinology clinic were recruited to follow either a carbohydrate-restricted diet or a calorie-restricted diet (15). The carbohydrate-restricted diet allowed less than 30 g of carbohydrate per day, with unlimited calories, protein, and fat. After two months, the 27 children (mean age of 12 years) following the carbohydrate-restricted diet lost an average of 5.2 ± 3.4 kg ($P < 0.001$) and decreased their BMI by 2.4 ± 1.3 points ($P < 0.001$). After two months, the 10 children following the calorie-restricted diet gained an average of 2.4 ± 2.5 kg and 1.0 point on the BMI value ($P < 0.001$). In this study, the carbohydrate-restricted diet was superior to a calorie-restricted diet for weight loss in obese school-aged children. Another study from the same clinic examined the effect of a carbohydrate-restricted diet on serum lipid profiles after 10 weeks in children aged 6 to 12 years (16). After 10 weeks, both the serum cholesterol and serum triglycerides showed significant improvements: −24.2 mg/dL in cholesterol and −56.9 mg/dL in triglycerides ($P < 0.02$ for both).

The effectiveness of a carbohydrate-restricted diet in obese children aged 12 to 18 years was tested in 11 community pediatric practices (17). A carbohydrate-restricted diet of less than 50 g of carbohydrate per day was used. A total of 38 teens completed the six-month study and 84% lost weight, ranging from −23.9 to +5.5 kg. There was also a significant decrease in mean BMI (from 34.9 to 32.5 kg/m^2).

Zeybek et al. examined the effect of a carbohydrate-restricted diet on cardiac function using echocardiography (18). Thirty obese children (mean age 12.2 years) were followed for six months on a low-carbohydrate, non–restricted-calorie diet providing less than 30% of the total calories from simple carbohydrates, with an exercise recommendation. The mean weight change was 5 kg ($P < 0.0001$), and 5 BMI units ($P < 0.0001$). The echocardiographic results showed that the low-carbohydrate diet led to improvements in subclinical right and left ventricular diastolic dysfunction (19).

The "ketogenic diet" is a low-carbohydrate diet developed in the 1920s for the treatment of children with seizures refractory to medical treatment (20). A modified "ketogenic diet," modeled after the carbohydrate-restricted diet used for weight loss has also been studied for seizure control (21). Twenty children, aged 3 to 18 years, with at least three seizures per week, who had been treated with at least two anticonvulsants, were enrolled and received the carbohydrate-restricted diet (10 g/day plus vitamin and calcium supplements) over a six-month period. After six months, it was found that 13 (65%) children had greater than 50% improvement in their frequency of seizures, and 7 (35%) children had greater than 90% improvement (four were seizure free). The diet was well tolerated, without adverse effects. The authors concluded that the modified "ketogenic diet" was an effective and well-tolerated therapy for intractable pediatric epilepsy.

Calorie Restriction

In calorie-restricted diets, calories are explicitly limited and instruction is given either to count calories or to follow a diet protocol that is low in calories. Calorie- and fat-reduced diets and balanced deficit diets generally do not achieve nutritional ketosis because they contain sufficient carbohydrate to prevent ketogenesis. While calorie-restricted diets will lead to weight loss, they do not lead to the same pattern of cardiometabolic risk reduction or lean tissue sparing as low-carbohydrate diets. In general, the 30% fat calorie-restricted diet will lower LDL-cholesterol, modestly impact triglycerides, and modestly raise HDL-cholesterol. Examples of popular calorie-restricted diet programs include Weight Watchers, Jenny Craig, and Nutrisystem.

Combination of Calorie Restriction and Carbohydrate Restriction (VLCD)

Very low calorie/low-carbohydrate diets (VLCD), also referred to as "supplemented fasting," are diets that provide between 300 and 800 kcal/day. VLCDs provide enough protein to meaningfully reduce lean tissue wasting and supply essential minerals and vitamins along with varying amounts of carbohydrates and fats (22). There are two general classes of VLCD: one consisting of common foods with dietary supplements of minerals and vitamins; the other consisting of a defined formula providing all nutrients as beverages, soups, and/or bars taken three to five times per day. The food-based VLCD consists mostly of lean meat, fish, and poultry, whereas the formula VLCD usually requires the addition of carbohydrate as sugar or modified starch to enhance palatability. The food-based VLCD provides a modest dose of fat inherent in the food choices, whereas fat is not always provided in the defined formula diets. Examples of formula-based VLCDs are Optifast, Medifast, Pro-Cal (R-Kane), and Robard New Direction.

A VLCD was included in a multidisciplinary weight-reduction program for children that extended over one year and included a hypocaloric diet, exercise, and behavior modification (23). Fifty-six overweight children (aged 7–17 years) were enrolled into the weight management program and 62.5% successfully completed the one-year program. There was a significant decrease in body weight and body fat, as assessed by weight determinations and skinfold measurements ($P < 0.0001$). The BMI decreased significantly, from 32.7 to 28.7 kg/m^2 ($P < 0.0001$). The authors concluded that a multidisciplinary weight-reduction program that combines a VLCD, followed by a balanced hypocaloric diet, with a moderate intensity, progressive exercise program, and behavior modification is an effective means for weight reduction in obese children and adolescents.

SIDE EFFECTS

There are two groups of side effects based on whether they occur early or late in the treatment process. VLCDs (400–800 kcal/day) probably have a higher incidence of side effects than does carbohydrate restriction using food (1200–1500 kcal/day) due to the lower calorie intake. During adaptation to carbohydrate restriction and nutritional ketosis, the most common side effects are weakness, fatigue, and lightheadedness. Although there is a modest reduction in peak aerobic performance in the first week or two of a VLCD, orthostatic symptoms occurring during normal daily activities are the result of the combination of diet-induced natriuresis and an inadequate sodium intake. These symptoms can be prevented by the addition of 2 to 3 g/day of sodium (taken as bouillon or broth, for example) in all patients not requiring continued diuretic medication, along with attention to adequate dietary potassium, with supplementation as needed. Of course diuretic medications may require downward adjustment during this period of naturesis.

After the first few weeks of adaptation to carbohydrate restriction, the most common side effects are constipation and muscle cramps. The constipation may result, in part, from the lower fiber content of dietary intake, but it is also exacerbated by dehydration. If increasing fluid intake to a minimum of 2 L/day does not resolve the constipation, then one teaspoon of milk of magnesia at bedtime, bouillon supplementation, or a carbohydrate-free fiber supplement can be used. Muscle cramps can occur either early or late in treatment and are more common in people with a history of diuretic medication use or prior heavy ethanol consumption. In almost all cases, the muscle cramps respond promptly to supplementation with one teaspoon of milk of magnesia at bedtime or 200 mEq/day of slow-release magnesium chloride, suggesting prior depletion of this essential mineral as the root cause. Excessively brisk deep tendon reflexes suggest hypomagnesemia in neurologically intact individuals.

CONCLUSION

Childhood obesity is at crisis levels; the current generation of children may die before their parents because of the comorbidities of excess adiposity. Many effective treatments are available including dietary and medical approaches, with a unifying theme of restricting sugar, carbohydrate, and caloric intake. Trained physicians developing comprehensive, individualized treatment plans can be extremely effective in assisting children to improve their health by treating this serious health problem.

ACKNOWLEDGMENT

The authors thank Wendy Scinta for reading and providing suggestions for this chapter.

REFERENCES

1. Olshansky SJ, Passsdssaro DJ, Hershow RC, et al. A potential decline in life expectancy in the United States in the 21st century. N Engl J Med 2005; 352:1138–1145.
2. http://www.cdc.gov/growthcharts/clinical_charts.htm. Accessed May 20, 2010.
3. Barlow SE; the Expert Committee. Expert Committee recommendations regarding the prevention, assessment and treatment of child and adolescent overweight and obesity: summary report. Pediatrics 2007; 120:S164–S192.
4. Joint FAO/WHO/UNU Expert Consultation on Protein and Amino Acid Requirements in Human Nutritional, 2002; Geneva, Switzerland. http://whqlibdoc.who.int/trs/WHO_TRS_935_eng.pdf. Accessed May 20, 2010.
5. Marshall WA, Tanner JM. Variations in the pattern of pubertal changes in boys. Arch Dis Child 1970; 45:13–23.
6. Marshall WA, Tanner JM. Variations in the pattern of pubertal changes in girls. Arch Dis Child 1969; 44:291–303.
7. Berkowitz RI, Fujioka K, Daniels SR, et al.; Sibutramine Adolescent Study Group. Effects of sibutramine treatment in obese adolescents: a randomized trial. Ann Intern Med 2006; 145(2):81–90.
8. Glaser Pediatric Research Network Obesity Study Group. Metformin extended release treatment of adolescent obesity: A 48-week randomized, double-blind, placebo-controlled trial with 48-week follow-up. Arch Pediatr Adolesc Med 2010; 164:116–123.
9. Vernon MC, Mavropoulos J, Transue M, et al. Clinical experience of a carbohydrate-restricted diet: effect on diabetes mellitus. Metab Syndr Relat Dis 2003; 1:233–237.
10. Vernon MC, Kueser B, Transue M, et al. Clinical experience of a carbohydrate-restricted diet for the metabolic syndrome. Metab Syndr Relat Dis 2004; 2:180–186.
11. Westman EC, Feinman RD, Mavropoulos JC, et al. Low-carbohydrate nutrition and metabolism. Am J Clin Nutr 2007; 86:276–284.

12. Nordmann AJ, Nordmann A, Briel M, et al. Effects of low-carbohydrate vs low-fat diets on weight loss and cardiovascular risk factors: a meta-analysis of randomized controlled trials. Arch Int Med 2006; 166(3):285–293.
13. Shai I, Schwarzfuchs D, Henkin Y, et al. Weight loss with a low-carbohydrate, Mediterranean, or low-fat diet. New Engl J Med 2008; 359(3):229–241.
14. Sondike SB, Copperman N, Jacobson MS. Effects of a low-carbohydrate diet on weight loss and cardiovascular risk factors in overweight adolescents. J Pediatr 2003; 142:253–258.
15. Bailes JR Jr, Strow MT, Werthammer J, et al. Effect of low-carbohydrate, unlimited calorie diet on the treatment of childhood obesity: a prospective controlled study. Metab Syndr Rel Dis 2003; 1:221–225.
16. Dunlap BS, Bailes JR Jr. Unlimited energy, restricted carbohydrate diet improves lipid parameters in obese children. Metab Syndr Relat Dis 2008; 6(1):32–36.
17. Siegel RM, Rich W, Joseph EC, et al. A 6-month, office-based, low-carbohydrate diet intervention in obese teens. Clin Pediatr (Phila) 2009; 48(7):745–749.
18. Zeybek C, Aktuglu-Zeybek C, Onal H, et al. Right ventricular subclinical diastolic dysfunction in obese children: the effect of weight reduction with a low-carbohydrate diet. Pediatr Cardiol 2009; 30(7):946–953.
19. Zeybek C, Celebi A, Aktuglu-Zeybek C, et al. The effect of low-carbohydrate diet on left ventricular diastolic function in obese children. Pediatr Int 2009 Aug 7 [epub ahead of print].
20. Freeman JM, Vining EP, Pillas DJ, et al. The efficacy of the ketogenic diet-1998: a prospective evaluation of intervention in 150 children. Pediatrics 1998; 102(6):1358–1363.
21. Kossoff EH, McGrogan JR, Bluml RM, et al. A modified Atkins diet is effective for the treatment of intractable pediatric epilepsy. Epilepsia 2006; 47(2):421–424.
22. Tsai AG, Wadden TA. The evolution of very-low-calorie diets: an update and meta-analysis. Obesity 2006; 14:1283–1293.
23. Sothern, Udall JN Jr, Suskind RM, et al. Weight loss and growth velocity in obese children after very low calorie diet, exercise, and behavior modification. Acta Paediatr 2000; 89(9):1036–1043.

12 Residential lifestyle modification programs for the treatment of obesity

Howard J. Eisenson and Eric C. Westman

INTRODUCTION

Obesity is understood to be fundamentally a problem of "energy imbalance," caused by habitual excess calorie consumption relative to the body's needs, typically exacerbated by a lack of exercise. Widely accepted guidelines promote "healthy lifestyle change" including prudent eating habits and regular exercise as the critical elements for improved weight control and better health (1). Unfortunately, interventions intended to promote these healthier behaviors typically demonstrate limited and temporary results (2). Most authorities agree that our modern environment, so conducive to excess food intake and insufficient physical activity, provides a serious impediment to the adoption of healthy eating habits and regular exercise (3). In light of this, it is interesting and perhaps surprising that "environmental modification" as a treatment for obesity has been little described, and little utilized.

In other domains, provision of a controlled environment for a defined period of time is well recognized as a way to transfer knowledge, promote practice, and instill new attitudes, habits, skills, and confidence. Recruits are sent to "boot camp" to learn military culture and to develop new competencies. New employees are often required to attend "orientation" activities—periods of time during which they are freed of other responsibilities and distractions, and expected to participate in intensive training and team building exercises to help them efficiently acquire skills essential for their new jobs. Those seeking to gain familiarity with a new language or culture know that nothing compares with an "immersion" experience in a setting where the new language is the dominant one, and the unfamiliar culture is manifest everywhere. Most of us have had the experience of spending years in a protected, in many ways, artificial setting—yet a wonderful environment for personal growth and for learning to achieve success in the "real world"—we called that place "college."

There are even a few examples of environmental or immersion treatment to address health needs. Best described are those in the mental health arena, such as residential treatment of severe psychological or behavioral problems and/or alcohol or other drug addiction (4). Extended periods of time in protected settings, or retreats, have long been utilized as a means of promoting personal growth and healing for those struggling with spiritual and emotional distress.

Although there are relatively few examples, and very few written descriptions, environmental, immersion, or residential treatment of obesity and sedentary lifestyles has been in use for many years (5–9). Durham, North Carolina is unique in being home to three of the best known and longest lasting such programs, the Rice Diet (RD, which began in 1939), the Duke Diet and Fitness Center (DFC, started in 1969 under the name "Dietary Rehabilitation Clinic"), and Structure House (SH, established in 1977) (Table 1). In this chapter, these three programs will be used to illustrate characteristics of what we will refer to here as residential treatment, including who the programs serve, how they work, and what results they have observed. We will also discuss the therapeutic potential of this mode of treatment and why we believe it warrants greater consideration in the continuum of strategies for the treatment of the very challenging twin disorders of obesity and poor physical fitness.

OVERVIEW OF RESIDENTIAL PROGRAMS

All three of the programs discussed here are designed to help participants accomplish weight loss and improved physical fitness, during the course of a residential experience that may extend over a period of weeks to months in a protected, retreat-like atmosphere. Consistent with guidelines published by the National Heart, Lung, and Blood Institute (NHLBI), they promote adoption of healthier habits of eating and physical activity (1). All provide dining facilities

Table 1 Brief Self-Descriptions of the Residential Weight Loss Programs in Durham, North Carolina

Duke Diet and Fitness Center (10)	Rice Diet (11)	Structure House (12)
"[The Duke Diet] is really a self-care plan . . . that can help you not only lose weight but also improve your overall quality of life. [It] has been developed and refined . . . by a team of professionals dedicated to educating and empowering the clients we serve, with the latest and most authoritative scientific information and time-tested practical tools"	"The Rice Diet is not just an eating plan. Rather it is what we call a dieta, which comes from the Greek word diaita, meaning way of life. We believe that in order to lose weight and keep it off, you must truly change the way you live . . . . There are four essential steps that guarantee success. The first step is doing the diet itself. The second step is becoming a mindful eater. The third step asks participants to make time for themselves each day to rest. The fourth step offers ways to create the support you need to stick to the diet and your new lifestyle"	"The key to the Structure House program is encompassed within Structured Eating®, a problem-solving strategy. Structured eating means eating nutritious food consumed in appropriate portions three times a day—the eating that you need to meet nutritional requirements and maintain the level of weight you desire. Four important strategies are part of the Structure House program: take responsibility, take control—and feel better about yourself; change your mind—and change your life; address your medical issues—and rest easy about your health; change how you exercise, and regain your joy in life"

serving three meals a day, seven days a week, and also offer a variety of evening and weekend activities. The Duke Diet and Fitness Center and Structure House provide on-site exercise facilities and instruction, and the Rice Diet encourages exercise using local resources. Importantly, all three programs aim to empower participants with the knowledge, self-awareness, skills, motivation, and confidence to enable them to maintain healthier habits of eating, physical activity, and self-care for life. Classrooms for large group lectures, smaller rooms for group discussions, and areas to demonstrate meal preparation are standard, as are examination rooms and small offices for private consultations. While we refer to all three of these as "residential" programs, only Structure House has residential facilities on the campus. Participants in the Rice Diet and in the Duke Diet and Fitness Center live in a variety of nearby accommodations, typically within a mile or two of the treatment center. Those attending from the local community may choose to live at home (Table 1).

Program participants are adults, ranging in age from the upper teens through advanced elderly. At the DFC, the average age is in the early 50s, approximately 60% female. Participants are mostly Caucasian, and they come primarily from larger population centers along the East coast, especially from New York, New Jersey, and Florida, though there is representation from across the United States, and internationally.

These programs are not inexpensive, with prices for first-time clients ranging from approximately $2400 at the DFC for a five-day stay (no lodging) to $9725 at SH (lodging included) for a four-week stay. All programs have lower weekly rates for returnees, for example, $825 per week (lodging not included) at the DFC, or $1574 per week at SH (lodging included), during the slower season (13,14). Most services are not typically covered by insurance, though certain program elements, especially medical services, may be covered by Medicare and sometimes by other payers. Program participants are advised that Internal Revenue Service (IRS) rules may allow deduction of expenses for treatment of obesity when medically indicated, and that medical savings accounts or flexible spending accounts may also be applicable. The typical patient is of upper socioeconomic status, though many attendees of more modest means are sponsored by family, friends, or employers, and some do make significant financial sacrifices in order to attend. The DFC program offers a very limited number of partial "scholarships" for deserving individuals who need financial assistance.

In all the programs clients vary greatly in their presenting weight, ranging from normal weight to very severely obese. At the DFC, the typical client is in the severe obesity range, with an average body mass index (BMI) of around 40, and with a low level of physical fitness. Many have the comorbidities commonly seen with obesity and inactivity. Particularly prevalent, as documented in recent reports from the DFC are diabetes/impaired fasting glucose (63.5%), hypertension (52.4%), hypertriglyceridemia (48%), obstructive sleep apnea (35.5%), impaired quality of sleep (84.7%), and presence of pain (83.4%) (15,16).

For each program, the number of clients "in residence" at any time varies with the season. At the Duke Diet and Fitness Center, the program "census" ranges from approximately 50 to 100. A typical length of stay at the DFC for a first time client is four weeks, though programs ranging from as little as five days to as long as three months are utilized. All three residential programs have a high percentage of return clients. The average length of stay for returnees tends to be shorter; at the DFC, return visits average two weeks in duration.

Specific staff components vary among the programs discussed here, but at the Duke Diet and Fitness Center includes registered dieticians (with one or more certified as diabetes educators); exercise physiologists, physical therapists, and other fitness professionals; licensed clinical social workers, psychologists, and other professional counselors; and physicians, nurses, nurse practitioners, and physician assistants. Ancillary staff include personnel in each of the following areas: food service, business office, client services (guest services, registration, and enrollment, etc.), facility management, housekeeping, security, marketing/public relations, and administration. Other professional consultative services are readily available in the local community as needed, including psychiatrists, cardiologists, and other medical and surgical specialties. Specialists in disciplines representative of "complementary medicine," for example, bodywork and acupuncture, are easily accessed.

THERAPEUTIC INTERVENTIONS

Diet

Prior to the 1980s, all three programs featured very low calorie dietary plans, approximately 800 calories per day or less. Subsequently, and at least in part, as a result of studies demonstrating that the lower weight achieved with very low calorie diets is rarely sustained, greater emphasis was placed on adoption of diets that represented a more moderate calorie restriction (17) (Table 2). Calorie intake recommendations are made on the basis of estimated daily requirements, as well as patient preference, and are intended to facilitate weight loss on the order of 1% to 1.5% of starting weight weekly, while avoiding hunger and providing sufficient energy to accommodate daily exercise. At the DFC, women typically follow a regimen of 1100 to 1300 calories per day; for men the usual intake is 1200 to 1600 calories per day. For most of their history all three programs featured a low fat, high carbohydrate diet. In recent years, dietary plans have become somewhat more liberal, with the Diet and Fitness Center adopting in 2002 a broader range of options for those desiring low carbohydrate meals. All three programs emphasize regular, planned meals, portion control, and reduced sodium consumption.

At the DFC, clients meet individually with dieticians at the start of their program. Their weight history, including previous dieting efforts, is reviewed. Their habitual eating and drinking habits (including alcohol consumption) are assessed, including types and quantity of food habitually eaten, frequency of eating out, consumption of snack foods, emotionally triggered eating, and the home eating "environment." In consultation with the dieticians, clients develop an eating plan for the week, and submit their menu in advance, each week. These menus are reviewed by dieticians to ensure that calorie content and nutrient balance are consistent with each client's nutritional plan. Menus are then revised as necessary to facilitate an appropriate rate of weight loss, to avoid hunger, and to ensure nutritional adequacy.

Exercise

All three programs teach clients the importance of regular physical activity—not only as a strategy to support weight loss and lasting weight control but also as an important determinant of overall health. The staffing, curricular time, and facilities specifically devoted to physical fitness vary among the programs, but in accord with guidelines from the Institute of Medicine and others, clients are generally encouraged to work toward 60 minutes of accumulated aerobic activity of moderate intensity, five to six days weekly, strength training two to three days per week, and regular flexibility activities (18,19). All the programs emphasize the importance of

Table 2 Characteristics of Residential Program Dietary Plans

Diet plan features	Duke diet and fitness (13)	Rice diet (14)	Structure house (15)
Principles	Wide variety, no "forbidden foods" Menu planning, regular meals, low fat proteins, whole grain, higher fiber carbs, limited consumption of saturated fat, use of "volumetric" principles (meals of lower energy density) in menu design	Phase I ("detox"—one week), first day Basic Rice Diet of grains and fruits only, then add vegetables, whole grain cereal or bread, and nonfat dairy. Phase II ("weight loss")—each week starts with one day of Basic Rice Diet, then 5 days of fruits, grains, veggies, nonfat dairy (soy, grain, or cow's milk), whole grain cereal or bread, and one day including protein source such as fish, more nonfat dairy, or organic eggs. Phase III maintenance plan same as phase II but more choice and flexibility	Emphasis on "Structured Eating"®: only 3 eating episodes occur each day, total calories consumed fall within a predetermined daily calorie goal, only nutritious food is consumed, and all food consumed is planned ahead of time
Typical daily calories	Women 1100–1300 Men 1200–1600, instructed to increased by approx 200 cal/day at home	Approx 1000 cal per day initially, gradually increasing to over 1200 per day	Minimum calories per day for weight loss of 1% per week determined by Miflin-St. Jeor equation for RMR, modified by activity factor
Typical dietary composition	40–45% carbs 30–40% fats 20–25% protein	70–90% carbs 5–10% fats 5–25% protein	Consistent with American Diabetes Association Exchange List
Sodium, daily	1500 mg	In Phases I and II 300–500 mg daily; in Phase III 500–1000	1500–2300 mg daily
Comments	Lower carb meal plans also available	Emphasis on "mindful eating"	Philosophy of "food as fuel" is emphasized. Food consumed outside the three planned daily meals serves purposes unrelated to nutrition and it is these calories that lead to problems with weight management

Abbreviation: RMR, resting metabolic rate.

an appropriate medical assessment prior to starting an exercise regimen, beginning slowly, and consistently practicing moderate intensity activity rather than high intensity activity.

For those who "hate exercise" or are unusually challenged, special attention is offered from treatment professionals to help identify and overcome obstacles to the adoption of an appropriate, more physically active lifestyle. For many clients, physical therapy consultation is recommended or required, for instance for those with chronic or acute musculoskeletal or neurologic concerns. At the DFC, the physical therapist is on-site, facilitating ease of referral, and coordination of care between the physical therapist and the fitness professional. Physical therapy consultation may involve one visit, or a series of several times weekly treatments extending over the duration of the patient's stay on the residential program. All facilities are accessible to people with disabilities.

At the DFC, in recognition of the fact that entering clients are of generally poor physical fitness and most are at increased risk for adverse cardiovascular and other events in association with exercise, a medical evaluation including a history and physical is performed on all prior to exercise clearance; many are required to undergo functional exercise testing prior to being given an exercise prescription and allowed to participate. Those whose evaluation suggests that they are at significantly increased risk may be required to undergo cardiology evaluation and additional diagnostic testing as recommended. Depending on the results of this evaluation, they may be required to exercise in a closely monitored setting (such as a supervised cardiac rehabilitation program in close proximity to the residential weight loss program), or may have other restrictions placed on their physical activity.

Fitness staff meet individually with each client to assess their current level of physical activity, their motivation, preferences, and available resources, their previous experiences with exercise, any significant injury history, current limitations in terms of endurance, strength, balance, coordination, and other relevant health history. In conjunction with the medical staff they design an exercise plan appropriate to the client's needs and preferences.

Behavioral Health

All three programs endeavor to help clients better understand their relationship with food, boost their self-care skills, and learn how to elicit effective support for their efforts. Well-described behavior modification principles are utilized to increase self-awareness, set realistic goals, anticipate and strategize around obstacles, and recover from setbacks (20). Monitoring/journaling is strongly encouraged including recording of weight, food consumption, and physical activity, as well as environmental/emotional factors associated with behaviors.

Prior to program acceptance, DFC clients are required to submit an application that is reviewed by the Behavioral staff. Those whose applications suggest major mental illness or major impairments in social function are further screened to ensure that they are under appropriate treatment and sufficiently stabilized so that clients will be able to participate safely and satisfactorily in the community environment of the residential program. Additional screening is conducted for active substance abuse and for eating disorders that may not be appropriate for this mode of treatment (for instance, anorexia, and in some cases active bulimia).

As in the Nutrition and Fitness areas, clients at the DFC meet individually with a Behavioral Health professional at the beginning of their stay. This meeting includes an assessment of psychological, emotional, and social health history and current level of function; an assessment of the patient's motivation for weight loss and lifestyle change and of their goals; and a review of personal attributes, experiences, attitudes, and behaviors, as well as family/social and environmental factors that may serve to enhance, or to impede accomplishment of their goals.

In all the residential programs, a wide range of psychoeducational classes as well as individual and group therapy services are available. Specialized behavioral health options are also available to assist participants in dealing with specific issues. For example, mindfulness training, career counseling, lifetime goals therapy, pain coping skills therapy, and family support training are designed to help participants make changes in aspects of their lives that will complement their work toward weight management goals.

The DFC includes a "lifestyle coaching" component administered by mental health professionals and certified coaches who provide ongoing support, encouragement, and assistance via phone and email contact with clients after they leave the residential program. Structure house (SH) also offers several options for participants who wish to continue receiving support after they leave the residential setting. Phone and Internet-based counseling are provided by the therapy staff, and participants are also invited to mail weight charts and self-reflection forms for staff review and feedback, every nine weeks at no additional cost.

Medical

At all three programs, participants undergo a thorough health review, physical exam, and a battery of routine lab tests at program entry. Further diagnostic testing or specialty consultation is arranged as necessary. This assessment establishes appropriate parameters for a safe and effective exercise regimen. It also serves to identify comorbidities of obesity/inactivity, as well as other medical issues to be addressed in implementing a lifestyle change intervention. Several conditions may be affected, even over the very short term, by changes in diet and exercise, and need careful monitoring (notably diabetes and hypertension) and often, medication adjustment. Other conditions, if undiagnosed, untreated or inadequately treated, are likely to interfere with the patient's function and ability to practice optimal self-care, including sleep apnea, other causes of chronic fatigue, shortness of breath, chronic pain, impaired balance and mobility, edema and skin breakdown, and mood and anxiety disorders. Depending on the time available, and the patient's interest, these issues may be addressed during the residential program. Alternatively, recommendations are given for follow-up at home.

When clients are taking medications that might interfere with their weight loss efforts, therapeutic substitutions are implemented as appropriate, often in consultation with the patient's regular primary care provider or psychiatrist. After admission, patients present for a weekly check in to assess weight loss and to monitor overall program progress. During the last week of their stay, blood tests are repeated and patients have an exit interview with one of the medical providers. At that time final lab results are reviewed, overall progress and plans for home are assessed, the medication list is reviewed, and patients are advised regarding appropriate further medical follow-up at home. A discharge summary is prepared and sent to all patients as well as (with patient approval) to their primary physician, to aid in coordination of care.

Interdisciplinary Teamwork

At the DFC, each client is discussed by the multidisciplinary team in a treatment staff meeting during the client's first week on program. High-risk features of the patient's history are shared, and a plan of treatment is outlined. When special challenges or needs are identified, or when program progress seems impaired, patients are discussed again in weekly clinical staff meetings and additional interventions or support added as appropriate (Table 3).

SHORT-TERM RESULTS

Several investigations have been conducted by the residential programs described here, assessing changes in weight, lipids, and diabetic control. These studies reported on changes observed in program participants during the course of a typical four-week program admission.

Table 3 Example Day at the Duke Diet and Fitness Center

7:45–9 a.m.	Breakfast: selection of egg white omelets, cereals, breads, yogurts, and fruit or choice of daily special entrée
8:30–9 a.m.	Guided meditation
9–10:30 a.m.	Choice of fitness classes "No impact" deep water aerobics Step or low impact aerobics "Fit and functional" strength training Stretching Spinning
11–11:45 a.m.	Nutrition lecture: "volumetric eating"
12:00–1 p.m.	Lunch: daily special lunch entrée (meat or vegetarian) or choice of sandwich options, salad bar, soup, steamed vegetables, baked potato, cottage cheese, yogurt, and fruit
1–2:30 p.m.	Lipid discussion: review of lab results with doctor
2:30–3:30 p.m.	Restaurant eating: strategies to prepare for a guided restaurant experience
4–5 p.m.	Survival skills for preventing relapse class, Yoga, or Tai Chi
5–6:15 p.m.	Dinner: choice of two daily special entrees or choice of four standard entrees, including vegetarian, chicken, fish, or pasta. Vegetable and/or salad and fruit are always available
6:30–8 p.m.	Evening activities: may include volleyball, movies, games, bowling, dancing, or attendance at special local events

Table 4 Admission Client Characteristics–Duke Diet and Fitness Center

Characteristics	Database review (mean ± SD)	Chart review (mean ± SD)
n	539	68
Age (years)	49.3 ± 15.1	50.6 ± 14.2
Female (percent)	64.0	54.4
Caucasian (percent)	96.0	94.1
Body weight (kg)	115.6 ± 34.3	129.6 ± 40.2
Body mass index (kg/m^2)	40.8 ± 10.1	43.9 ± 11.4

Duke Diet and Fitness Center—Weight Loss and Lipids

A database review at the DFC examined weight loss over the course of a three- to four-week admission in 539 first time program participants who had a baseline, final week, and at least one interim weight available (21). The mean age of clients was 49.4 years, 62.9% were female and 95.7% were Caucasian (Table 4). The overall mean admission weight was 117.2 kg. The overall mean admission BMI was 41.4 kg/m^2. Men weighed more than women at admission (Fig. 1).

Body weight decreased by 5.4% over the 24-day interval between recording of the admission and discharge weights: from 115.6 kg to 109.4 kg ($P < 0.001$). Men lost more weight than women, even after adjusting for their greater baseline body weight. After 24 days, men lost 8.3 kg (SD = 3.4) on average compared with 5.1 kg (SD = 2.2) for women, $P < 0.001$ (Fig. 2). When measured as percent body weight, men lost 6.0% (SD = 2%) and women lost 5.0% of body weight (SD = 2%), $P = 0.001$. All men lost weight: 93.4% lost ≥3% of body weight, 67.3% lost ≥5% of body weight. Ninety-eight percent of women lost weight: 86.3% lost ≥3% of body weight, 49.6% lost ≥ 5% of body weight. Weight loss was significantly associated with weight on admission ($P < 0.001$), age ($P < 0.001$), and gender ($P < 0.001$).

Another analysis of short-term changes in weight at the Diet and Fitness Center also included changes in lipid profiles (22). A chart review was performed during September to December 2000 and November 2002 to January 2003. Clients were included if their length of stay was at least 24 days, and there were complete body weight and serum lipid records from admission to discharge. The records of 68 patients were suitable for study. On the first full day of the admission, height and weight were measured. Two serum lipid panels were obtained after overnight fasting: one on the second morning of admission, and the other during the last week of their stay. In most cases, clients had been consuming the program meals for 24 to 36 hours prior to the first "admission" blood test. Because this analysis uses a "pre–post" design and the

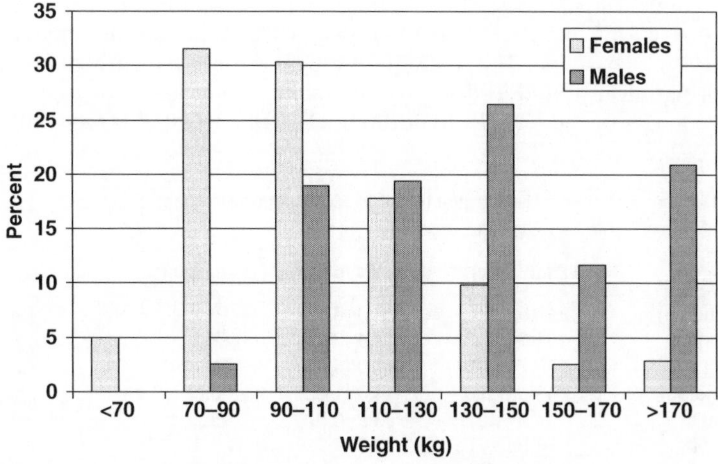

Figure 1 Duke Diet and Fitness Center admission weight distribution by gender ($n = 539$).

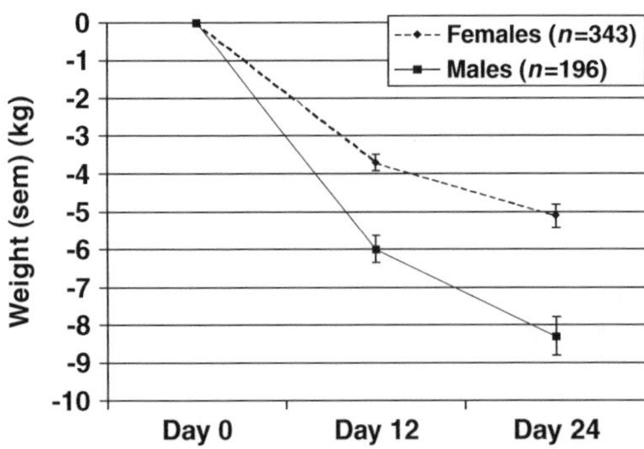

Figure 2 Effect of a comprehensive residential lifestyle modification program on body weight ($n = 539$).

comparison of interest was the change from baseline to 24 days, a paired t-test was used to test for statistical significance of change in outcomes.

There was a decrease in body weight of 5.3% over the 24 days from 130.1 to 123.2 kg ($P < 0.001$). There was a trend for men to lose more weight than women (5.3% vs. 4.4%, $P = 0.07$), but this trend was no longer present after adjusting for the greater weight in men at baseline. Over the 24-day period between baseline and final lipid profile measurements, there was an 18.1% reduction in total cholesterol ($P = 0.001$), a 22.1% reduction in low-density lipoprotein (LDL) cholesterol ($P = 0.001$), a 24.1% reduction in triglycerides ($P < 0.001$), a 3.0% decrease in high-density lipoprotein (HDL) cholesterol ($P < 0.001$), and a 15.2% reduction in cholesterol/HDL ratio ($P < 0.001$) (Table 5). Men had a greater reduction in total cholesterol, LDL cholesterol, triglycerides, and cholesterol/HDL ratio than women even after adjusting for percent change in body weight (Table 6). Lipid changes did not differ as a function of age.

Structure House—Weight Loss, Lipids, and Diabetic Control

A study at Structure House assessed changes in weight, lipids, HbA1c, and diabetes medications following a four-week behavioral weight loss intervention tailored to the needs of patients with type 2 diabetes (23). Participants were 55 adults (69% female; mean age 56.6 years) with type 2 diabetes and obesity (mean BMI 44.5). In addition to the core weight loss program, participants received individual consultation and classes designed to assist in achieving and sustaining glycemic control. Weight, lipids, glucose, HbA1c, and diabetes medications were assessed at the start of the program and during the fourth week (posttreatment). t-Tests were conducted to examine changes in risk factors and descriptive analyses were used to characterize medication changes. Statistical tests were used to determine whether baseline HbA1c levels influenced treatment outcomes. On average, participants lost 5.6% of their starting weight, with other reductions as follows: triglycerides 222.3 to 153.5, cholesterol 185.3 to 142.3, fasting glucose 143.2 to 118.3, HbA1c 7.5% to 6.9%. At posttreatment, 64% of the sample achieved HbA1c < 7, compared with 49% at baseline. The average number of diabetes medications prescribed to participants was significantly reduced at posttreatment, and at least one diabetes medication was withdrawn for 42% of the sample. In addition, 31% of participants were able to lower the

Table 5 Effect of a Comprehensive Residential Lifestyle Modification Program at the Duke Diet and Fitness Center on Fasting Serum Lipids ($n = 68$)

Test	Admission	24 days	Change (%)
Total cholesterol (mg/dL)	217.6 (34.0)	178.3 (32.7)	−18.1
LDL cholesterol (mg/dL)	131.5 (30.0)	102.4 (27.2)	−22.1
Triglycerides (mg/dL)	189.7 (110.1)	144.0 (62.6)	−24.1
HDL cholesterol (mg/dL)	49.5 (12.3)	48.0 (11.2)	−3.0
Cholesterol/HDL ratio	4.6 (1.2)	3.9 (0.9)	−15.2
Triglyceride/HDL ratio	4.3 (3.7)	3.3 (1.7)	−23.3

$P < 0.001$ comparing admission to 24-day values.

Table 6 Effect of Gender on the Percentage Changes in Fasting Lipid Profile at the Duke Diet and Fitness Center

Test	Males (%) ($n = 31$)	Females (%) ($n = 37$)	P value
Total cholesterol	−23.7	−12.1	<0.001[a]
LDL cholesterol	−30.4	−13.6	<0.001
Triglycerides	−25.5	−10.1	<0.01[a]
HDL cholesterol	−4.2	−5.8	0.67
Cholesterol/HDL ratio	−19.5	−5.1	<0.001[a]
Triglyceride/HDL ratio	−19.5	−3.1	0.01[a]

[a]These differences remained statistically significant after adjusting for weight change.

dose of at least one medication. Overall, individuals with higher baseline HbA1c responded equally well to the intervention compared with those with lower baseline HbA1c.

LONGER TERM RESULTS

Structure House—Weight Loss at One Year and Association with Binge Eating Status at Baseline

A study at Structure House examined response to weight loss among morbidly obese severe binge eaters (24). Participants were 117 adults (72% female, mean BMI 42.9) who completed the four-week cognitive behaviorally based residential treatment program and provided complete data for the study variables, including pre and posttreatment weight and height, Gormally Binge Eating Scale, Beck Depression Inventory, Weight Efficacy Lifestyle Scale, and one-year weight. ANOVAs were used to analyze the effect of binge eating (BE) status (none–mild; mild–moderate; moderate–severe) on changes in weight, depressive symptoms, and eating self-efficacy during treatment and changes in weight at one year. Of 117 participants, 27% reported none–mild BE, 30% reported mild–moderate BE, and 43% reported moderate–severe BE. There were no significant group differences in pretreatment BMI; however, depressive symptoms and self-efficacy worsened with increasing BE severity. Neither posttreatment nor one year weight losses were impacted by pretreatment BE severity. At one year, average percent weight losses from pretreatment were as follows: BE none–mild = 12.2%, BE mild–moderate = 15.7%, BE moderate–severe = 13.7%. Participants in the most severe BE group reported the greatest degree of improvement in depressive symptoms and eating self-efficacy.

Diet and Fitness Center—Weight Loss and Quality of Life at One Year

A study at the Duke Diet and Fitness Center assessed weight loss and quality of life (QOL) one year following a four-week residential weight loss program in a consecutive sample of clients enrolling over a six-month period (22). Pre and posttreatment (four weeks) weights were available for 150 clients (56% female, mean baseline weight = 119.8 kg). Mean posttreatment (four weeks) weight loss was 4.6%. The initial sample was contacted ~ 1 year post program by telephone and/or email (mean = 329.2 days) to assess self-reported weight and QOL. Responses were received from 59 clients, or 39% of the total sample. Mean self-reported weight loss at one year was 10.5%. Of individuals for whom it was an issue, the ability to bend improved for 87%, mobility improved for 86%, self-consciousness about weight lessened for 68%, 80% reported reducing their clothing size, 85% reported improved QOL, 81% had improved confidence in following a healthy lifestyle, 81% noted improved stamina, and 81% reported an increased activity level since beginning treatment.

Discussion

There are several theoretical reasons to consider residential, environmental, or "immersion" lifestyle modification as a treatment strategy for obesity that does not respond to less intensive measures. Given the widely accepted belief that we live in an "obesigenic" environment, it seems reasonable to remove patients, at least for a time, from such an environment. With residential approaches to lifestyle change, clients are temporarily separated from many of the stresses, distractions, and temptations that challenge them in "the real world." They have elected to leave home, job, and school to immerse themselves in a protected setting where only healthy meals are provided, and where exercise opportunities abound and participation is expected. They join a "therapeutic community" of fellow participants who provide valuable acceptance and support, and who generously share with each other strategies, encouragement, empathy, and humor. The residential treatment setting effectively constitutes a "learning laboratory," or a safe haven, for those greatly challenged by the "real world" to become empowered to practice healthier habits.

Residential treatment also makes it possible to closely observe and encourage adherence to the therapeutic program, and to tailor the intervention as needed to increase the likelihood of long-term success. The setting allows monitoring not only of changes in weight but also adequacy of control of comorbidities commonly associated with obesity, notably hypertension, diabetes mellitus, and hyperlipidemia. Many medications, most commonly anti-diabetic and antihypertensive medications, are reduced or eliminated during the residential intervention as they are no longer needed. Issues that may impede the patient's self-care abilities, including chronic pain, fatigue, shortness of breath, musculoskeletal limitations, mood disorders, anxiety, stress, and other concerns are addressed by an interdisciplinary team as part of the assessment and plan of treatment.

The three programs described here have many features in common. Typical clients, while generally well off from a socioeconomic standpoint, are arguably among those most challenging to treat, with BMIs in the severe obesity range, with poor physical fitness, and with multiple associated comorbidities. Most participants report that they have tried many less intensive interventions before entering a residential program, and commonly report that their enrollment weight is their lifetime maximum. Despite the challenges these clients bring, the short-term weight loss regularly achieved during these interventions, most commonly a four-week stay, is medically significant, and remarkably consistent among the programs, averaging approximately 5% of starting weight. Significant short-term improvements in lipids and in blood sugar control are also reported.

The improvement in total cholesterol, LDL, and cholesterol/HDL ratio agrees with the usual improvement in fasting lipid profiles seen in other settings after weight loss (25). However, in the DFC study reported earlier, 10% of clients had an increase in serum triglycerides and 75% had a reduction in HDL cholesterol. This "adverse" lipid response early in a weight loss intervention has been documented in the literature for low-fat, high-carbohydrate diets, but the HDL will typically return to, or exceed, the baseline level after six months (26). Because serum triglycerides are increasingly implicated as a risk factor for coronary heart disease, individualization of the dietary recommendations is being considered to minimize this response (27). From other research, hypertriglyceridemia may be lessened by a reduction in dietary carbohydrate, incorporation of lower glycemic index foods, increase in dietary protein, or increase in monounsaturated fats (28,29).

While our strong perception is that participants in all three programs typically report impressive short-term improvements in multiple domains of physical fitness, this has not been objectively examined and is an important subject for study.

An accumulating body of evidence suggests that obesity surgery is the most effective strategy for those suffering from severe obesity (26). However, many obese individuals do not wish to undergo surgery; others may be receptive to the idea, but lack insurance coverage or may be judged inappropriate candidates for surgery; still others are considering surgery but wish to attempt intensive lifestyle efforts to avoid surgery if possible, to better prepare themselves for surgery, and to enhance their surgical results.

The programs described here all provide on their web sites, in their newsletters, and in their books, vignettes and testimonials from numerous grateful clients, including many who have kept off major amounts of weight over the years and claim major and lasting improvements in all domains of their lives. However, it is a legitimate criticism of these interventions that little objective data are available to quantify such longer term results. Relatively small studies, limited by self-report bias and modest rates of response, suggest that there is, on average, fairly good maintenance of weight loss one-year postprogram and that there may also be lasting improvements in QOL. More and better quality studies are challenging to accomplish, especially given that most participants in these programs do not reside permanently in the local area, and a high proportion of these participants are not seen again after their first admission. However, more rigorous evaluations of longer term outcomes are clearly needed, with a focus on what elements of the interventions are most effective, and for what kinds of patients.

Even in the absence of robust long-term outcome studies, it is clear to those of us working in the residential therapeutic settings that this mode of treatment routinely provides, at the very least, a "remission" from the physical and emotional burdens of obesity and related health concerns. Indeed, for some patients residential treatment proves to be a form of "rescue therapy" for those in physical or psychological crisis from complications of their obesity—people for whom the usual recourse might be an even more expensive hospital stay, with little if any emphasis on long-term weight control, and little expectation of achieving it. Almost universally, program participants report that they are well satisfied with a reduced calorie dietary regimen; almost universally they experience significant short-term weight loss and report improvements in physical function. Those experiencing significant psychosocial distress prior to program entry typically report feeling better by the time of discharge, and encouraged regarding their future prospects for improved health. We believe that this experience of success is vital in engendering feelings of competence, self-efficacy, and realistic hope, and that residential treatment should be given serious consideration as a therapeutic tool for those seriously challenged by medically significant obesity, poor physical conditioning and related health issues, and who have not achieved needed results from less costly and intensive interventions.

CONCLUSION

Residential programs are the most intensive lifestyle modification approach to the treatment of obesity, and can play an important component of a "stepped care" approach to treatment. Of particular importance is the fact that almost all patients experience short-term benefit and that there is little or no risk. This nearly universal experience of success may well prove to be an important contributor to confidence and motivation, both of which are described as characteristics of individuals likely to succeed with long-term health behavior changes (30). It is important that further research be conducted to assess the outcomes described here over a longer term, and with patients who are more diverse racially, ethnically, and socioeconomically. Extraction of those elements of the residential interventions that are key to their effectiveness will be critical if less intensive, and more practical and affordable formats are to be developed.

ACKNOWLEDGMENTS

We wish to acknowledge Gerard J. Musante, PhD, Anna Stout, PhD, and Katie Rickel, PhD, all of Structure House, who contributed information on the Structure House program, and Francis A. Neelon, MD with the Rice Diet, who contributed information on that program.

REFERENCES

1. The Expert Panel on the Identification, Evaluation and Treatment of Overweight in Adults. Clinical guidelines on the identification, evaluation, and treatment of overweight and obesity in adults; executive summary. Am J Clin Nutr 1998; 68:899–917.
2. Wadden TA, Butryn ML, Byrne KJ. Efficacy of lifestyle modification for long-term weight control. Obes Res 2004; 12:151S–162S.
3. Hill JO, Peters JR. Environmental contributions to the obesity epidemic. Science 1998; 280:1371–1374.
4. Smith LA, Gates S, Foxcroft D. Therapeutic communities for substance related disorder. Cochrane Database Syst Rev 2006; 25(1):CD005338.
5. Kempner W, Newborg BC, Peschel RI, et al. Treatment of massive obesity with rice/reduction diet program. Arch Intern Med 1975; 135:1575–1584.
6. Nelius SJ, Heyden S, Hansen JP, et al. Lipoprotein and blood pressure changes during weight reduction at Duke's Dietary Rehabilitation Clinic. Ann Nutr Metab 1982; 26(6):384–392.
7. Sjostrom M, Karlsson AB, Kaati G, et al. A four week residential program for primary health care patients to control obesity and related heart risk factors: Effective application of principles of learning and lifestyle change. Eur J Clin Nutr 1999; 53(suppl 2):s72–s77.
8. Malcolm R, Von JM, O'Neil PM, et al. Update on the management of obesity. South Med J 1988; 81(5):632–639.

9. Shapiro JR, Stout AL, Musante GJ. "Structure-size me:" Weight and health changes in a four week residential program. Eat Behav 2006; 7(3):229–234.
10. Eisenson HJ, Binks M. The Duke Diet. New York: Ballantine Books, 2007:3.
11. Rosati KG, Rosati R. The Rice Diet Solution. New York: Berkley Books, 2006:20–23.
12. Musante GJ. The Structure House Weight Loss Plan. New York: Fireside, 2007:8–9.
13. www.dukehealth.org/services/diet_and_fitness/programs/fees. Accessed December 13, 2009.
14. www.structurehouse.com/reservations.html. Accessed December 13, 2009.
15. Wachholtz A, Binks M, Suzuki A, et al. Sleep disturbance and pain in an obese residential treatment-seeking population. Clin J Pain 2009; 25(7):584–589.
16. Suzuki A, Binks M, Sha R, et al. Serum aminotransferase changes with significant weight loss: Sex and age effects. Metabolism 2010; 59(2):177–185.
17. Wadden TA, Sternberg JA, Letizia KA, et al. Treatment of obesity by very low calorie diet, behaviour therapy, and their combination: A five year perspective. Int J Obes Relat Metab Disord 1989; 13(suppl 2):39–46.
18. Brooks GA. Chronicle of the Institute of Medicine physical activity recommendations: How a physical activity recommendation came to be among dietary recommendations. Am J Clin Nutr 2004; 79:921s–930s.
19. Okay DM, Jackson PV, Marcinkiewicz M, et al. Exercise and obesity. Prim Care 2009; 36(2):379–393.
20. Poston WSC, Foreyt JP. Successful management of the obese patient. Am Fam Physician 2000; 61:3615–3622.
21. Eisenson H, Westman E, Knowles J, et al. Effect of a comprehensive residential lifestyle modification program for obesity. Obes Res 2003; 11(Suppl):A147.
22. Binks M, Ostbye T, Eisenson H, et al. Physical and quality of life outcomes one year following participation in a residential lifestyle change program. Obes Res 2005; 13(suppl):A76.
23. Pells J, Stout A, Rodrigues-Diaz M, et al. Rapid improvements in hemoglobin A1c and cardiometabolic risk factors during intensive lifestyle intervention among individuals with obesity and type 2 diabetes. Obesity 2009; 17(supp 2):S280.
24. Pells J, Rodriguez-Diaz M, Stout A, et al. Response to weight loss treatment among severe binge eaters who are morbidly obese: Implications for an integrative, intensive, residential treatment model. Obesity 2009; 17(supp 2):S279.
25. Dattilo AM, Kris-Etherton PM. Effects of weight reduction on blood lipids and lipoproteins: A meta-analysis. Am J Clin Nutr 1992; 56:320–328.
26. DeMaria EJ. Bariatric surgery for morbid obesity. N Engl J Med 2007; 356(21):2176–2183.
27. Parks EJ, Hellerstein MK. Carbohydrate-induced hypertriglycerolemia: Historical perspective and review of biological mechanisms. Am J Clin Nutr 2000; 71:412–433.
28. Ludwig DS. The glycemic index. Physiological mechanisms relating to obesity, diabetes, and cardiovascular disease. JAMA 2002; 287:2414–2423.
29. Yancy Jr WS, Olsen MK, Guyton JR, et al. A low-carbohydrate, ketogenic diet versus a low-fat diet to treat obesity and hyperlipidemia. Ann Intern Med 2004; 140:769–777.
30. Rollnick S, Mason P, Butler C. Health Behavior Change—A Guide for Practitioners. London: Churchill Livingstone, 2001.

13 Current research and future hope

Frank L. Greenway and Steven R. Smith

INTRODUCTION

This chapter will review some of the current research into treatments of obesity and discuss the future of obesity research. The current research on obesity will be divided into diet and lifestyle change, dietary herbal supplements, pharmaceuticals, and surgery and devices. Obesity is the last of the chronic diseases to be defined as such. The future of obesity research can be predicted from the research in other chronic diseases such as hypertension and diabetes. Since the tools available today are more sophisticated than in prior decades, it is likely that treatment of obesity will advance faster than what we have seen in the past with other diseases like hypertension.

DIET AND LIFESTYLE

Combined Diet and Lifestyle Research

Promoting diet and lifestyle intervention has been a priority of the National Institutes of Health (NIH). The Diabetes Prevention Trial enrolled 3234 subjects with impaired glucose tolerance into an intensive lifestyle group, a group treated with metformin 850 mg twice a day and a usual care group. The intensive lifestyle group lost 7% of body weight and exercised 150 min/wk. The study was stopped prematurely at an average follow-up period of 2.8 years. The intensive lifestyle intervention caused a 58% reduction in the conversion from impaired glucose tolerance to diabetes compared with the usual care group. Metformin reduced the conversion to diabetes by 31% (1). Interestingly, the Finnish Diabetes Prevention Trial confirmed that diet and lifestyle reduced the conversion from impaired glucose tolerance to diabetes by 58% compared with control (2). The primary medical concern surrounding obesity is its association with diabetes and other cardiovascular risks. These diabetes prevention studies have emphasized the importance of diet and lifestyle interventions to the treatment of obesity and underscore the recommendations in obesity treatment guidelines, which suggest diet and lifestyle should be the basis of any obesity treatment program (3).

Commercial Weight Loss Programs

Commercial weight loss programs have traditionally been advertising-driven and either unable or reluctant to share results with the scientific community. This is changing. Weight Watchers published a two-year trial performed at six academic centers, which randomized 211 subjects to the Weight Watchers program and 212 subjects to self-help. The subjects had a body mass index (BMI) of 27 to 40 kg/m^2 lost 4.3 $\pm$ 6.1 kg (4.6% initial body weight) in the Weight Watchers group and 1.3 $\pm$ 6.2 kg (2% initial body weight) in the self-help group at one year, and at two years, the weight losses were 2.9 $\pm$ 6.5 kg and 0.2 $\pm$ 6.5 kg, respectively, by intent to treat analysis (4). A similar study was performed at a single site, which randomized 35 subjects to the Jenny Craig program and 35 subjects to self-help. At one year, the group randomized to Jenny Craig lost 6.6 $\pm$ 10.4 kg (7.1% initial weight loss) and the self-help group lost 0.7 $\pm$ 5.5 kg (0.7% of initial weight loss) (5). The difference in the two programs is that Weight Watchers uses a group format for delivering behavior change instruction, whereas Jenny Craig uses individual counseling and calorie-controlled portions. These two large commercial weight loss programs are the only ones that have subjected their programs to a randomized clinical trial by an outside group, but now that a trend has been set, it would not be unexpected for other programs to follow suit, since this information is essential to referring physicians.

Exercise

Exercise has been known to be of help with weight maintenance, but adding exercise to a weight loss program gives, at best, only a marginal increase in weight loss (6). The reasons for this have been obscure, but recent research has shed some light on the issue. The Dose Response to Exercise in Women (DREW) study evaluated exercise in postmenopausal women at 50%, 100%, and 150% of the NIH recommended levels. Although exercise increased weight loss to the degree expected in the 50% and 100% groups, the 150% group had a compensatory increase in food intake that defeated the increase in physical activity (7). Thus, although more physical activity increased fitness and seemed to have additional health benefits, exercise in excess of the recommended 8 kcal/kg/wk has little incremental benefit for weight loss.

Diet

There has been a controversy regarding the best diet for obesity with some advocating a low-carbohydrate diet and others advocating a low-fat diet (8). This controversy has had proponents and detractors on both sides of the issue, at least since the 1970s when the first Atkins' diet book was published. It now appears, as is often the case, that the answer is more complex than a single diet that is best for all individuals with obesity. Cornier et al. developed two groups of obese, nondiabetic women, one with fasting insulin values above 15 mcU/mL (insulin resistant) and the other with fasting insulin values below 10mcU/mL (insulin sensitive). Both groups had insulin sensitivity characterized using a frequently sampled insulin glucose tolerance test and were randomized to a low-carbohydrate (40% carbohydrate and 40% fat) or to a low-fat (60% carbohydrate and 20% fat) diet. The insulin sensitive group lost more weight on the high-carbohydrate diet (13.5% $\pm$ 1.2% initial body weight vs. 6.8% $\pm$ 1.2%, $P < 0.002$). The insulin resistant group lost more weight on the low-carbohydrate diet (13.4% $\pm$ 1.3% vs. 8.5% $\pm$ 1.4%, $P < 0.04$) (9). Since insulin resistance is more common in the face of obesity, it is not surprising that many studies have found a greater weight loss in subjects with obesity treated with a low-carbohydrate diet than with a high-carbohydrate diet.

Those who treat obesity have observed for some time that any treatment one uses seems to have responders and nonresponders. This has prompted the hypothesis that, like diabetes that is divided into type 1 and type 2, there are also different types of obesity. The differential response to macronutrient composition of the diet, depending on the degree of insulin sensitivity, is the first example that this hypothesis may indeed be so. This raises the question as to why some individuals with obesity are insulin sensitive while others are insulin resistant. Research into the obesity virus seems to be shedding some light in this area.

Adenovirus AD-36 was first reported coincident with the increase in the prevalence of obesity that began about 1980 (10). Adenovirus AD-36 has been shown to cause obesity in chickens, rodents, and marmosets (which are primates) (11). The prevalence of neutralizing antibodies to AD-36 are 30% in individuals with obesity and only 11% in lean, but even in the lean, the antibody positive individuals are heavier than antibody negative ones (12). When identical twins are discordant for the AD-36 virus, the antibody positive twin is significantly heavier (12). Adenovirus AD-36 appears to cause obesity in a similar manner to thiazolidinedione (TZD) drugs that stimulate peroxisome proliferator–activated receptor (PPAR) gamma. The *E4orf-1* gene of the AD-36 virus seems to activate PPAR gamma in human and rodent adipocytes causing an increase in adipogenesis and an increase in insulin sensitivity characteristic of small fat cells (13). Thus, adenovirus AD-36 may be one reason for the insulin sensitive obesity.

Another interesting dietary intervention is methionine restriction. Methionine restriction increases life span in rats by 30%, similar in magnitude to calorie restriction, but does so while increasing food intake and reducing body weight (14). Epner et al. treated eight patients with cancer who were not cachectic with a methionine restricted diet for 8 to 39 weeks (mean 17 weeks) (15). Protein was supplied in the form of a commercial methionine deficient medical food, Hominex-2. The diet was not restricted in calories. Only methionine was restricted to 2 mg/kg/day. The only side effect appeared to be an average weight loss of 0.5 kg/wk, which occurred despite a 20% increase in dietary calories. Albumin and prealbumin remained normal suggesting that the weight loss was not associated with malnutrition. Methionine is an essential amino acid, but in the presence of adequate homocysteine (demethylated methionine), normal cells can make methionine by remethylating homocystine. Cancer cells are less able to remethylate methionine and methionine deficiency increases apoptosis in cancer cells (16). In addition, methionine deficiency inhibits thymidylate synthase and acts synergistically with 5-fluro-uricil in treating cancer (17). Further research is clearly needed and is presently in progress.

Nevertheless, a methionine deficient diet holds some promise as an intervention that will allow weight loss without calorie restriction, while inhibiting cancer growth and prolonging life.

Lifestyle

Clearly, recording of dietary intake, activity, and other eating-related activities are associated with weight loss and are a major component of success of behavior modification or lifestyle strategies (18). Unfortunately, although recording of dietary intake does help to reduce food intake and induce weight loss, the accuracy of self-recorded intake or physical activity is dismal in subjects with obesity. In one study, subjects with obesity ate 50% more than recorded and exercised 50% less (19). Increasing the accuracy of self-reported energy intake and energy expenditure is essential to the study of obesity and judging the effectiveness of interventions. Doubly labeled water has been the gold standard to measure energy intake and expenditure in a free-living environment, but it is too expensive for general use (19). There have been attempts to develop new techniques for measuring food intake. One of these methods involves photography of the meal and plate waste using cellular phones with data transfer capability in a free-living environment. The accuracy of this method was within 5% and 7%, a great improvement over self-report (20). Likewise, attempts have been made to quantitate energy expenditure. Sensors to measure movement and posture on various areas of the body have been called Intelligent Device for Energy Expenditure and Activity. This device, which depends on computer analysis of the data collected, gives estimates of energy expenditure in agreement with metabolic chamber studies at an accuracy of greater than 95% (21). Thus, although these new devices may still be more expensive than self-report, reasonably accurate methods to judge food intake and physical activity that are less expensive than doubly labeled water are being developed. Clearly, more accurate estimates of food intake and energy expenditure will add to our knowledge of these areas and hopefully contribute to progress in lifestyle modification research.

Summary

The importance of diet and lifestyle change in preventing diabetes and causing weight loss gives credence to recommendations that lifestyle and diet be the basis for all weight loss programs. Commercial weight loss programs that use diet and lifestyle change to treat obesity have recently allowed third parties to conduct randomized clinical trials testing the program safety and efficacy. This line of research should prove useful to both potential clients and to the physicians who advise them. New research in exercise has shown that at levels of exercise above that recommended by the NIH, further increases in fitness, but the advantage to weight loss starts to be lost due to a compensatory increase in food intake. The controversy regarding the optimal macronutrient composition for a weight loss diet is probably an artifact of the difference in weight loss response related to insulin sensitivity. Preliminary evidence suggests that insulin sensitive obese lose more weight on a high-carbohydrate diet while those who are insulin resistant lose more weight to a low-carbohydrate diet. A methionine restricted diet may have value in the future, but more research is clearly needed. New devices to quantitate food intake and energy expenditure may advance lifestyle research by increasing the accuracy of the presently used self-report.

DIETARY HERBAL SUPPLEMENTS

Caffeine and Ephedrine

Caffeine and ephedrine was a prescription combination drug in Denmark between 1990 and 2002 but was taken off the market due to reports that raised safety concerns. Other stimulant anorectics for the treatment of obesity like phentermine and diethylpropion were removed from the European market for safety concerns around the same time but were reinstated after a year or two later on appeal. Caffeine with ephedrine was not reinstated in Denmark, but held an 80% market share while it was approved, even when fenfluramine was available (22). Ephedra is an herb used in tea consumed by some ethnic populations. Since ephedra was in the food chain prior to 1994, it was classified as a dietary herbal supplement in the United States, which is regulated like a food. Ephedra and ephedra combined with caffeine were removed from the U.S. market in 2004 by the Food and Drug Administration (FDA), which classified it as an adulterant (23). This decision was based on adverse event reports and a review of the literature by Shekelle et al. (24). This report documented the efficacy of ephedrine and ephedra combined with caffeine. There were no serious adverse events in the controlled trials that lasted up to six months, and there were a total of approximately 1000 subjects in those combined trials. There was a 2.2- to 3.6-fold increase in side effects in the ephedra-treated groups compared with placebo consisting of psychiatric, autonomic, gastrointestinal symptoms, and heart palpitations (24). Ephedra consists of four isomers, the most active of which is ephedrine (22). Ephedrine is still available by prescription and, although it does not have an indication for the treatment of obesity, could still be used by a physician off-label combined with caffeine. The dose of caffeine and ephedrine used in the combination pill approved for obesity treatment in Denmark was caffeine 200 mg and ephedrine 20 mg (equivalent to 25 mg ephedrine HCl) three times a day (22). The symptoms of stimulation seen initially in the trial to register caffeine and ephedrine as prescription obesity drug in Denmark returned to placebo levels by eight weeks in a similar manner to the tolerance one builds up to the stimulation associated with coffee when one drinks it daily (22).

Fucoxanthin

Fucoxanthin is the major carotenoid in edible seaweed such as *Undaria pinnatifida*. When fed to rodents fucoxanthin increased uncoupling protein 1 in white adipose tissue and reduced fat accumulation compared to a control (25). Fucoxanthin is effective at a lower dose when combined with medium chain triglycerides and fish oil (26,27). Although the animal studies look promising, human studies have not yet been published. Nevertheless, fucoxanthin is being promoted as a dietary supplement for the treatment of obesity.

Hoodia gordonii

H, gordonii, a succulent that grows in Africa, has been used by Bushmen to decrease appetite on long treks across the desert. The active ingredient is a steroidal glycoside called P57. When P57 is injected into the third ventricle of animals, it increases the ATP content of the hypothalamic tissue by 50% to 150% ($P < 0.05$) and decreases food intake by 40% to 60% over 24 hours ($P < 0.05$) (28). Phytopharm, which is developing Hoodia, reports on its website a 15-day study in 19 overweight males who were randomized to P57 or placebo. Nine subjects in each group completed the study and there was a 1000 kcal/d reduction in food intake that was statistically significant and a decrease in body fat with good safety (29). *H. gordonii* seems to hold promise as a safe and effective treatment of obesity. However, since Phytopharm is still developing Hoodia and since this succulent is rare and difficult to grow in captivity, the presently marketed products claiming to contain Hoodia have no proven effectiveness.

Astaxanthin

Astaxanthin is the red carotinoid that gives the pink color to salmon. Astaxanthin occurs normally in algae and is eaten by crustaceans that are food for salmon. Astaxanthin has been shown to decrease body weight in rats fed a high-fat diet. This reduction in weight gain was accompanied by a reduced liver weight, reduced liver fat, and reduced cholesterol and triglycerides in plasma (30). Astaxanthin appears to increase carnitine palmitoyltransferase-I activation in muscle, shifting metabolism to fat oxidation with a sparing of glycogen (31). This metabolic shift increases the time of exercise to exhaustion by a factor of two and increases fat loss with preservation of lean tissue (32). Astaxanthin, although promising for the treatment of obesity and athletic performance, has only been tested in rodents and human studies have yet to be published.

Cissus quadrangularis

C. quadrangularis is a commonly used folk medicine in India, Africa, and Asia for a variety of purposes. Oben et al. have published three papers on the use of *C. quadrangularis* for the treatment of obesity in humans. The first study compared *C. quadrangularis* standardized to 2.5% phytosterols and 15% soluble plant fibers combined with green tea extract (22% epigallocatechin gallate and 40% caffeine), niacin-bound chromium, selenium (0.5% L-selenomethionine), pyridoxine, folic acid, and cyanocobalamin compared with placebo in a double-blind trial with 123 subjects.

In this eight-week study, subjects with obesity lost 7.2% of initial body weight compared with 2.5% for placebo and 6.3% for the overweight subjects ($P < 0.05$). Body fat and waist circumference were also reduced ($P > 0.01$). There were significant reductions in low-density lipoprotein (LDL) cholesterol, triglycerides, C-reactive protein, glucose, and a significant increase in high-density lipoprotein (HDL) cholesterol compared with placebo (33). The second study compared *C. quadrangularis* standardized to 5% ketosteroids to placebo in 64 subjects with obesity. The placebo group gained 1% of initial body weight over six weeks compared with a loss of 4% in the *C. quadrangularis* group. Adverse events were greater in the placebo group (34). In the third study, *C. quadrangularis* standardized to 2.5% ketosteroids (150 mg) was compared to *C. quadrangularis* with *Irvingia gabonensis* standardized to 7% albumin (250 mg) or a placebo given twice a day for 10 weeks. At the end of 10 weeks, the placebo group lost 2.1% of initial body weight compared with 8.8% in the *C. quadrangularis* group and 11.9% in the *C. quadrangularis* combined with *I. gabonensis* group. Both treatment groups lost more weight than placebo and the combination group lost more weight than the group taking *C. quadrangularis*. There were corresponding changes in body fat, waist circumference, total cholesterol, LDL cholesterol, and blood sugar (35).

Functional Food

Functional foods are foods that have a specific health function separate from their use as foods. Dietary fiber, which is also called fermentable fiber or resistant starch, is one example (36). Resistant starch is fermented in the colon to form butyrate, which stimulates the colonic L-cells to produce the satiety hormones peptide YY (PYY) and glucagon-like peptide-1 (37). These hormones mediate the reduction in body fat seen in resistant starch-fed animals, and feeding resistant starch to humans results in elevation of these same hormones (38). Another example of a functional food is 1,3-diacylglycerol, which is used as a cooking oil and sold under the trade name Econa™. Although there are small amounts of this diglyceride in all vegetable oils, the product is made enzymatically so the oil contains 70% 1,3-diglyceride. The lack of a free fatty acid at the 2 position makes it impossible for the body to store, and it is oxidized in the liver instead (39). The fatty acids on the 1,3-diglyceride have the same caloric value as the free fatty acids on triglyceride, but 1,3-diacylglyceride decreases appetite in addition to increasing fat oxidation (40,41). One double-blind study randomized 131 overweight and obese subjects to food containing triglyceride or 1,3-diacylglyceride for 24 weeks. The body weight and body fat decreased by 3.6% and 8.3%, respectively, in the 1,3-diacylglyceride group and 2.5% and 5.6%, respectively, in the triglyceride group ($P < 0.04$) (38). A five-month study in children between 7 and 17 years of age showed similar results (42). Although these functional foods give between 1% and 2.5% greater weight loss than placebo, using functional foods in combination may give clinically significant weight losses.

Summary

Caffeine combined with ephedrine is no longer available as a dietary herbal supplement. Ephedrine is still a prescription medication, but since it is the starting product to make illegal methamphetamine, it is being treated as a controlled substance making it more difficult to use it off-label for the treatment of obesity. Fucoxanthin, Hoodia, and astaxanthin all have very promising animal studies, but human studies are sparse to nonexistent. Hopefully, human studies will be available in the near future. *C. quadrangularis* has three studies, all by the same group, showing weight losses equivalent to the prescription obesity medications approved for long-term use. Functional foods are a new category of treatments of obesity that give small weight losses in excess of placebo, but, due to their safety, it is probable that used in combination, they could result in clinically significant weight losses.

PHARMACEUTICALS

Cannabanoid-1 Receptor Antagonists

Although many pharmaceutical companies have a cannabanoid-1 (CB-1) receptor antagonist in development, rimonabant is the representative of this class that has progressed furthest in development. Sanofi, the company developing rimonabant, completed its New Drug Application

(NDA), and the results were presented to an FDA advisory panel in June of 2007. The advisory panel unanimously recommended against approval due to increased risks of suicidal ideation and a possible increase in the prevalence of seizures. Seizures were seen in the preclinical studies of rimonabant and may represent an adverse event unique to that drug. Suicidal ideation, however, is probably a class effect of CB-1 antagonists (43). Marijuana, which stimulates the CB-1 receptor increases food intake ("munchies") while causing euphoria and relaxation. It is not difficult to imagine that blocking this receptor will create a decrease in food intake, depression, and anxiety. Rimonabant was approved in Europe and several other countries. Although Sanofi withdrew its U.S. NDA after the FDA advisory panel rendered its decision, Sanofi was continuing to support further studies that might allow a return to the FDA with new data to support a positive risk benefit assessment. In October of 2008, rimonabant was removed from the European market due to a doubling of psychiatric adverse events in those treated with the drug. Since that decision, Sanofi halted its ongoing clinical trials. Rimonabant in the phase 3 studies gave weight loss that was similar to sibutramine, but rimonabant seems to have a beneficial effect on insulin resistance-associated endpoints, in addition to the weight loss it engenders (43). The bar for safety in regards to obesity drugs seems to be very high at the U.S. FDA, and it seems clear that all CB-1 antagonists will have difficulty attaining approval in the U.S., if any achieve approval at all.

Lorcaserin

Lorcaserin is a serotonin agonist, specific to the 5-HT_{2C} receptor. Fenfluramine was a nonspecific agonist of this receptor that is metabolized to nor-dexfenfluramine, which has a greater affinity for the 5-HT_{2B} receptor, the receptor associated with heart valve pathology, than serotonin itself (44). Thus, lorcaserin has the potential to replace fenfluramine in the phentermine–fenfluramine combination without the risk of heart valve pathology. Lorcaserin was evaluated in a 12-week phase 2 dose-ranging study. A total of 459 subjects with a BMI between 29 and 46 kg/m^2 and an average weight of 100 kg were randomized into a double-blind trial comparing placebo against 10 and 15 mg given once daily and 10 mg given twice daily (20 mg/d). The placebo group gained +0.32 kg ($N = 88$ completers) compared to –1.8 kg with 10 mg/d ($N = 86$), –2.6 kg with 15mg/d ($N = 82$), and –3.6 kg with 10 mg twice daily (20 mg total) ($N = 77$). Side effects that were more in the active treatment groups than in placebo were headache, nausea, dizziness, vomiting, and dry mouth. No cardiac valvular changes were noted (45). Thus, lorcaserin appears to have no greater efficacy than existing obesity medications, so its potential seems to lie in its possible use in a drug combination.

Cetilistat

Cetilistat is a lipase inhibitor like orlistat and appears to give similar efficacy. A 12-week trial randomized 442 subjects to cetilistat 60, 120, or 240 mg three times a day (t.i.d.) or to placebo. Cetilistat gave a dose-related weight loss that was significant compared with placebo, and the 240 mg t.i.d. group lost 4.1 kg. Adverse events were similar to orlistat, but seemed to occur at a reduced frequency (46).

Tesofensine

Tesofensine is a norepinephrine, dopamine, and serotonin reuptake inhibitor being developed for the treatment of Parkinson's and Alzheimer's diseases for which weight loss was noted in the clinical trials (47). A 24-week trial randomized 203 subjects with obesity to 0.25, 0.5, 1 mg or placebo once a day. The percent weight losses were 6.8%, 11.4%, 12.7%, and 2.3%, respectively (48,49). This efficacy is greater than the presently approved obesity pharmaceuticals.

Bupropion–Naltrexone

Bupropion (BUP) is known to activate melanocortin pathways, and naltrexone (NAL) is an antagonist of the opioid receptor, a receptor on the proopiomelanocortin (POMC) neurons in the hypothalamus that inhibit the secretion of POMC. It was hypothesized that combining BUP with NAL would give sustained weight reduction over a longer period and give more weight loss. Synergy of BUP and NAL was first demonstrated electrophysiologically in hypothalamic slices and confirmed using food intake in lean and obese mice. A clinical trial randomized 238 obese subjects to BUP (300 mg) + NAL (50 mg), BUP (300 mg) + placebo (P), NAL (50 mg) + P, or P + P for up to 24 weeks. The BUP group lost 4.5% of body weight compared with 6.8% in the BUP + NAL group at 24 weeks. The NAL and P + P groups lost 2.2% and 0.9%, respectively, at 16 weeks, and the NAL + BUP group was continuing to lose weight at 24 weeks in contrast to the BUP group. The side effects present in 10% or more of the BUP + NAL group and greater than placebo were nausea, headache, dizziness, and insomnia (50). BUP + NAL in a time-released formulation (Contrave®) is presently in phase 3 trials for the treatment of obesity.

Bupropion–Zonisamide

A time-released formulation of BUP and zonisamide is being developed for the treatment of obesity (Empatic®). A clinical trial randomized 226 obese subjects to placebo, BUP 300 mg/d, zonisamide 400 mg, and the combination. This six-month study gave body weight losses of −0.4%, −3.6%, −6.6%, and −9.2%, respectively. The BUP–zonisamide group lost 12% of initial body weight at 48 weeks. Adverse events with a prevalence greater than 10% included insomnia, nausea, fatigue, upper respiratory infection, headache, and anxiety (51).

Phentermine–Topiramate

A combination of phentermine 15 mg/d and topiramate 100 mg/d is being developed for the treatment of obesity and will be called Qnexa®. A six-month study in 200 subjects gave an −11.4 kg weight loss in the phentermine–topiramate group and a –2.3 kg weight loss in the placebo group. More than half of the phentermine–topiramate subjects lost 10% of their initial body weight. The dropout in the phentermine–topiramate group was 8% compared with 38% in the placebo group (52).

Pramlintide–Leptin

The combination of leptin and pramlintide gives synergistic weight loss in mice with diet-induced obesity. A trial in humans gave 180 mg of pramlintide subcutaneously twice a day for two weeks and the dose was increased to 360 mg twice a day for an additional two weeks. Subjects lost 4.3% of their body weight in those four weeks and were then randomized to continue pramlintide alone, receive leptin 5 mg subcutaneously twice a day alone or receive leptin plus pramlintide. After 24 weeks of treatment weight losses were 8.4%, 8.2%, and 12.7% in the pramlintide, leptin, and the combination, respectively. The major side effect was nausea, and this was usually mild to moderate with improvement with time (53).

SURGERY AND DEVICES

Surgery

Surgical treatment is the only obesity treatment that has been shown to decrease mortality, possibly, because it is the only obesity therapy that enforces the maintenance of a weight loss for more than a decade of a magnitude necessary to document a decrease in mortality (54). Not only has Roux-en-Y gastric bypass been shown to result in better weight loss and a reduced number of failures compared with laparoscopic gastric banding, laparoscopic gastric bypass is as safe as the open procedure with lower morbidity (55,56). Two new procedures are being evaluated—the transoral gastroplasty and the duodenal sleeve gastrectomy. Transoral gastroplasty is performed with a set of transoral endoscopically guided staplers that are used to create a stapled restrictive pouch along the lesser cure of the stomach. The weight loss at six months in 26 morbidly obese subjects was 24 kg, or 46% of excess body weight (57). The laparoscopic gastric bypass, the accepted standard for obesity surgery, was compared over three years with the laparoscopic sleeve gastrectomy. The sleeve gastrectomy gave more satiety and greater weight loss at both time points (58). Although longer-term follow-up is clearly needed, sleeve gastrectomy could become the preferred operation in the future. One of the perceived advantages of the gastric bypass is that it alters gut-derived satiety hormones like PYY. A recent study shows that the sleeve gastrectomy reduces ghrelin to a greater extent than the gastric bypass and gives similar increases in PYY (59).

Devices

Despite the advances in surgery for obesity, research has been active in devices that might obviate the need for surgery. One such device is the duodenal–jejunal bypass sleeve. This is a laparoscopically placed cage that sits in the pyloris with a 60-cm plastic sleeve attached that prevents food from coming in contact with the duodenum and upper jejunum. In an initial trial with 12 subjects, 4 of whom had diabetes, the sleeve gave a 26% loss of excess weight over 12 weeks, and those who had diabetes were able to eliminate their hypoglycemic medications while experiencing improvement in their levels of glycohemoglobin (60). Gastric pacing is another device area that has experienced an increase in research activity. The present gastric pacemakers block vagal transmission and are associated with a mean weight loss of 14.2% of excess body weight over six months, but the weight loss is quite variable with 25% losing over 25% of their excess body weight over the six-month period (61).

FUTURE HOPE

History of Obesity and Chronic Disease Research

As physicians, we believe the goal of research into obesity or other chronic diseases is to develop better treatments and ultimately a cure as a means of improving the quality of life for those afflicted with the disease. The bench-to-bedside principle of medical research still applies today as it did in time of William Osler (62). Discoveries in the clinic will stimulate laboratory investigations whereas laboratory discoveries will stimulate clinical trials.

Obesity is the chronic disease that has been most recently recognized as such. Obesity was considered to be bad habits prior to the 1985 NIH Consensus Conference (63). This late recognition of obesity as a chronic disease is the reason that drugs developed prior to 1985 were tested and approved for up to 12 weeks of use. It was believed that one could develop a new habit or extinguish an old one over that period of time. Obesity in that era was likened to learning to ride a bicycle, and one should be able to take the training wheels off a bicycle after 12 weeks or less of practice. Since obesity is the most recent of the chronic diseases to be recognized, we can learn the probable future of obesity research by observing the progress of research in other chronic diseases that preceded it.

The initial treatments of chronic diseases have been dietary. Diets limited to 10 g of carbohydrate and 2400 kcal/d were typical for the treatment of the type 1 diabetic patient in the era prior to the discovery of insulin (64). The rice diet was the basis for the most successful treatment of hypertension prior to the advent of effective antihypertensive drugs (65). Although the first treatments for chronic diseases were dietary, the first effective treatments have traditionally been surgical. Malignant hypertension resulted in death within six months when treated with dietary therapy alone, but the use of surgical sympathectomy reduced this figure by half (66). Pancreatic islet transplant is still the only cure for type 1 diabetes (67). Coronary artery bypass surgery for coronary atherosclerosis is still used today, as is gastric bypass and other operations for obesity (68,59).

Safe and effective antihypertensive medications have essentially eliminated the need for surgery in the treatment of hypertension. It is the hope and expectation that safe and effective drug treatments for obesity will also eliminate the need for obesity surgery in the future. The first effective medications for hypertension in the 1940s worked upstream on the central nervous system or on the sympathetic nerves to control blood pressure, like reserpine or ganglionic blocking drugs. Because of their associated side effects and their mode of action far from the blood vessels that mediate blood pressure, these drugs had side effects and are rarely used today. Ganglionic blocking agents interfered with the ability of the eye to focus, caused impotence, ileus, and peptic ulcer disease whereas reserpine caused depression (69).

Hydrochlorothiazide, which causes the loss of salt into the urine, was introduced in the 1950s and is still in use today (70). As the number of blood pressure medications increased, combination therapy became the norm and some combinations with component medications affecting different control points in the same pathway give more than additive reductions in blood pressure (71). With the multiple medication combinations now available to treat hypertension, it is the rare circumstance when good control of blood pressure cannot be obtained with well-tolerated medication combinations. This situation can be anticipated to occur in the future for obesity medication.

The second advance, in addition to combination therapy for hypertension, was the development of drugs that act on the blood vessels themselves. By having a mode of action on the blood vessels, spillover of side effects to other systems becomes less likely. For example, angiotensin receptor blockers act directly on blood vessels and are almost devoid of adverse events.

At present there is a limited arsenal of medications with which to treat obesity. In fact, there are only two drugs approved by the FDA for use in the United States without time limitations, based on the indications in the package insert. Approval of these drugs was based on one- to two-year trials. Orlistat, which causes a loss of fat in the stool can be likened to a thiazide diuretic in the treatment of hypertension, which causes a loss of sodium into the urine. As with thiazides, due to their safety and proven efficacy, orlistat is likely to remain an obesity treatment option even as more effective medications are developed. Sibutramine, the only other medication without time limitations on use in the treatment of obesity, acts on the central nervous system. Although sibutramine is effective and reasonably well tolerated, its targeting of the central nervous system increases the risks of unintended adverse events in other systems. Symptoms like dry mouth may be only an annoyance, but the blood pressure elevation associated with sibutramine has created much concern in the medical community. It seems likely that sibutramine will become relegated to use in unusual circumstances for the treatment of obesity, much as alpha methyl dopa, an antihypertensive drug with actions in the central nervous system and once a popular treatment of hypertension is now reserved for unusual circumstances.

Developing drugs for the treatment of obesity comes with some special challenges. First, the drugs that have been used for the treatment of obesity have been accompanied by a litany of safety problems. This started with the first drug to be used for the treatment of obesity, thyroid hormone, which caused hyperthyroidism (72,73). Dinitrophenol was associated with cataracts, neuropathy, and even death by hyperthermia (74,75). Amphetamine was addictive, and aminorex, an amphetamine derivative with a noradrenergic mechanism, was removed from the European market for primary pulmonary hypertension that carried 50% mortality (76,77). More recently, fenfluramine was removed from the market due to its association with cardiac valvulopathy, phenylpropanolamine was removed due to the risk of hemorrhagic stroke, and ephedra was removed due to systemic adrenergic stimulation (24,78,79). This history has raised the bar for insuring the safety of obesity medications. Obesity is a risk factor for cardiovascular disease and diabetes, but the risks are low in the short-term, making the U.S. FDA intolerant of all but minimal risks. In fact, rimonabant, which was approved in Europe, was denied approval by the U.S. FDA due to an increased risk of suicidal ideation and seizure activity (43).

The second challenge is, unlike medications for the other chronic diseases, obesity drugs are rarely covered by third party payers. Thus, the cost of obesity drugs is borne by the patients, and price becomes a much greater constraint to sales than when medical insurance reimburses the costs. As safer and more effective drugs are developed for treating obesity, it is likely that patients will want access to these medications and their demand will prod insurance companies to include obesity drugs in the covered benefits. Until the potential consumers are willing to pay a higher premium for insurance that covers obesity medications, any improvement in the reimbursement landscape is likely to remain slow. Phentermine, a drug that is labeled for short-term use and has the DEA designation class IV suggesting addiction potential, albeit low, has consistently outsold the combined sales of the two drugs (sibutramine and orlistat) approved for the treatment of obesity without time limitations on use, suggesting the importance of pricing (80).

The Ideal Obesity Drug

Epidemiologic studies have shown that weight loss increases mortality despite weight loss being associated with a reduction in cardiovascular risk factors (81,82). This paradox was explained by the reanalysis of the Tecumseh and Framingham studies, both of which measured skinfold thicknesses as a measure of body fat, in addition to body weight. This reanalysis showed that mortality increased by 30% for every standard deviation of weight loss but decreased by 15% for every standard deviation of fat loss (83). Thus, a loss of fat seems to confer health while a loss of lean tissue is unhealthy. Although an increased amount of body fat is a recognized mortality risk, visceral fat, the intra-abdominal fat that drains through the liver, is a greater mortality risk due to its association with insulin resistance (84). Visceral fat and insulin resistance are associated with hypertension, dyslipidemia, and diabetes, the major cardiovascular risks associated with obesity (85). Therefore, the ideal obesity drug would give substantial weight loss that was safe and well tolerated. Also, this ideal drug would give preferential loss of fat tissue and visceral fat in particular. This ideal drug may actually be a combination of drugs due to the redundant nature of control mechanisms for chronic diseases.

Approaches to Obesity Research

Empiric observations have been the most common impetus for progress in obesity research. Coleman, for example, discovered a mouse that was massively obese due to a spontaneous mutation. He was able to demonstrate that its obesity was due to the lack of a receptor by parabiosis experiments (86). These observations eventually lead to the discovery of leptin (87). Progressing from empirical observations to physiologic explanations, and then to molecular approaches that define the mechanism has been the most common pathway of discovery in obesity. Physiologic observations leading directly to new treatment has occurred less commonly, but Cone was able to demonstrate that mu opioid receptors exist on POMC neurons in the arcuate nucleus of the hypothalamus (88). These mu opioid receptors were subsequently shown to reduce the secretion of POMC. The cleavage products of POMC are alpha melanocyte-stimulating hormone and an opioid. These observations lead to the combining of BUP, a stimulator of POMC, with NAL, an inhibitor of the mu opioid receptor, and a time-released formulation of BUP and NAL is now in phase 3 drug development for the treatment of obesity (50). The human genome has now been sequenced and put in the public domain (89). This opens the possibility of moving from genes and the molecular basis of disease to physiology and then to new treatments. Thus, there is potential for much more rapid advances in the treatment of obesity than existed when antihypertensive medications were developing.

MOLECULAR APPROACHES

There has been an explosion of new technologies that have not only increased the sensitivity of clinical analyte detection but have also increased the numbers of analytes that can be detected in a single biological sample. This is true not only for the measurement of hormones in blood, but also for the measurement of metabolites of pathways, vitamins, and the circulating products of cell lysis. These tools can be used not only to tell whether a drug engages a target, but can also be used to diagnose subtypes of obesity. This has the potential to revolutionize the way that we diagnose, and therefore treat, obesity.

One example of this technology is the bead-based immunoassay. These allow for the measurement of dozens of hormones in a single blood sample. In fact, most only require 50 μL or less of blood and are as accurate and precise as the classical ELISA or RIA. Sensitivity is occasionally a limitation (Table 1).

The major advances, however, have been in genome-based molecular approaches and technologies. For example, this kind of technological development is already changing the way in which we view cancer and cancer therapy. Widespread and inexpensive genetic testing leads to improved treatments of breast cancer and the identification of those women at increased risk. The rarity of genes where mutations lead to major effects has stymied the field of obesity research, but new discoveries such as the *FTO* gene make it more likely that our genetic knowledge base will develop beyond the random candidate single nucleotide polymorphism (SNP) analyses where the results are so often nonreproducible. Sequencing the genome *of an individual* is not that far away and promises to increase the power to identify genetic variation in genes that influence not only body weight but also other important subphenotypes such as energy metabolism, propensity to binge eat, capacity for burning fat, etc. The promise of this kind of research is that treatments might be better tailored toward the specific causes. This field, called pharmacogenomics, should tip the risk/benefit ratio in a favorable direction by enhancing the prospects of a successful treatment and reduce the risk of treating patients with the "wrong" drug. When the genetic science is fully developed, in other words, when we

Table 1 Molecular Approaches in Obesity Research

Sample type	Analysis	Classical measurement	New technology
Blood	Hormones, cytokines	RIA, ELISA[a]	Multiplex bead–based immunoassays
	Metabolites	Enzyme-based assays	Mass spectrometry–based metabolomics
	mRNA	Northern blots	Gene expression level[b]
	Protein/enzyme	Western immunoassay	Proteomics
	Gene variation	DNA "SNPs"[c]	Whole genome sequencing—GWAS
	Genomic modification	None	Epigenome analysis[c]
Tissues	mRNA	None	Gene expression level[b]
	Protein	None	Proteomics, multiplex bead–based immunoassays
	Protein	None	Tissue arrays
	Metabolism	None	Stem cell isolation for metabolic studies

[a]RIA, radioimmunoassays; ELISA, enzyme linked immunosorbent assay.
[b]New techniques for gene expression include quantitative reverse-transcriptase polymerase chain reaction (qRT-PCR) and various platforms for near-whole genome "transcriptome" analysis.
[c]See text for a discussion.
GWAS, genome-wide association studies; SNP, single nucleotide polymorphism.

know which genes are responsible for what subtypes of obesity, the diagnostic technologies will already be available to roll this into the clinic.

Another example of how a new technology promises to revolutionize is the microarray (transcriptome). Microarray analysis allows for the measurement of essentially every gene that is expressed in a sample. This kind of analysis can be used for peripheral blood mononuclear cells or any tissue to identify which genes are upregulated and which genes are downregulated in a given condition. The cost of this technology has dropped dramatically leading to clinical utility in cancer. For example, knowing the pattern of gene expression in biopsy specimens from cancers leads to a more precise diagnosis as compared to histopathological analysis alone. Furthermore, the pattern of genes expressed predicts responses to specific kinds of treatments. We are just now beginning to see this kind of analysis in patients with obesity where the promise will lead to better strategies for the diagnosis and treatments which are specific for a person's "subtype" of obesity.

The new field of epigenomics is charging ahead. The epigenome refers to modification of the DNA or the proteins that fold and coil the DNA (90). The best studied is the methylation of cytosines in the DNA backbone. These modifications occur in regions known as CpG islands and modify the expression of genes (i.e., turn them on or off). There is growing evidence that these DNA modifications might predispose persons to the risk of obesity, just like for mutations in the classic ATGC nucleotides (SNPs) (91). When the important regions of the genome are identified, a simple blood sample could identify a specific subtype of obesity—another type of genetic testing—as a means of improving patient care.

Not all new technologies are genetic, however. A few others deserve mention. *Metabolome* (92,93) and *lipidome* (94) refer to the overall pattern of metabolites and lipids in the blood. Mass spectrometry methods allow for the simultaneous detection of hundreds to thousands of analytes in blood or urine.

So how might all of these data points fit together to help us in the treatment of obesity? Will we require genomics, epigenomics transcriptomics, proteomics, metabolomics, and lipidomics? Probably not. We are generally optimistic that the research process will lead us to a small group of analytes that capture the complexity of a person's diagnostic pattern. Alternately, there may be more "power" and/or precision in measuring multiple analytes simultaneously. New statistical techniques such as advanced principal components analysis, cluster analysis, or FOREL can reduce a multidimensional dataset into two or three dimensions making the subgrouping of subjects into discrete diagnostic categories much easier (95). Pathway analysis of transciptome data or metabolome data may identify metabolic pathways where a specific therapy can be applied. At this point, all we can say is that the tools and techniques are in place to move us toward a molecular diagnostic paradigm in obesity—this is the clear trend in most other diseases such as cancer (96,97).

The major barrier to the adoption of these technologies is cost. Payors seem willing to pay for these kinds of technologies such as magnetic resonance imaging and positron emission tomography scans when a patient is diagnosed with cancer. Obesity and metabolic disorders are very different, even though the risk of dying from obesity can be very high for some patients. For example, it is difficult for the average physician to get paid for the measurement of two of the most important metabolic hormones insulin and adiponectin. Both have strong positive predictive values for disease and can be used to gauge the effectiveness of a therapy like TZDs; however, it is difficult to convince payors of the value of these tests when the economics are difficult to quantify. We believe that one likely scenario is that one of these molecular technologies will become cost effective by identifying a subpopulation of patients with obesity that will be super-responders to a specific drug therapy. If one of these tests could identify even 5% of the population who would lose 25% body weight—with a drug that that typically produces 5–10% body weight loss—that would make the test much more attractive from a cost perspective. Thus, pharmacogenomics or "personalized medicine" (98) is one way to get payors to reimburse the molecular testing, not paying for pharmacotherapy of patients with obesity that are unlikely to respond and paying for pharmacotherapy of patients with obesity that are likely to respond. This scenario is a double-edged sword because this approach might be used to deny treatment to patients who might benefit from a drug.

To summarize, new molecular technologies and approaches will revolutionize the diagnosis of obesity and influence pharmacotherapy. Picking the "winning horse" in this race is no easy task, but it is almost certain that one of them will be a winner.

ADVANCED CLINICAL ENDPOINTS

When testing a new drug for obesity, the simplest approach is to see if the drug causes weight loss. This is a long and expensive process requiring hundreds of participants and months of treatment. An alternate approach is, after confirming that the drug is safe and tolerated in multiple-dose phase 1 studies, to test for effects on resting or 24-hour energy expenditure (99), hepatic lipid, food intake, or other behaviors such as binge eating. These kinds of advanced clinical endpoints may provide early clues in short-term studies to a drug's efficacy and stimulate the investment in a subsequent "classic" clinical phase 2 testing paradigm. The danger in these intermediate proof-of-concept studies studies is twofold. An ambiguous outcome where a drug gives some positive result but not a definitive answer can slow decision making and stall the development of a good drug. Alternately, a negative result for a "noisy" measure, as is often the case for measuring food intake, does not absolutely mean that the drug will be ineffective in a longer clinical study. Newer technologies such as whole body nuclear magnetic resonance (100) may be more precise than existing technologies. This may lead the measurement of changes in body energy stores (body fat) as opposed to the measurement of body weight; measuring body weight is often noisy because of changes in body water. With some caveats, the drug development field has a love–hate relationship with Advanced Clinical Endpoints. The advantages of these measures in developing obesity drugs (justifies the investment, reveals new pharmacodynamic properties of a target) do not always outweigh the disadvantages (slow, often not definitive). A full discussion is beyond the scope of this chapter but suffice it to say that Advanced Clinical Endpoints can be helpful in drug development if used carefully and judiciously (Table 2).

An alternate view of Advanced Clinical Endpoints is that they can reveal beneficial effects of a drug. For example, magnetic resonance spectroscopy can be used to measure fat in the liver as a surrogate for biopsies. Some obesity drugs may have direct effects on the liver or modulate areas in the brain that control liver metabolism. Many of the newer obesity targets are likely to have weight-loss independent effects on insulin secretion or insulin resistance (101). This makes the measurement of insulin sensitivity particularly important. Many of these measures are not practical in large numbers of subjects. The more invasive studies can often make up for this limitation as they are more precise. It is critical to know in advance the test–retest stability of a

Table 2 Clinical Approaches in Obesity Research

Measurement		Technology
Food intake		Single meal or 24-hour inpatient testing
"		Telephone- or internet-based diet intake assessment
Hunger		VAS or fMRI[a]
Energy expenditure		Doubly labeled water (DLW[b]), hood (indirect) calorimetry[c]
Spontaneous physical activity		Pedometers, accelerometers or DLW REE
Body composition		Weight, DEXA, MRI, qNMR
Fat distribution	Visceral adipose tissue	CT scanning or MRI
	Intermuscular adipose tissue	"
	Epicardial adipose tissue	"Also echocardiography
Fat oxidation during a meal		Stable isotope
Gastric emptying		Stable isotope or acetamenophen appearance
Gut peptide secretion		Indwelling IV catheter and special blood specimen handling procedures
Vascular reactivity		Brachial artery flow mediated dilatation
"		Peripheral arterial tonometry
"Ectopic" lipid	Intramyocellular or intrahepatic lipid	Magnetic resonance spectroscopy (MRS)
Exercise parameters		VO_2 max
"		31P MRS
Blood pressure		24-hour ambulatory blood pressure monitoring
Insulin sensitivity		Euglycemic-hyperinsulinemic clamp, FSIGTT, oGTT[d]
Tissue effects		Microdialysis of adipose tissue to measure lipolysis
"		Adipose tissue, liver or muscle biopsy

[a]Visual analog scales and functional MRI, respectively {leptin}.
[b]$D_2{}^{18}O$
[c]Measures REE only.
[d]Frequently sampled intraveneous glucose tolerance test, oral glucose tolerance test.
CT, computed tomography; DEXA, dual energy X-rays absorptiometry; FSIGTT, frequently sampled intravenous glucose tolerance test; MRI, magnetic resonance imaging ; oGTT, oral glucose tolerance test; qNMR, quantitative nuclear magnetic resonance; REE, resting energy expenditure.

measure, i.e., precision, before including these measures. This is important not only to reduce sample size and cost but also to be able to trust the negative result.

Conclusions

We are presently experiencing a proliferation in obesity research. The declaration of obesity as a chronic disease and not just bad habits was not nearly as powerful as the discovery of leptin, a hormone that is genetically absent in a small minority of rodents and humans. The response of leptin deficient obesity with weight loss to the replacement of leptin, more than anything else, convinced the scientific community that obesity is a chronic physiologic problem worthy of study. This interest and scientific exploration has resulted in new discoveries that impact obesity treatment. This chapter has reviewed some of these advances in diet, lifestyle, and exercise therapy. Although dietary herbal supplements have little to offer at present, there are promising treatments still needing further research. Not only are obesity surgeries advancing, but new devices, based on the physiology of obesity surgery, are also making surgical strategies less invasive. The stimulation of obesity research has resulted in a better understanding of obesity pathophysiology, and several new drugs, many of them combination pharmaceuticals, are in the later stages of drug development. We are in a new era of scientific tools and technology. The human genome has been sequenced, and we have sophisticated molecular tools in addition to advanced physiologic endpoints that we did not previously have. This places obesity in a situation that predicts much more rapid progress in reaching the goal of a safe and effective treatment than was the case for other chronic diseases like hypertension. Thus, there is hope for returning those who suffer from the disease to a healthy and socially acceptable weight in the foreseeable future. The safety and efficacy of these various treatment modalities vary. Diets and herbs, which are classified by the FDA as foods are the least risky, medications and devices are intermediate in risk, surgery carries the highest risk, but the efficacy is greater for long-term maintenance of weight loss as the risk increases. Hopefully, the expected progress will provide new treatments that increase efficacy and reduce risk for the same degree of efficacy.

REFERENCES

1. Knowler WC, Barrett-Connor E, Fowler SE, et al. Reduction in the incidence of type 2 diabetes with lifestyle intervention or metformin. N Engl J Med 2002; 346(6):393–403.
2. Tuomilehto J, Lindstrom J, Eriksson JG, et al. Prevention of type 2 diabetes mellitus by changes in lifestyle among subjects with impaired glucose tolerance. N Engl J Med 2001; 344(18):1343–1350.
3. Clinical Guidelines on the Identification, Evaluation, and Treatment of Overweight and Obesity in Adults–The Evidence Report. National Institutes of Health. Obes Res 1998; (suppl 2):51S–209S.
4. Heshka S, Anderson JW, Atkinson RL, et al. Weight loss with self-help compared with a structured commercial program: a randomized trial. JAMA 2003; 289(14):1792–1798.
5. Rock CL, Pakiz B, Flatt SW, et al. Randomized trial of a multifaceted commercial weight loss program. Obesity (Silver Spring) 2007; 15(4):939–949.
6. Pavlou KN, Krey S, Steffee WP. Exercise as an adjunct to weight loss and maintenance in moderately obese subjects. Am J Clin Nutr 1989; 49(suppl 5):1115–23.
7. Church T, Earnest C, Blair S. Dietary overcompensation across different doses of exercise. Obesity 2007; 15(suppl):A17.
8. Shai I, Schwarzfuchs D, Henkin Y, et al. Weight loss with a low-carbohydrate, Mediterranean, or low-fat diet. N Engl J Med 2008; 359(3):229–241.
9. Cornier MA, Donahoo WT, Pereira R, et al. Insulin sensitivity determines the effectiveness of dietary macronutrient composition on weight loss in obese women. Obes Res 2005; 4:703–709.
10. Wigand R, Gelderblom H, Wadell G. New human adenovirus (candidate adenovirus 36), a novel member of subgroup D. Arch Virol 1980; 64(3):225–233.
11. Atkinson RL. Viruses as an etiology of obesity. Mayo Clin Proc 2007; 82(10):1192–1198.
12. Atkinson RL, Dhurandhar NV, Allison DB, et al. Human adenovirus-36 is associated with increased body weight and paradoxical reduction of serum lipids. Int J Obes (Lond) 2005; 29(3):281–286.
13. Rogers PM, Fusinski KA, Rathod MA, et al. Human adenovirus Ad-36 induces adipogenesis via its E4 orf-1 gene. Int J Obes (Lond) 2008; 32(3):397–406.
14. Orentreich N, Matias JR, DeFelice A, et al. Low methionine ingestion by rats extends life span. J Nutr 1993; 123(2):269–274.
15. Epner DE, Morrow S, Wilcox M, et al. Nutrient intake and nutritional indexes in adults with metastatic cancer on a phase I clinical trial of dietary methionine restriction. Nutr Cancer 2002; 42(2):158–166.
16. Lu S, Hoestje SM, Choo E, et al. Induction of caspase-dependent and -independent apoptosis in response to methionine restriction. Int J Oncol 2003; 22(2):415–420.
17. Lu S, Chen GL, Ren C, et al. Methionine restriction selectively targets thymidylate synthase in prostate cancer cells. Biochem Pharmacol 2003; 66(5):791–800.
18. Wadden TA, Berkowitz RI, Womble LG, et al. Randomized trial of lifestyle modification and pharmacotherapy for obesity. N Engl J Med 2005; 353(20):2111–2120.
19. Lichtman SW, Pisarska K, Berman ER, et al. Discrepancy between self-reported and actual caloric intake and exercise in obese subjects. N Engl J Med 1992; 327(27):1893–1898.
20. Martin CK, Han H, Coulon SM, et al. A novel method to remotely measure food intake of free-living individuals in real time: the remote food photography method. Br J Nutr 2008; 11:1–11.
21. Zhang K, Pi-Sunyer FX, Boozer CN. Improving energy expenditure estimation for physical activity. Med Sci Sports Exerc 2004; 36(5):883–889.
22. Greenway FL. The safety and efficacy of pharmaceutical and herbal caffeine and ephedrine use as a weight loss agent. Obes Rev 2001; 2(3):199–211.
23. Cockey CD. Ephedra banned. AWHONN Lifelines 2004; 8(1):19–25.
24. Shekelle PG, Hardy ML, Morton SC, et al. Efficacy and safety of ephedra and ephedrine for weight loss and athletic performance: a meta-analysis. JAMA 2003; 289(12):1537–1545.
25. Maeda H, Tsukui T, Sashima T, et al. Seaweed carotenoid, fucoxanthin, as a multi-functional nutrient. Asia Pac J Clin Nutr 2008; 17(suppl 1):196–199.

26. Maeda H, Hosokawa M, Sashima T, et al. Effect of medium-chain triacylglycerols on anti-obesity effect of fucoxanthin. J Oleo Sci 2007; 56(12):615–621.
27. Maeda H, Hosokawa M, Sashima T, et al. Dietary combination of fucoxanthin and fish oil attenuates the weight gain of white adipose tissue and decreases blood glucose in obese/diabetic KK-Ay mice. J Agric Food Chem 2007; 55(19):7701–7706.
28. MacLean DB, Luo LG. Increased ATP content/production in the hypothalamus may be a signal for energy-sensing of satiety: studies of the anorectic mechanism of a plant steroidal glycoside. Brain Res 2004; 1020(1–2):1–11.
29. Phytopharm. Hoodia factfile. [cited October 1, 2007]. http://www.phytopharm.co.uk/hoodiafactfile/. Accessed November 6, 2008.
30. Ikeuchi M, Koyama T, Takahashi J, et al. Effects of astaxanthin in obese mice fed a high-fat diet. Biosci Biotechnol Biochem 2007; 71(4):893–899.
31. Aoi W, Naito Y, Takanami Y, et al. Astaxanthin improves muscle lipid metabolism in exercise via inhibitory effect of oxidative CPT I modification. Biochem Biophys Res Commun 2008; 366(4):892–897.
32. Ikeuchi M, Koyama T, Takahashi J, et al. Effects of astaxanthin supplementation on exercise-induced fatigue in mice. Biol Pharm Bull 2006; 10:2106–2110.
33. Oben J, Kuate D, Agbor G, et al. The use of a Cissus quadrangularis formulation in the management of weight loss and metabolic syndrome. Lipids Health Dis 2006; 5:24.
34. Oben JE, Enyegue DM, Fomekong GI, et al. The effect of Cissus quadrangularis (CQR-300) and a Cissus formulation (CORE) on obesity and obesity-induced oxidative stress. Lipids Health Dis 2007; 6:4.
35. Oben JE, Ngondi JL, Momo CN, et al. The use of a Cissus quadrangularis/Irvingia gabonensis combination in the management of weight loss: a double-blind placebo-controlled study. Lipids Health Dis 2008; 7:12.
36. Keenan MJ, Zhou J, McCutcheon KL, et al. Effects of resistant starch, a non-digestible fermentable fiber, on reducing body fat. Obesity (Silver Spring) 2006; 14(9):1523–1534.
37. Zhou J, Hegsted M, McCutcheon KL, et al. Peptide YY and proglucagon mRNA expression patterns and regulation in the gut. Obesity (Silver Spring) 2006; 4:683–689.
38. Greenway F, O'Neil CE, Stewart L, et al. Fourteen weeks of treatment with Viscofiber increased fasting levels of glucagon-like peptide-1 and peptide-YY. J Med Food 2007; 10(4):720–724.
39. Rudkowska I, Roynette CE, Demonty I, et al. Diacylglycerol: efficacy and mechanism of action of an anti-obesity agent. Obes Res 2005; 13(11):1864–1876.
40. Taguchi H, Nagao T, Watanabe H, et al. Energy value and digestibility of dietary oil containing mainly 1,3-diacylglycerol are similar to those of triacylglycerol. Lipids 2001; 36(4):379–382.
41. Kamphuis MM, Mela DJ, Westerterp-Plantenga MS. Diacylglycerols affect substrate oxidation and appetite in humans. Am J Clin Nutr 2003; 77(5):1133–1139.
42. Matsuyama T, Shoji K, Watanabe H, et al. Effects of diacylglycerol oil on adiposity in obese children: initial communication. J Pediatr Endocrinol Metab 2006; 19(6):795–804.
43. Christensen R, Kristensen PK, Bartels EM, et al. Efficacy and safety of the weight-loss drug rimonabant: a meta-analysis of randomised trials. Lancet 2007; 70(9600):1706–1713.
44. Fitzgerald LW, Burn TC, Brown BS, et al. Possible role of valvular serotonin 5-HT(2B) receptors in the cardiopathy associated with fenfluramine. Mol Pharmacol 2000; 57(1):75–81.
45. Smith SR, Prosser W, Donahue D, et al. APD356, an orally-active selective 5HT2c agonist reduced body weight in obese men and women. Diabetes Metab 2006; 55(suppl 1):A80.
46. Kopelman P, Bryson A, Hickling R, et al. Cetilistat (ATL-962), a novel lipase inhibitor: a 12-week randomized, placebo-controlled study of weight reduction in obese patients. Int J Obes (Lond) 2007; 31(3):494–499.
47. Astrup A, Meier DH, Mikkelsen BO, et al. Weight loss produced by tesofensine in patients with Parkinson's or Alzheimer's disease. Obesity (Silver Spring) 2008; 16(6):1363–1369.
48. Sjodin A, Gasteyger C, Nielsen A-LH, et al. The effects of tesofensine on body composition in obese subjects. Int J Obes 2008; 32(suppl 1):S83.
49. Astrup A, Madsbad S, Breum L, et al. Effect of tesofensine on bodyweight loss, body composition, and quality of life in obese patients: a randomised, double-blind, placebo-controlled trial. Lancet 2008; 372(9653):1906–1913.
50. Greenway FL, Whitehouse MJ, Guttadauria M, et al. Rational design of a combination medication for the treatment of obesity. Obesity (Silver Spring) 2009; 17(1):30–39.
51. Greenway FL, Anderson JW, Atkinson RL, et al. Bupropion and zonisamide for the treatment of obesity. Obes Res 2006; 14(suppl):A17.
52. Gadde KM, Yonish GM, Foust MS, et al. A 24-week randomized controlled trial of VI-0521, a combination weight loss therapy, in obese adults. Obesity (Silver Spring) 2006; 14(suppl):A17.

53. Roth JD, Roland BL, Cole RL, et al. Leptin responsiveness restored by amylin agonism in diet-induced obesity: evidence from nonclinical and clinical studies. Proc Natl Acad Sci U S A 2008; 105(20):7257–7262.
54. Sjostrom L, Narbro K, Sjostrom CD, et al. Effects of bariatric surgery on mortality in Swedish obese subjects. N Engl J Med 2007; 357(8):741–752.
55. Angrisani L, Lorenzo M, Borrelli V. Laparoscopic adjustable gastric banding versus Roux-en-Y gastric bypass: 5-year results of a prospective randomized trial. Surg Obes Relat Dis 2007; 3(2):127–132; discussion 132–133.
56. Nguyen NT, Hinojosa M, Fayad C, et al. Use and outcomes of laparoscopic versus open gastric bypass at academic medical centers. J Am Coll Surg 2007; 205(2):248–255.
57. Moreno C, Closset J, Dugardeyn S, et al. Transoral gastroplasty is safe, feasible, and induces significant weight loss in morbidly obese patients: results of the second human pilot study. Endoscopy 2008; 40(5):406–413.
58. Himpens J, Dapri G, Cadiere GB. A prospective randomized study between laparoscopic gastric banding and laparoscopic isolated sleeve gastrectomy: results after 1 and 3 years. Obes Surg 2006; 16(11):1450–1456.
59. Karamanakos SN, Vagenas K, Kalfarentzos F, et al. Weight loss, appetite suppression, and changes in fasting and postprandial ghrelin and peptide-YY levels after Roux-en-Y gastric bypass and sleeve gastrectomy: a prospective, double blind study. Ann Surg 2008; 247(3):401–407.
60. Rodriguez-Grunert L, Galvao Neto MP, Alamo M, et al. First human experience with endoscopically delivered and retrieved duodenal-jejunal bypass sleeve. Surg Obes Relat Dis 2008; 4(1):55–59.
61. Camilleri M, Toouli J, Herrera MF, et al. Intra-abdominal vagal blocking (VBLOC therapy): clinical results with a new implantable medical device. Surgery 2008; 143(6):723–731.
62. Golden RL. William Osler at 150: an overview of a life. JAMA 1999; 282(23):2252–2258.
63. Health implications of obesity. National Institutes of Health Consensus Development Conference Statement. Ann Intern Med 1985; 103(1):147–151.
64. Banting FG. Pancreatic extracts in the treatment of diabetes mellitus: preliminary report. Can Med Assoc J 1922; 12(3):141–146.
65. Kempner W. Treatment of hypertensive disease with rice diet. Am J Med 1948; 3:545.
66. Platt R, Gilchrist R, Wilson C, et al. Discussion on sympathectomy in hypertension. Br Heart J 1948; 10(4):293–297.
67. Gliedman ML, Tellis VA, Soberman R, et al. Long-term effects of pancreatic transplant function in patients with advanced juvenile-onset diabetes. Diabetes Care 1978; 1(1):1–9.
68. Song YB, On YK, Kim JH, et al. The effects of atorvastatin on the occurrence of postoperative atrial fibrillation after off-pump coronary artery bypass grafting surgery. Am Heart J 2008; 156(2): 373.e9–e16.
69. DeQuattro V, Li D. Sympatholytic therapy in primary hypertension: a user friendly role for the future. J Hum Hypertens 2002; (suppl 1):S118–S123.
70. Rapoport A, Evans BM, Wong H. Some short-term metabolic effects of chlorothiazide in hypertensives on a rice diet. Can Med Assoc J 1959; 81:984–990.
71. McMahon FG. Efficacy of an antihypertensive agent. Comparison of methyldopa and hydrochlorothiazide in combination and singly. JAMA 1975; 231(2):155–158.
72. Putnam J. Cases of myxoedema and acromegalia treated with benefit by sheep's thyroids. Am J Med Sci 1893; 106(2):125–148.
73. Gardner DF, Kaplan MM, Stanley CA, et al. Effect of tri-iodothyronine replacement on the metabolic and pituitary responses to starvation. N Engl J Med 1979; 300(11):579–584.
74. Masserman J. Dinotrophenol. Its therapeutic and toxic actions in certain types of psychobiologic underactivity. JAMA 1934; 102:523.
75. Colman E. Dinitrophenol and obesity: an early twentieth-century regulatory dilemma. Regul Toxicol Pharmacol 2007; 48(2):115–117.
76. Bartholomew AA. Amphetamine addiction. Med J Aust 1970; 1(24):1209–1214.
77. Kramer MS, Lane DA. Aminorex, dexfenfluramine, and primary pulmonary hypertension. J Clin Epidemiol 1998; 51(4):361–364.
78. Connolly HM, Crary JL, McGoon MD, et al. Valvular heart disease associated with fenfluramine-phentermine. N Engl J Med 1997; 337(9):581–588.
79. Kernan WN, Viscoli CM, Brass LM, et al. Phenylpropanolamine and the risk of hemorrhagic stroke. N Engl J Med 2000; 343(25):1826–1832.
80. Stafford RS, Radley DC. National trends in antiobesity medication use. Arch Intern Med 2003; 163(9):1046–1050.
81. Andres R, Muller DC, Sorkin JD. Long-term effects of change in body weight on all-cause mortality. A review. Ann Intern Med 1993; 119(7 pt 2):737–743.

82. Pi-Sunyer FX. A review of long-term studies evaluating the efficacy of weight loss in ameliorating disorders associated with obesity. Clin Ther 1996; 18(6):1006–1035.
83. Allison DB, Zannolli R, Faith MS, et al. Weight loss increases and fat loss decreases all-cause mortality rate: results from two independent cohort studies. Int J Obes Relat Metab Disord 1999; 23(6):603–611.
84. Troiano RP, Frongillo EA Jr, Sobal J, et al. The relationship between body weight and mortality: a quantitative analysis of combined information from existing studies. Int J Obes Relat Metab Disord 1996; 20(1):63–75.
85. Kissebah AH, Krakower GR. Regional adiposity and morbidity. Physiol Rev 1994; 74(4):761–811.
86. Coleman DL, Hummel KP. Effects of parabiosis of normal with genetically diabetic mice. Am J Physiol 1969; 217(5):1298–1304.
87. Halaas JL, Gajiwala KS, Maffei M, et al. Weight-reducing effects of the plasma protein encoded by the obese gene. Science 1995; 269(5223):543–546.
88. Cone RD, Cowley MA, Butler AA, et al. The arcuate nucleus as a conduit for diverse signals relevant to energy homeostasis. Int J Obes Relat Metab Disord 2001; (suppl 5):S63–S67.
89. Manolio TA, Brooks LD, Collins FS. A HapMap harvest of insights into the genetics of common disease. J Clin Invest 2008; 118(5):1590–1605.
90. Novik KL, Nimmrich I, Genc B, et al. Epigenomics: genome-wide study of methylation phenomena. Curr Issues Mol Biol 2002; 4(4):111–128.
91. Weaver IC, Cervoni N, Champagne FA, et al. Epigenetic programming by maternal behavior. Nat Neurosci 2004; 7(8):847–854.
92. Griffin JL, Vidal-Puig A. Current challenges in metabolomics for diabetes research: a vital functional genomic tool or just a ploy for gaining funding? Physiol Genomics 2008; 34(1):1–5.
93. Lawton KA, Berger A, Mitchell M, et al. Analysis of the adult human plasma metabolome. Pharmacogenomics 2008; 9(4):383–397.
94. Gross RW, Han X. Lipidomics in diabetes and the metabolic syndrome. Methods Enzymol 2007; 433:73–90.
95. Ptitsyn A, Hulver M, Cefalu W, et al. Unsupervised clustering of gene expression data points at hypoxia as possible trigger for metabolic syndrome. BMC Genomics 2006; 7:318.
96. Segal E, Friedman N, Kaminski N, et al. From signatures to models: understanding cancer using microarrays. Nat Genet 2005; 37:S38–S45.
97. Raetz EA, Moos PJ. Impact of microarray technology in clinical oncology. Cancer Invest 2004; 22(2):312–320.
98. Ginsburg GS, McCarthy JJ. Personalized medicine: revolutionizing drug discovery and patient care. Trends Biotechnol 2001; 19(12):491–496.
99. Redman LM, de Jonge L, Fang X, et al. Lack of an effect of a novel beta3-adrenoceptor agonist, TAK-677, on energy metabolism in obese individuals: a double-blind, placebo-controlled randomized study. J Clin Endocrinol Metab 2007; 92(2):527–531.
100. Napolitano A, Miller SR, Murgatroyd PR, et al. Validation of a quantitative magnetic resonance method for measuring human body composition. Obesity (Silver Spring) 2008; 16(1):191–198.
101. Zhou L, Sutton GM, Rochford JJ, et al. Serotonin 2C receptor agonists improve type 2 diabetes via melanocortin-4 receptor signaling pathways. Cell Metab 2007; 6(5):398–405.

14 Legal aspects and issues related to bariatric medical practice

James L. Bland

Basic to the practice of bariatric medicine, and medicine in general, there are a number of legal situations and related concerns that must be understood. This chapter will attempt to list, and illuminate, many of these areas and related questions. However, the material contained herein should not be considered as legal advice. In general, the information provided is basic in all states. States, however, must be considered as individual entities for the purpose of what applies through state law. Therefore, all legal issues must be understood or utilized on the basis of that state's interpretation of any given situation. Because of this, it is wise to establish a professional contact with a local attorney to ask questions if the need arises. This information reflects the opinions of the writer, on the basis of many years of medical and legal practice, and is thought appropriate for the reader's consideration.

The following few paragraphs briefly touch on what will be discussed in more detail as this chapter unfolds. Several of the issues discussed will also be evaluated in other chapters, by other authors, with more specific "use in practice" recommendations. These important topics should be studied and if used must be put into place based on proper background knowledge. Therefore, any duplication of information in this presentation should be looked on as reinforcing and refreshing your understanding.

Bariatric medical practice shares the same basic legal elements of any professional medical practice. However, there are a number of legal issues that are more germane to bariatrics than in most other medical specialties. For example, the practice of bariatrics often includes dispensing prescription drugs and supplements in the office setting. This practice brings into play a number of legal requirements that, if not met, can lead to disaster. Then, the use of anorectic drugs in a different manner than that mentioned in the label (off-label use), literally demands that the practitioner gives and receives "informed consent" authorization from the patient. In recent events, there are at least two states, and perhaps more, that are showing major concern regarding the off-label use of anorectic medications. Those states want to strictly limit the time those medications can be used to the "few weeks" mentioned in the label. Considerable measures are currently being developed and presented to educate state boards on these and related issues. However, it is important for the practitioner to secure information as to what rules his or her state follows in the prescriptive use of these medications.

Professional liability insurance continues to be a "must." However, it is true that bariatric medical practice enjoys a very low amount of exposure when compared to other medical specialties. Your insurance policy, regardless of the insurance company issuing the policy, is full of "small print" issues that may be adverse to you. Read your policy in its entirety! Related issues to liability insurance coverage will be discussed in more detail in a later section.

When a physician decides to add bariatrics to an existing medical practice or to do bariatric medicine, ab initio, or otherwise as a full-time practice, a major issue must be dealt with at the beginning . . . . who will pay for your medical charges, the patient or a health insurance company? This area of concern must be thoroughly thought out and a course of action put into place. Herein lay a number of legal issues, including the potential for charges of fraud against the physician! Fraud is not "malpractice" and is not covered under any medical liability insurance policy. This is not a simple decision and will be considered later in much greater detail.

In this chapter you will also find brief outlines of basic legal information related to the important topic of negligence and related nightmares. An attorney, who is also a friend, will be an excellent resource to review any issue that you wish to explore. He, or she, should be able to at least help you determine if what you are doing, or propose to do, is acceptable in your state. Keep in mind that state law may be significantly different on a given issue in your state as compared to my state. Thus, the need to review your legal materials with an attorney in your area is important.

Bariatric medicine is a specialty practice whose time has very definitely arrived. The alarming increase in obesity in most countries has created such increased morbidity and mortality that even the politicians are now recognizing that this major health issue must be addressed! Prepare yourself with proper fundamental basic bariatric education (and keep up to date) to practice in this very important medical specialty!

The sections that follow will begin with presentations that first discuss those legal issues which are perhaps unique to bariatric medicine. After these are developed, they will be followed by legal principles, in general, that are important to review in any legal setting. The topics are not considered in any order of importance and a careful reading, and study, of each section is important to understand the entire scenario.

BARIATRIC PROFESSIONAL LIABILITY INSURANCE

Even though liability involving medical bariatrics is, and has been, at a lower level of exposure than most other medical specialty practices, the necessity for this coverage remains very important. Coverage for bariatric practice is generally included in most liability policies. However, as will be discussed later in this section, there are possible exceptions. From a cost concern, one would be wisely directed to consider liability insurance providers that may be associated with a professional organization of which you are a member. The American Society of Bariatric Physicians has developed this kind of relationship over a number of years and insurers so related will probably be less expensive and offer better bariatric coverage. Do your own due diligence in securing this important foundational necessity.

Read and study your professional liability policy. Do it early, rather than wishing at a later date that you had done so. If you do not understand any section in your policy, ask for help! If any referral is made to attachments, make sure that they are included with the policy. Often, they are absent. Look for words or phrases that may exclude bariatric practice specifically, or weight management and treatment of obesity in general. Some insurance plans have these exclusions either specifically delineated or clothed in an ambiguity. If unsure, get help.

Look for certain coverage provisions in your policy. Secure inclusive coverage for product liability. Look for "moonlighting exceptions" or other related business activity exclusions. Keep in mind that some states limit, control, or prohibit the sale of supplements in a physician's office. If requested in your policy, state the approximate percentage of your practice that is devoted to bariatrics.

Review the insurance coverage of any and all professional persons working for you (e.g., physician, nurse practitioner, or physician assistant). Can they be covered under your policy, depending on their job, or must they be covered under separate policies? Do you have multiple practice locations? Look for specific herbal recommendation exclusions (e.g., Florida).

Always remember that a good relationship with your patient is probably your best insurance! Maintaining true, objective concern for your patient is perhaps your best deterrent to a legal action for an adverse event. The patient who feels that you do care will generally not pursue an action unless the damages are terrible. In the event that a professional liability action arises, the following comments become very important. Promptly notify your insurance carrier. Do not alter any record related to the patient in question. Do not call or talk to the plaintiff and remember that "loose lips sink ships." Do not release narrative reports written by you unless told to do so by your attorney. Do not release copies of medical records without appropriate requests in writing.

Discuss facts with your insurance carrier representative and do not hide information or falsify comments. Record and report significant adverse incidents related to an injured or dissatisfied patient—this is probably a requirement that will be found in your policy. By far, the great majority of such events will never be addressed to an attorney. However, if an insurer has this requirement in your policy and an adverse event does occur, and is recognized by you and not reported, the insurer at a later date, when an action is filed, may choose to deny coverage! Be careful! Do not allow your ego to create an uncaring or defensive attitude in any related legal proceeding. This can, and often does, sink you in the courtroom.

TO FILE, OR NOT FILE, INSURANCE CLAIMS FOR BARIATRIC CARE

This is perhaps the most important and basic decisions to be made in establishing a medical bariatric practice! This issue will be developed in other areas of this book, but there are certain essential legal understandings that are very important. This is one area that has landed many physicians in truly "hot legal water" when an investigator came to call.

In my area of the country, I am not aware of any health insurance policy that covers bariatric medical care. I understand that this is true in almost all of the United States, with certain exceptions where medical bariatric care has been provided by an employer. If you desire to provide bariatric coverage and file to accept assignment from your patient's insurance plan, you should take the time to learn if coverage is afforded by that policy. If it is excluded then this presents an additional issue for you to decide how to handle.

The health insurance issue is a primary concern for every physician! It must be so, because the misuse of an insurance claim could result in a legal disaster! The most commonly used word to describe this potential situation is "fraud"! This can result when a claim is presented that cloaks a bariatric visit as something else that is covered. Also remember that there is no professional liability policy that covers you for fraud!

I understand that most medical bariatric physicians choose not to accept health insurance in their practice. This opinion is based on conversations with innumerable physicians throughout the United States. They are very happy with this arrangement, and are very glad for once in their professional lives, not to have to deal with a health insurance company! However, as obesity becomes more and more in the forefront of American medical concerns, this may cause a change in the health insurance industry and coverage may be afforded. When, and if, that happens, then additional thought must be given as to accept or not accept insurance coverage. Almost, without exception, all these physicians provide a "Super Bill" (or "Super Receipt") that includes all information necessary for the patient to, on their own, attempt to request reimbursement from their insurance company.

Then, there are physicians who do bill the health insurance company for bariatric care. However, those physicians prepare their medical records to reflect that they are treating the comorbid conditions, especially those related to metabolic syndrome. Then, this information is used on the insurance form for payment request. You will encounter physicians who are comfortable with this approach. After all, the treatment of obesity and weight management are the major important issues affecting care for metabolic syndrome comorbid conditions.

When you have the opportunity, take the time to discuss issues such as health insurance with other bariatric physicians. There is no absolute line, other than fraud, that is clear cut in this basic area. In any case, do your homework well and do not be caught uninformed when dealing with health insurance companies. Some physicians will take the time to specifically write to each insurer in his or her practice (especially if it is a mixed medical and bariatric practice) asking whether that insurance covers primary bariatric practice. Herein lies another gray area of just what a primary bariatric practice provides. Is it a weight management center or a treatment center for the metabolic syndrome?

In any case, your patient must be clearly informed about your payment policy! Some practitioners provide a small document to this effect that the patient is required to sign. From a legal point of view, the more "paper" the better! It is truly amazing what patients will forget.

Another basic premise in your care for a bariatric patient, is asking yourself the question, "what was the primary purpose of the office visit"? That is truly a thought-provoking question. In this answer lies the wisdom of how to proceed. Obviously, there is major comfort in avoiding all possible questions of impropriety. This mental gymnastic can also affirm your resolve and direction if you choose to complete insurance claims. An important issue to keep in mind as you decide how to handle, or not handle, insurance claims relates to the care provided for your bariatric patient. Do you require the patient to be seen weekly, twice a month, or monthly—and for how long? It would not take an astute insurer very long to ask questions if claims for treatment for a comorbidity were presented too frequently. An insurance profile of your practice is an automatic "happening" with all insurers!

If your practice is a mixed practice with both medical bariatric visits and other medical-related issues, this presents an additional basic question. That is, do you use the same chart for a patient in your practice for both primary care issues and bariatric problems? Strong consideration should be given to preparing two different charts for that patient. Color coding charts tend to help in keeping the type practice care provided clear and separate. This certainly provides evidence that you are not co-mixing visit purposes for insurance filing. Some physicians, who practice as a corporate entity, go as far as establishing a different corporate entity for their bariatric practice—generally this is seen in a mixed primary and bariatric practice. Other physicians will provide bariatric medicine on certain days, or hours, in a week, and provide the other part of their practice during other periods. Some in a mixed practice will delineate certain rooms and waiting areas for use by bariatric patients.

BARIATRIC OFFICE PRESCRIPTION DISPENSING

Many medical bariatric offices provide an in-house dispensary for medications used in treating their bariatric patients. This provides several distinct advantages for the physician and the patient. The physician is totally aware of the quality of the drugs that are used. The cost to the patient is generally significantly lower than if purchased at a local pharmacy. You will frequently find that some physicians will actually furnish the medication without extra cost to the patient because of the low wholesale price paid for the drug. And today, a major factor in favor of providing this service in-house is to prevent the cost and travel for the patient to line up at a drug store counter. I am not aware of any insurance company that pays for anorectic medications, so insurance claims do not present an issue. This also eliminates loose talk from a pharmacist as to what "doctor" is or is not doing in their practice, without understanding the nature of the specialty! This area of bariatric medical practice will be discussed in other sections of this book, but certainly is always an area that must be totally above-board and conform to state law!

Before beginning a bariatric in-house dispensary, you must carefully do your homework! The first basic question relates to whether or not it is allowed in your state. You may find that the dispensary practice is controlled by the State Board of Pharmacy or the Medical Board, or both! Do not guess, find these answers. Then you should have contact with your State and Federal Drug Enforcement agencies to learn what record keeping is required, as well as other extremely important issues such as what must be included on a dispensed bottle label, the type of container allowed, and where and how these drugs are kept and protected in your office. Also check to see if your state requires a state sales tax on dispensed drugs, and/or supplements.

Each state also has specific requirements as to how a prescriptive in-house drug is dispensed, from the beginning to the actual transfer to the patient. You must know what is required! Most will require an actual written prescription to be prepared and filed. Then, when the filled medication is ready to be handed to the patient, who can do this? Many states require the physician to be that person! Some states will require that the written prescription be physically handed to the patient, allowing that patient to get it filled at some other place, or hand it back to the "in-house" person to be filled. These are simple concerns but very important!

BARIATRIC LEGAL MINEFIELDS

The following are issues that are very important in a bariatric practice, as well as in any medical practice. They are here listed as a reminder of what constitutes every day concerns in the practice of medicine. This listing is obviously not an entire compilation but relates to those issues of daily importance.

1. Inadequate record documentation.
2. Incomplete history and physical examination.
3. Failure to monitor, or have monitored, a patient who also has other diseases, such as hypertension, diabetes, heart disease, or psychological problems.
4. Inadequate laboratory testing and failure to act on laboratory results!
5. Medication prescribing when the use is medically improper or otherwise contraindicated.
6. Beware of fostering drug dependency.
7. Failure to follow state law in prescribing controlled drugs when inadequate weight loss has been documented or established.
8. When thought appropriate, failure to secure written informed consent that is understood by the patient.

9. Failure to warn.
10. Be very careful to avoid a charge of assisting in "street diversion" of a controlled substance.
11. Adverse medication reactions.
12. "Off-label" prescribing without appropriate informed consent from the patient. Here, also be aware of your state's current posture on the use of these drugs for longer periods than described in the Physicians' Desk Reference or product label.
13. In a very low-calorie diet, failure to follow established guidelines requiring physician contact and the use of appropriate supplements and laboratory follow-up!

Always remember that proper and adequate documentation is an absolute necessity! The little extra time expended can pay dividends in time, costs, and emotional tranquility in the event a legal question arises.

LEGAL "DEFINITIONS" AND COMMENTS

The following definitions and related comments relate to legal procedures that one will generally encounter in the event that a medical liability complaint is made against a physician. The first definition will relate to "negligence" and what factors are involved in this haunting word! Following this material will be presentations that may be used as a review for a few legal scenarios that are commonly encountered.

STANDARD OF CARE

In earlier years, the acceptable standard of care was primarily considered a local standard that did not compare medical care given to what may have been provided on a larger scale. This is no longer the law, as the standard of care is now a national standard. Appropriate care is based on knowledge and skill learned via formal education, personal experience, and staying informed through many sources. It reflects what is medically and scientifically reasonable. An average degree of skill and care as exercised by members of the same specialty provides the foundation. An acceptable standard does not require the absolute best care available but does require that the care given is acceptable and practiced by reasonable practicing physicians. A good example of what is meant by an acceptable standard of care is simplified by an analogy. For example, suppose that, from where I live, I wanted to travel by auto to Atlanta. Consulting a map, there are a number of routes that would get me there. One or more may get me there quicker than the others selected, but they would all get me there in a reasonable period of time. All of these roads are equivalent to an acceptable standard of care. However, if I chose a road that carried me from my home in South Carolina down through Florida, or up through North Carolina on my way to Atlanta, those routes would certainly represent a deviation from an acceptable standard of care.

NEGLIGENCE—THE THEORY OF LIABILITY

Negligence Must Be Proved for a Liability Action to Prevail

The Four Essential Elements of Negligence

1. **DUTY—**To treat a patient within an acceptable standard of medical care.
2. **BREACH OF DUTY OWED**—Must show that a duty owed was not done or not completed.
3. **CAUSATION**—The breach of duty must be a proximate cause in bringing about an injury. It does not have to be the only cause of an injury.
4. **DAMAGES**—Must prove that a damage, or damages, actually resulted from the causation of an injury, during the breach of a duty owed. This element must be shown to complete the "four elements" of Negligence. Without all four elements in place, negligence has not been proven! However, keep in mind that damages may only be "nominal" in extent. When a damage is converted to monetary compensation, the amount may be small, or "nominal." Even when only a nominal damage has been proved, this will complete the "four element" requirement and may be an open door for the plaintiff to sue for "punitive damages."

LEGAL DEFENSES TO A MEDICAL NEGLIGENCE CHARGE

The following comments are among the most common bases that are used in developing a defense to a medical negligence complaint. At least one, or more, may become very important as a fundamental response.

1. A duty was satisfied.
2. No breach in a duty owed.
3. No proximate cause proven.
4. No damages resulted.
5. Mistake—not negligence.
6. Statute of limitations has run.
7. In a state or federal tort claims act, the complaint was not filed on time.
8. Informed consent was obtained.
9. Informed refusal was understood.
10. Contributory negligence by the plaintiff.
11. Comparative negligence by the plaintiff.
12. Previous release.
13. Previously tried in a different court or state.
14. "Not me"—It was someone else who was responsible! The "empty chair" defense. (A major reason that frequently several defendants are named to avoid the empty chair defense.)
15. Counter claim against the plaintiff.
16. Cross claim to bring in an unnamed defendant.
17. Contribution by others.
18. "Good Samaritan" statutes.
19. Utilize "mediation" opportunities. Some states require this prior to a trial.
20. Arbitration, rather than a trial.

PUNITIVE DAMAGES

To be awarded punitive damages, gross negligence must generally be proven! This infers that the negligence was above and more egregious than simple negligence. Concepts used to assert that gross negligence occurred include conduct departure from an acceptable standard of care that is "willful and wanton", or a "conscious disregard" for the required Standard of Care.

There are times when egregious conduct results in only nominal damages. However, even if only nominal damages are shown, this can open the door to a major punitive damage award against the physician. More often than not, a punitive damage award relates to a negative demeanor and attitude of the defendant physician!

BURDEN OF PROOF

The "burden of proof" is the degree and amount of proof required for a court or jury to find for the plaintiff in a legal action.

1. **MORE PROBABLE THAN NOT**—This is the standard in most civil actions, including medical negligence cases. When the term "preponderance of evidence" is used, it has the same meaning. This generally means 50% plus.
2. **CLEAR AND CONVINCING**—Used in more serious civil cases including a claim and complaint for "punitive damages."
3. **BEYOND A REASONABLE DOUBT**—The "burden" of proof in a criminal case.

In actual legal practice, more often than not, the jury uses the "clear and convincing" burden of proof without a clear understanding between this and the less proof requirement of the "more probable than not" standard. This is the most probable reason that the great majority of medical negligence cases that go to trial are found for the defendant physician rather than for the plaintiff!

RISK PREVENTION BASIC PRINCIPLES

1. Become consciously aware of the bariatric "minefield" problem issues.
2. Become proactive with your bariatric patients. They will do better, and you will sleep better.

3. Stay up to date in your bariatric practice and teach your employees bariatric principles important to the practice.
4. Maintain your educational foundation by keeping up with important medical issues and clinical information.

NEGLIGENCE—CONTRIBUTORY VS. COMPARATIVE?

In the not too distant past, some degree of negligence by the patient involved in a professional liability action made it very difficult for the patient to pursue a medical malpractice action. This was considered contributory negligence by the patient, and by operation of law, could bar a lawsuit. In recent years, most states have enacted comparative negligence statutes that allow a suit to go forward, but to apportion what percentage of fault was related to the patient and what percentage was related to the physician. Generally, only if the percentage of comparative negligence is equal by percentage assignment will a suit be bared. Otherwise, the physician, if found at fault, would be responsible for his or her percentage of the total damages due the patient.

AFFIDAVITS AND EXPERT TESTIMONY

Many states now require an affidavit from a separate physician attesting to the probability of negligence by the defendant. This must be included as an attachment to the formal complaint before the summons and complaint can be filed and result in the "birth" of the lawsuit. The physician who gives an affidavit may or may not be a medical expert for the plaintiff and may not surface again during the progression of the action. However, a named medical expert may be the physician who prepares the affidavit. This affidavit attests that the affiant believes that a departure from an accepted standard of medical care has occurred and damages have resulted.

INFORMED CONSENT AND REFUSAL

A nurse, or other responsible person, can review and explain an informed consent form with included information. However, it is the physician's responsibility to make sure that the patient understands the consent form and signs the form along with the patient. Many bariatric practices rely on a variety of informed consent, or refusal, forms that cover various aspects of provided care. This perhaps is not an absolute need, but the greater the evidence that a patient understood and agreed to a given treatment option, the easier it can be to provide a very strong defense for the physician.

DEPOSITIONS AND RELATED SUGGESTIONS

A deposition is a very important aspect of preparation in a medical liability lawsuit. It is a "discovery "tool used after a suit has been filed. In rare instances, a judge may allow a "discovery only" deposition to be taken before a lawsuit is filed. It may be done for discovery purposes only, or for use at trial. The standard deposition is a face-to- face confrontation. However, it may be videotaped, for use in trial or it may be taken via the telephone. In any case, a court reporter is a part of the deposition team and will administer the oath, or affirmation, for truthful answers. The court reporter will also prepare the deposition as a written transcript. The deposition is designed, and carried out, in such a manner to learn information so important to proper progression of a legal action. If the physician is the defendant and is served a notice to have his or her deposition taken, major preparation must take place! The physician's attorney will go over, and over, and over the facts in the case with the physician. One cannot be overprepared for this important event, as therein lays an early opportunity to end a case. However, if the physician's ego gets in the way, this presents an open door for the opposing attorney to create significant problems for the defendant. Be prepared!

The following considerations are important to remember when a physician is being deposed. These suggestions are equally important in all depositions, whether or not the physician is the defendant, a fact witness, or an expert witness.

1. If you do not remember or recall an event, say so! Do not guess! Problems can quickly arise when an answer constitutes a guess or an inaccurate recollection.

2. You may carry the patient's chart into the deposition room for your use. However, beware of carrying in any narrative or report generated by you. Also, any written summary of events should first be cleared with your attorney. Any other notes should also be first shown to your attorney prior to the deposition. Do not allow the opposition to gain an early unfair advantage! You can be assured that all notes, summaries and narratives will become evidence if you have them with you during the deposition. An excellent rule to follow is to show all materials to your attorney prior to bringing them into the deposition room. What you may think is unimportant may present a totally different legal connotation!
3. If the deposition is held at the physician's office, be very careful that adjacent rooms are either clear of any material related to the case in plain sight, or simply close the doors! Opposing attorneys will wander about during a break and will often go into open rooms. Materials in those rooms, which can be easily seen without plundering, are fair game and can be added sources of questions to you during the deposition. Even an open journal on your desk or table that relates to a legal issue in the involved deposition can present major problems when the deposition is resumed after the break.
4. Show, or refer to, any document during the deposition and it will generally go into evidence.
5. During any break in the deposition, be very careful of what you say to anyone, especially your attorney. When you return to the table, you may be reminded that you are still under oath, and may be asked for the content of the conversation during the break.
6. Do not become argumentative with the opposing attorney. Your attorney will generally sense this type of situation and will be able to do, or say, something that will give you a moment or so to regroup your thoughts.
7. Your attorney will raise objections to certain questions, generally under a comment as to the "form" of the question, the content or a host of other reasons. At that time, you would be instructed (generally) to go ahead and answer the question over the objection. Most of the answers to the "objected to questions" would not survive for trial purposes but could be used for other discovery investigations.
8. If you do not understand a question, ask for it to be repeated.
9. If you need a break during the deposition, ask for it.
10. If you do not know the answer, do not speculate with an answer that might hurt your cause.
11. Do not answer more than was asked in the question.
12. Do not volunteer information, unless previously discussed with your attorney.
13. The opposing attorney will generally be very cordial and "nice" during the early part of the deposition. This helps to set you up and get you off guard for later questions! That attorney is not your friend!
14. Try to stay relaxed! A slow deep breath, now and then, will be a great help.
15. If the case goes to trial and you testify in person, then the answers in your deposition can be used as an impeachment tool if your answers in court differ from the answers you gave in the deposition.
16. Be very careful in admitting that a book or article is authoritative! Such an admission on your part may turn around and "bite you."
17. Do not talk "down" to a patient, attorney, or jury! This will result in greater costs!
18. Always request a copy of your transcribed deposition for your review, corrections and signature prior to it becoming the accepted version for legal purposes. The court reporter, or your attorney, will provide you a copy with an approved errata page for you to make correction comments. Reading your own deposition is a very interesting event and it is not unusual to find answers that were not complete, or confusing. Often you will find misspelled medical words by the court reporter that may change the entire meaning of a comment. Review the document carefully and make appropriate corrections. As long as there is an appropriate reason (which you must also state on the errata page) you can record certain changes that you made to the document. Generally, you have 30 days from the time of receipt of the transcript to do your corrections and return it to the sender. If you do not complete it on time, then by operation of law, the original without corrections will become the version that is used.

FACT "VS." OPINION WITNESS

1. **FACT WITNESS**—What you know and/or have in your medical record is presented during a deposition, or at trial.
2. **OPINION WITNESS**—When you state an opinion, based on facts, either real or those in a given hypothetical situation, "That to a reasonable degree of medical certainty your opinion (whatever it is) is more probable than not, the correct observation or answer."
3. **OPINION WITNESS FEES**—If you are not the defendant in a lawsuit action, and you are in a deposition, or at trial, as a fact witness (or expert), if you are asked to give an "opinion" in addition to just facts, you are at that time an "opinion witness" and entitled to a much larger and appropriate fee! Attorneys will frequently ask you opinion questions without giving you the above information. When you give an "opinion", you open the door for greater involvement of your time in the case. You become an "expert witness."
4. **EXPERT WITNESS**—Generally expert witness is not the treating physician or fact witness. This witness is employed by an involved attorney, either for the plaintiff or the defendant, and is to provide information in the legal setting related to the departure, or nondeparture, from an Acceptable Medical Standard of Care. The fees for this work are agreed on by the expert and the attorney, generally before becoming involved in the case.

"THOSE WORDS!!"—POSSIBILITY, PROBABALITY, ALWAYS, NEVER

The above words are commonly used in medical records and narratives. Often, the physician does not give much concern to their use because they are such commonly used words and terms. However, from a legal standpoint they have totally different meanings and can become the basis of major conflicts.

1. **POSSIBILITY—**Almost anything may be possible.
2. **PROBABLE OR PROBABLITY**—Generally, this means "more likely than not"!
3. **ALWAYS AND NEVER**—Be very careful in using these words! In most situations, other than taxes and death, they do not exist. The misuse of either word in a document could become a major "headache" in a legal setting.

The active practice of bariatric medicine can be, and for most involved practitioners is, the most personally rewarding medical practice in existence today! The expressed feelings of appreciation and the changes that occur in the lives of patients because of your help, is without equal in the general practice of medicine.

However, the most important requirement for the bariatric medical practitioner is to maintain an up to date educational background! It is such a great feeling to attend Continuing Medical Education meetings and leave with the feeling that you look forward being able to put into practice on Monday morning those new, or changed, clinical approaches that you just learned.

The purpose of this "chapter" was to provide discussion and listing of the more important issues that are germane fundamentals in a bariatric practice and present legal definitions and related comments to create at least a basic familiarity with the more commonly encountered legal scenarios. It would not be unusual for the reading of certain sections in the latter part of this presentation to be an excellent treatment for insomnia. It is hoped that, if a need arises, the included material will give you some basic information that you may quickly need!

Appendix A
Notes on nutrition for bariatricians

Jeffrey D. Lawrence

A full discussion of human nutrition is beyond the scope of this book. However, it is important to emphasize that bariatricians must have a good understanding of basic nutritional science. It does not make any sense to just reduce caloric intake without any regard to maintaining adequate levels of the various essential nutrients. While obesity has been shown to be important factor for many medical conditions, nutritional deficiencies alone can cause many medical problems. Many of these conditions are life altering or threatening. The following outline covers some basic nutritional information. I suggest checking one of the many nutrition textbooks for a more complete discussion.

Lastly, the information below is basic normal nutrition. When we manipulate the macronutrients to achieve weight loss, we must adjust all of the micronutrients. With very low-calorie, protein-sparing diets, for example, micronutrient supplementation is required. With low-fat diets there must be adequate amounts of essential fatty acids and fat-soluble vitamins. Low carbohydrate diets must have adequate water-soluble vitamins, minerals, and fiber.

ENERGY REQUIREMENTS

RDA—Men: 2300 to 2900 kcal/day; women: 1900 to 2200 kcal/day

Basal

Resting Metabolic Rate (RMR)—energy expended resting in bed, in the morning, at the time of fasting, and in ambient conditions. Correlates with gender (women lower), lean body mass (more muscle = higher RMR), slight decline with age, and correlates with body temperature (biomarker?). Largest component of energy needs (60–70%).

Resting Energy Expenditure (REE)—energy expended at rest and in ambient conditions (not necessarily fasting, before noon). Used by World Health Organization, differs less than 10% from RMR, used interchangeably.

Physical Activity

Energy expenditure due to occupation has declined; recreational activity is now an important determinant. Energy requirement is proportional to body weight; however, obesity is associated with lower activity level. Second largest component of energy requirements (20–40%).

Thermic Effect of Food

Metabolic rate increases after eating, maximum at one hour. Energy expenditure small (10–15% of total).

Other Determinants of Energy Needs

Age—Lean body mass declines beyond early adulthood at 2% to 3% per decade, one factor in calculating REE.

Gender—Ten percent difference of REE per unit weight between men (higher) and women due to increased muscle mass of men.

Growth—Except for first year of life, small component.

Body size—Large bodies require more energy per unit of time for activities which involve moving mass over distance (e.g., walking).

Climate—Requirements increase when physically active in extreme heat. Exposure to cold conditions may also increase needs due to increased muscle activity or shivering.

Special Requirements

Pregnancy—increased need of 300 kcal/day
Lactation—increased need of 500 kcal/day
Disease states—malabsorption, infection, trauma, and surgery will increase needs variably.

Calorie

Kilocalorie (kcal)—the amount of heat necessary to raise 1 kg of water from 15°C to 16°C. Note: We do not eat calories, we eat food. All food is not burned for energy.

DIETARY STANDARDS

Recommended Dietary Allowances (RDAs)

The levels of intake of essential nutrients that, **on the basis of scientific knowledge**, are judged by the Food and Nutrition Board of the National Research Council to be adequate to meet the known nutrient needs of 97% to 98% **healthy persons**. They are amounts intended to be consumed as part of a normal diet. If they are met through diets with a variety of foods from diverse food groups rather than by supplementation, such diets are likely to be adequate in other nutrients for which RDAs cannot currently be established. **RDAs are neither minimal requirements nor necessarily optimal levels of intake**. Rather, RDAs are safe and adequate levels of intake (with built-in margins of safety to account for the variability in requirements among people) with regard to the knowledge about a nutrient. RDAs generally **allow substantial storage** to cover periods of reduced intake or increased needs. The RDAs are set to meet the needs of 97% to 98% of individuals in that group. The RDA values for nutrients were, in the past, revised on a regular basis by the Food and Nutrition Board of the National Research Council (NRC) and published in book form. It was last done in 1989.

U.S. Recommended Daily Allowances (U.S. RDA)

Started in 1974 by the U.S. Food and Drug Administration (U.S. FDA) to be used for labeling only. Unlike the RDA, it used a single standard for everyone older than 4 years. There were separate values for infants, toddlers, and pregnant and lactating women. They are dated and no longer used.

Daily Values and Percent Daily Values (DVs and % DV)

Introduced for labeling purposes only. The purpose was to allow people to compare processed foods. Data for the macronutrients, fat, carbohydrates, and protein that are the sources of energy and for cholesterol, sodium, potassium, and vitamins A and C, which do not contribute calories. In 2006, the amount of trans-fatty acids was added. The DV is based on a 2000-calorie daily intake.

Dietary Reference Intakes (DRIs)

This standard is an ongoing effort by the National Research Council to create a set of reference values that can be used for planning and assessing diets for healthy populations and for many other purposes. They will replace the periodic revisions of the RDAs. Their first report, "Dietary Reference Intakes for Calcium, Phosphorus, Magnesium, Vitamin D, and Fluoride," was published by the National Academy Press in March 1998. The DRIs refer to daily intakes averaged over time and are classified as follows:

EAR (Estimated Average Requirement)—Intake that meets the nutrient need of 50% of individuals in that group.

AI (Adequate Intake)—Average observed or experimentally derived intake by a defined population or subgroup that appears to sustain a defined nutritional state, such as normal circulating nutrient values, growth, or other functional indicators of health. AI is expected to exceed the EAR and possibly the RDA.

RDA (Recommended Dietary Allowance)—See definition above; this is the value to be used in guiding individuals to achieve adequate nutrient intake. It is a "target" intake. Remember that nutrient intake less than the RDA does not necessarily mean that the criterion for adequacy has not been met. RDA is generally defined as EAR + 2 standard deviations.

UL (Tolerable Upper Intake Level)—The maximum intake by an individual that is unlikely to pose risks of adverse health effects in almost all (97–98%) individuals.

Acceptable Macronutrient Distribution Ranges (AMDR)—Healthy range of intake for carbohydrates, fat, and protein (expressed as percentage of total daily calories) that are sufficient to provide adequate nutrients while reducing the risk of chronic disease.

45% to 65% of daily calories from carbohydrate
10% to 35% of daily calories from protein
20% to 35% of daily calories from fat
5% to 10% of daily calories from linoleic acid (omega 6)
0.6 to 1.2% of daily calories from alpha-linolenic acid (omega-3)

There are DRIs for water, all vitamins, minerals, electrolytes, antioxidants, protein, fats, and carbohydrates. The complete tables can be viewed at many web sites.

NUTRIENTS

Macronutrients

Defined as the principal dietary sources of energy.

1. **Proteins**—RDA (Men: 63 g/day; women: 50 g/day). Furnish amino acids required to build and maintain body tissues. Several times more protein is turned over daily within the body than is ordinarily consumed, indicating that reutilization of amino acids is a major feature of protein metabolism. As an energy source they are equivalent to carbohydrates, providing 4 kcal/g.
   a. Dietary sources—Meat, poultry, fish, milk, legumes (soybeans, peanuts, peas, beans, lentils), and cereals (much lesser amount of protein per serving, but important because of total quantity consumed).
   b. Digestion
      Stomach: (Pepsin) Proteins → Polypeptides
      Small intestine:
      (Carboxypeptidase) Polypeptides, dipeptides → Amino acids
      (Trypsin, chymotrypsin) Proteins, polypeptides → Amino acids
      (Enterokinase) activates trypsinogen
      (Aminopeptidase) Polypeptides, dipeptides → Amino acids
      (Dipeptidase) Dipeptides → Amino acids
   c. Requirements—based on the following:
      Nitrogen balance—The difference between measured nitrogen intake and the amount excreted in urine, feces, sweat, and other minor losses is measured. Data are extrapolated to zero balance point for adults, or to defined positive balance for children to allow for growth.
   d. Essential amino acids
      Leucine
      Isoleucine
      Valine
      Tryptophan
      Phenylalanine
      Methionine
      Threonine
      Lysine
      Histidine (in infants only, adults can synthesis it)
   e. Deficiency—Rarely occurs as an isolated condition. It usually accompanies energy and other nutrient deficiencies from insufficient food intake.
      Primary
      1. Protein/calorie. malnutrition (marasmus)
      2. Protein malnutrition with adequate calories (kwashiorkor)

Secondary—illness
1. Inflammatory bowel disease
2. Chronic renal failure
3. Intestinal malabsorption
4. Malignancy

f. Excess—No current firm evidence that increased levels are harmful, other than obesity.
g. High-protein diets can be an important part of weight management programs. Current literature suggests increased satiety, increased thermogenesis, and protection of lean body mass with 30% protein diets.

2. **Carbohydrates**
RDA ($\geq$ 50% of daily calories, 250 g in a 2000-cal diet) As a macronutrient, it is an important source of energy. Provides 4 kcal/g, as does protein.
   a. Sugar
      Monosaccharides—glucose, fructose
      Disaccharides—Sucrose = glucose + fructose (table sugar)
      Maltose = glucose + glucose
      Lactose = glucose + galactose (milk sugar)
   b. Complex carbohydrates
      Starches—polymers of glucose
      Dietary fiber
      Soluble—pectins, gums, mucilages; found primarily in fruits and vegetables, can hold water and form gels, can act as substrate for fermentation by colonic bacteria (apples, oranges, carrots, oats)
      Insoluble—cellulose and some hemicellulose (bran layer of cereal)
      Lignin—a noncarbohydrate that is often included in fiber determinations, provides structure to the woody parts of plants
   c. Dietary sources—most originate in foods of plant origin, lactose is an exception (milk). Plants such as cereal grains are major source.
   d. Digestion
      Mouth: (Salivary amylase) starch → disaccharides
      Small intestine: (Pancreatic amylase) Starch → Maltose
      (Sucrase): Sucrose → Glucose + Fructose
      (Maltase): Maltose → Glucose
      (Lactase) Lactose → Glucose + Galactose
   e. Deficiency: Dietary fiber—constipation, possible increase in incidence of colon cancer.
   f. The fructose problem

There has been a large increase in the amount of dietary fructose consumption, coming largely from added sucrose (glucose + fructose) and high fructose corn syrup to foods and drinks.

This increase of fructose load to the liver disturbs glucose metabolism and the glucose uptake pathways and leads to an enhanced rate of de novo lipogenesis and triglyceride synthesis. These changes may underlie the induction of insulin resistance and metabolic syndrome.

3. **Fats**
RDA: 5% to 30% of daily calories, <67 g in a 2000-calorie diet. Aid in transport and absorption of the fat-soluble vitamins, depress gastric secretion, slow gastric emptying, add palatability to the diet, and reduce feeling of satiety. Energy-dense source of fuel, with 9 kcal/g.
   a. Dietary sources—More than one-third of the calories consumed by most of the people in the United States is provided by fat. Animal products in particular contribute more than half the fat, three-fourths of the saturated fat, and all of the cholesterol. **Ground beef has been found to be the single largest contributor to fat in the U.S. diet**. Eggs supply the most cholesterol. Grains, nuts, and animal and vegetable oils are some of the good sources of fats.
   b. Nonpolar—mainly esters of fatty acids, insoluble in water, enter metabolic pathways only after hydrolysis.
      Triglycerides—three fatty acids + glycerol

c. Polar

Fatty acids – polar component is a negatively charged carboxyl ion. More than 90% have even number of carbons.

Classification:

Short-chain fatty acid (FAs) (<6 carbons)

Medium-chain FAs (6–10 carbons)

Long-chain FAs (12 or more carbons)

Saturated—no double bonds

RDA ($\leq$ 10% of daily calories)

Palmitic acid and stearic acid are major ones.

Monounsaturated—single double bond

Polyunsaturated—more than one double bond

Essential fatty acids—prevent deficiency symptoms and cannot be synthesized by humans. They carry fat-soluble vitamins.

Linoleic acid

The primary **omega-6 fatty acid**. It does not have the properties of the **omega-**3 fatty acids.

Deficiency causes dermatitis and poor growth.

α-Linolenic Acid

The primary **omega-3 fatty acid**. It is converted to a hormone-like substances that reduce inflammation

Deficiency causes neurological changes (numbness, paresthesias, weakness, inability to walk, blurring of vision)

(Both are 18 carbon unsaturated fatty acids.)

Cholesterol—polar component is an alcohol. RDA (<300 mg/day)

With phospholipids, it is a major component of all cell membranes; a precursor to steroid hormones of adrenal and gonadal origin and of the bile acids. Amount of fat ingested, especially saturated fatty acids, affects serum levels. Cholesterol intake in the diet has a lesser but appreciable effect.

Phospholipids—see the previous text

Olestra: This is not a fat. It is a sucrose polyester which has the taste and properties of fat and is not absorbed in the gastrointestinal tract.

d. Digestion

Stomach: (Gastric lipase) Emulsified fats → Glycerol + Fatty acids

Small intestine: (Pancreatic lipase) Fats → Glycerol + Mono and diglycerides + Fatty acids

(Intestinal lipase) Fats → Glycerol +Glycerides + Fatty acids

(Bile) Accelerates action of pancreatic lipase, emulsifies fat, neutralizes chyme, and stabilizes emulsions

e. Deficiencies (essential fatty acids)—dermatitis, alopecia, and fat-soluble vitamin deficiencies.

f. Trans-fatty acids. Hydrated polyunsaturated fats. Created by food chemists to solidify liquid fats and increase shelf life of fat containing processed food (e.g., cookies 90%, fatty snacks 50%). Have been related to cardiovascular disease. Should be eliminated or at least markedly reduced in the diet.

Micronutrients

1. **Vitamins**—Thirteen organic molecules needed in the diet in tiny amounts. They can serve two functions in the body. In small amounts they serve as catalysts, increasing the speed of a chemical reaction without being used up by that reaction. In large doses (above a body's demand) they can act like drugs or chemicals causing other, sometimes significant, effects. Original theory as "Vital Amines" has been discredited.

   a. Fat soluble—are absorbed with other lipids, need bile and pancreatic juice for efficient absorption. Are stored in various body tissues, notably fat.

   Vitamin A (retinol, B-carotene) (retinoids)

   RDA—(Men: 1000 RE (retinol equivalents)/day) (Women: 800 RE/day) 1/2 cup of cooked spinach and 1/2 carrot.

Carotenoids are provitamins, converted by the body to A.

Dietary sources: Preformed vitamin A from foods of animal origin (liver, fat from milk and eggs). Carotenoids from carrots, dark green leafy vegetables. Fortified foods. Cooking increases bioavailability but overcooking decreases.

Digestion: Absorbed: Small intestine

Stored: 90% in liver

Deficiency : Ocular—night blindness, corneal lesions (xeropthalmia); cutaneous—follicular hyperkeratosis "goose flesh" (keratin plugs), dry, scaly, rough skin.

Excess: Nausea, vomiting, fatigue, diplopia, alopecia, dryness of mucous membranes, desquamation, and death; carotenoids, even in large amounts, are safe because of limited conversion to active vitamin A; skin may turn yellow, however.

Vitamin D (Calciferol)

RDA—(5 μg/day = 200 IU) 2 cups of fortified milk and 1 oz of salmon or brief exposure of face, arms, and hands to sunlight. There is a strong suggestion that the RDA for vitamin D in the far northern and southern hemispheres should be 50 μg = 2000 IU due to the lack of exposure to ultraviolet (UV) light.

Calcitrol (most active form of D) stimulates synthesis of calcium-binding protein in intestine, promoting calcium absorption.

Dietary sources: Vitamin D (cholecalciferol) is a provitamin formed in the skin by the action of UV rays from sunlight. It is also found in fish liver oils. Milk and many dairy products are fortified with D2 (ergosterol). It is remarkably stable and does not deteriorate with heating.

Absorbed: Small intestine.

Stored: Liver, skin, brain, bones.

Deficiency: Children—rickets; Adults—osteomalacia.

Excess: Calcification of soft tissues like kidney (including stones), lungs, tympanic membrane (deafness), also headache, nausea.

Vitamin E (tocopherols, tocotrienols)

RDA—(Men: 10 α-tocopherol equivalents; women: 8 α-tocopherol equivalents) 1 tbs corn oil, 1.5 cups of milk, and two avocados.

An antioxidant, vitamin E protects cellular and subcellular membranes from deterioration by scavenging free radicals that contain oxygen. Is currently under study in preventing aging effects of environmental toxins and the triggering of some forms of carcinogenesis.

Dietary sources: Seed oils, especially wheat germ oil; stable with cooking (in water) except deep fat frying; freezing also destroys.

Absorbed: Small intestine (inefficiently); stored: liver and fat

Deficiency: Uncommon; peripheral neuropathy

Excess: Low toxicity, possibly bleeding associated with warfarin use.

Vitamin K (phylloquinone (K1) and menaquinone (K2))

RDA—(Men: 80 μg/day, women: 65 μg/day) 50 g broccoli, 66 g cabbage, 200 g green beans. Antihemorrhagic factor: acts as cofactor for carboxylase in the liver in the formation of prothrombin, among other proteins. Warfarin drugs antagonize the action of vitamin K.

Dietary sources: Green leafy vegetables, especially broccoli, cabbage, turnip greens, and lettuce. A significant amount is formed by the intestinal flora of the lower intestinal tract. Fairly resistant to heat, not destroyed by ordinary cooking methods.

Absorption: Small intestine, requires bile and pancreatic juice.

Storage: Liver.

Deficiency: Associated with lipid malabsorption or destruction of intestinal flora by antibiotics. Liver disease which prevents utilization produces deficiency. Newborns are susceptible because of poor placental transfer and failure to establish intestinal bacteria which produce vitamin K.

Excess: Excessive doses of synthetic K have produced kernicterus in infants.

b. Water soluble—Most are components of essential enzyme systems, are not normally stored in the body in appreciable amounts, and excreted in the urine.

Thiamin (B_1)

RDA—(Men: 1.5 mg/day, women: 1.1 mg/day) 3 oz of lean pork and 1.5 cups of roasted peanuts.

Coenzyme in phosphate forms vital to tissue respiration. Strongly linked to carbohydrate metabolism.

Dietary sources: Lean pork, wheat germ, and organ meats. Cooking losses highly variable, depending on cooking time, temperature, and quantity of water.

Absorption: Actively transported in the acid medium of the proximal duodenum. Can be inhibited by alcohol.

Storage: Liver

Deficiency: Seen most frequently in alcoholics, clinical signs most often involve nervous (dementia) and cardiovascular systems. Beriberi includes mental confusion, muscle wasting (dry beriberi), edema (wet beriberi), peripheral paralysis, tachycardia, and enlarged heart.

Excess: No known toxic effects.

Riboflavin (B_2)

RDA—(Men: 1.7 mg/day, women: 1.3 mg/day) 1.5 oz of beef liver and 3 cups of fruit-flavored low-fat yogurt.

Discovered as a yellow-green fluorescent pigment in milk, is a component of the coenzyme flavin adenine diphosphate (FAD) important in energy production.

Dietary sources: Milk, cheddar cheese, cottage cheese, organ meats, and eggs. Heat, oxidation, and acid stable but disintegrates in alkali or UV light. Little lost in the cooking and processing of food.

Absorption: Actively absorbed in the proximal small intestine.

Storage: Not stored in any great amount, must be supplied in the diet regularly.

Deficiency: Usually associated with deficiencies of other water-soluble vitamins. Photophobia, lacrimation, burning–itching eyes, soreness, and burning of the lips and the tongue. Cheilosis (fissuring of lips) and angular stomatitis (cracks in the skin at the corners of the mouth).

Excess: No known toxicity.

Niacin (nicotinic acid and nicotinamide) (B_3)

RDA—(Men: 19 mg NE/day) (niacin equivalents) (women: 15 mg NE/day) Average daily intake: 41 mg NE (men), 27 mg NE (women)

Acts as coenzyme in oxidation/reduction.

Dietary sources: Lean meats, poultry, fish, and peanuts. Resistant to heat, light, air, acids, and alkalis—small amount may be lost in cooking water.

Niacin can be synthesized from tryptophan with vitamin B_6 as a cofactor.

Absorption: Small intestine

Storage: Very little storage

Deficiency: Pellagra: (4 Ds = dermatitis, dementia, diarrhea, and death), tremors, and sore tongue. Seen on highly inadequate diets with little niacin and inadequate protein.

Excess: Large doses of niacin (1–2 g tid) can cause histamine release with flushing, also liver toxicity.

Vitamin B_6 (pyridoxine, pyridoxal, pyridoxamine)

RDA—(Men: 2.0 mg/day; women: 1.6 mg/day) 5 oz of liver and 12 oz of chicken.

Coenzyme in transamination and other reactions related to protein metabolism.

Dietary sources: Yeast, wheat germ, pork, glandular meats, whole grain cereals, and oatmeal. Unstable in light; losses in freezing, 36% to 55%.

Absorption: Upper small intestine

Storage: Muscle (up to 50% of stores)

Deficiency: Rare, medications [isoniazid, Birth Control Pills (BCPs)] can interfere with metabolism. Malaise, depression, and glucose intolerance. With severe deficiency, convulsions.

Excess: Seen in premenstural syndrome (PMS) treatment studies; ataxia and severe sensory neuropathy.

Folic acid

RDA—(Men: 200 μg/day, women: 180 μg/day) 3 oz of fried beef liver and 3/4 cup of white baked beans. Women of reproductive age planning to conceive—400 μg/day to prevent neural tube defects).

Important role in RNA and DNA synthesis/function.

Dietary sources: Liver, kidney beans, lima beans, and fresh dark green leafy vegetables (spinach, asparagus, broccoli). Losses occur with storage of vegetables at room temperature and during processing at high temperatures.

Absorption: Folate broken down, then actively absorbed in the small intestine.

Storage: In the form of methyltetrahydrofolic acid.

Deficiency: Alteration of DNA metabolism, therefore, affects rapidly dividing cells—red blood cells, leukocytes; epithelium of stomach, intestine, vagina, and cervix. See poor growth, megaloblastic anemia, glossitis, and gastrointestinal tract disturbances.

Excess: No toxicity reported in adults.

Vitamin B_{12} (cobalamin)

RDA—(2.0 pg/day) 2 oz of canned tuna and 4 oz of beef hamburger.

Essential for the normal function of all cells, DNA synthesis, affects myelin formation.

Dietary sources: Animal protein foods, liver, kidney, milk, eggs, cheese, fish, and muscle meats.

Absorption: Hydrochloric acid in the stomach releases cobalamin from its peptide bonds, binds with the intrinsic factor, and then is absorbed in the ileum. **There is a problem of poor absorption in patients after bariatric surgery because of reduced stomach HCl.**

Storage: Liver and kidney before release to bone marrow and other tissues.

Deficiency: Megaloblastic anemia, glossitis, hypospermia, and degeneration of central and peripheral nerves (seen as numbness, tingling, and burning of the feet with stiffness and weakness of the legs).

Excess: No known toxic effects.

Pantothenic acid

RDA—(Level not determined but 4–7 mg estimated) 3 oz of beef liver and 6 cups of low-fat yogurt with fruit.

Constituent of coenzyme A essential to many areas of cellular metabolism.

Dietary sources: Present in all plant and animal tissues, egg yolk, kidney, liver, and yeast. A total of 33% lost in cooking and 50% lost in milling of flour.

Absorption: Small intestine.

Storage: Little known.

Deficiency: No deficiency disease observed in humans.

Excess: No serious toxic effects known.

Biotin

RDA—(Not known, but 30–100 μg/day estimate).

Coenzyme for reactions involving gluconeogenesis, synthesis and oxidation of fatty acids, and purine synthesis.

Dietary sources: Protein bound in most natural foods, significant amount synthesized by intestinal bacteria. Kidney, liver, egg yolk, soybeans, and yeast. Stable to heat, soluble in water and alcohol. *Absorption*: Readily absorbed; taken up by liver, muscle, and kidney.

Storage: Little is known.

Deficiency: Dry scaly dermatitis, pallor, alopecia, nausea; long-term anticonvulsant drugs interfere with biotin transport.

Excess: No known toxic effects.

Vitamin C (ascorbic acid)

RDA—(60 mg/day) One orange, "spear" fresh broccoli, one grapefruit.

Antiscorbutic vitamin, has multiple functions as either a coenzyme or a cofactor, can lose and take on hydrogen, helps iron absorption, and is involved in collagen formation, and promotes resistance to infection via immunologic function of leukocytes, interferon production, or integrity of the mucous membrane. Findings related to prevention and cure of the common cold are controversial. It is an important antioxidant.

Dietary sources: Fresh acidic fruits and vegetables (citrus fruits, fresh leafy vegetables, and tomatoes). It is easily destroyed by oxidation particularly with heat and alkali. Cooking should be rapid, in little water, and food served immediately. Refrigeration and quick freezing help retain vitamin.

Absorption: Small intestine; between 20 and 120 mg absorption, 90%; at high intakes (12 g) only 16%.

Storage: Adrenals, kidney, liver, and spleen, in equilibrium with serum.

Deficiency: Scurvy, swollen and inflamed gums, loosening teeth, dryness of the mouth and eyes, loss of hair, dry itchy skin, failure of wound healing, and possible gallstone formation.

Excess: Diarrhea from osmotic effect of unabsorbed vitamin; excreted in the urine, can give a false + test for sugar. In amount greater than 10× the normal amount may inhibit absorption of vitamin B_{12}.

Vitamin-like factors

Other food factors that have some but not all of the characteristic of vitamins. Their role is unclear. Requirements are unclear.

Choline: As phosphatidylcholine it is a structural element of membranes, a precursor of sphingolipids, and promoter of lipid transport. As acetylcholine it functions as a neurotransmitter and as a component of platelet-activating factor. DRI varies with age. Has been used in very high doses to alleviate symptoms of tardive dyskinesia and Huntington disease. Has been used with some success to diminish short-term memory loss in Alzheimer's disease.

Others: Carnitine, Myo-inositol, pyrroloquinoline, quinone, ubiquinones, and the bioflavonoids.

2. **Minerals**

Constitute 4% to 5% of body weight (40% calcium)

a. Calcium

RDA—(1200 mg/day through age 24; 800–1200 mg thereafter).

Four cups of milk and 3 cups of yogurt with fruit.

Functions in building and maintaining bone and teeth, as well as cell membrane stabilization, role in membrane transport, important in nerve transmission, and blood clotting.

Dietary sources: Dairy products, dark green leafy vegetables, sardines, and canned salmon.

Absorption: Duodenum and proximal jejunum in acidic medium; vitamin D stimulates absorption.

Storage: Nonexchangeable skeletal pool; exchangeable pool in trabeculae of bone. Stored in the form of hydroxyapatite crystals.

Deficiency: Bone deformities (osteoporosis, osteomalacia), tetany, hypertension

Excess: With high levels of vitamin D may lead to excessive calcification of bone and soft tissues, can interfere with iron absorption if taken at same time.

b. Magnesium

RDA—(Men: 350 mg/day, women: 280 mg/day) 3 cups of chili with beans and 1 cup of roasted cashews.

Intracellular cation, acts as a cofactor in more than 300 metabolic processes.

Dietary sources: Seeds, nuts, legumes, and unmilled cereal grains; lost during refining and processing.

Absorption: Most in jejunum, but all along small intestine.

Storage: 60% in bone, 26% in muscle.

Deficiency: Tremor, muscle spasms, personality changes, anorexia, and possible cardiac arrhythmias.

Excess: With normal renal function, is excreted; with compromised renal function, can see nausea, vomiting, hypotension, and hypotonia; may progress to respiratory depression and asystolic arrest.

c. Phosphorus

RDA—(Same as calcium, 800–1200 mg/day) 4 cups of milk and two grilled cheese sandwiches.

One of most essential elements, 80% bound as calcium phosphate crystals in bone and teeth; many functions—DNA, RNA, ATP, CAMP.

Dietary sources: Meat, poultry, fish, eggs, and dairy products.

Absorption: Mostly as inorganic phosphate; organic phosphate hydrolyzed in the acid environment of the proximal jejunum for absorption. Vegetarian diets contain mainly phytate which is poorly digested in humans.

Storage: Bone, every cell in body.

Deficiency: From decreased production of ATP; there can be various neuromuscular, skeletal, hematologic, and renal abnormalities.

Excess: Can lower blood calcium level.

d. Iron

RDA—(Men: 10 mg/day, women: 15 mg/day) 6 oz of beef liver and 1/4 cup of clams.

Constituent of hemoglobin, myoglobin.

Dietary sources: Liver, oysters, shellfish, kidney, heart, and lean meat.

Absorption: Small intestine, heme iron highly absorbed; nonheme iron absorption can be influenced by presence of vitamin C.

Storage: Ferritin and hemosiderin (spleen, liver, and bone marrow).

Deficiency: Most common nutritional deficiency. Most common cause of anemia among children and women of childbearing age. Manifested by a hypochromic, microcytic anemia, corrected by iron supplementation.

Excess: Seen with hereditary hemochromatosis. Recent studies do not support relationship between high serum ferritin and risk of heart disease.

e. Zinc

RDA—(Men: 15 mg/day, women: 12 mg/day) 1/4 cup of pacific oysters and 9 oz of ground beef.

Known to participate in reactions involving synthesis or degradation of major metabolites.

Dietary sources: Meat, fish, poultry, and milk.

Absorption: Small intestine, not well understood.

Storage: All tissues.

Deficiency: Short stature, hypogonadism, and mild anemia; delayed wound healing, alopecia, skin lesions, and zinc responsive night blindness.

f. Iodine

RDA—(150 μg/day) 1/2 tsp of iodized salt and four slices of bread.

Integral part of thyroid hormone.

Dietary sources: Seafood and iodized salt.

Absorption: Easily in small intestine.

Storage: Primarily in the thyroid gland; also in mammary tissue.

Deficiency: Cretinism (severe deficiency during gestation and early postnatal growth) and goiter.

Excess: Goiter can be seen in long-term excesses.

g. Selenium

An antioxidant—no comprehensive table for content in food; present in brazil nuts, seafood, and kidney.

h. Copper

Normal constituent of blood, component of many enzymes.

Deficiency causes microcytic, hemochromic anemia followed by neutropenia, leukopenia, and bone demineralization. Wilson's disease is characterized by accumulation of excess copper in body tissues from genetic defect in liver synthesis of ceruloplasmin.

i. Manganese
Found in tissues rich in mitochondria, is a component of many enzymes.
Dietary sources: Found in whole grains, legumes, nuts, and tea.
Deficiency: Causes weight loss, transient dermatitis, and slow growth of hair.

j. Fluoride
Essential because of its beneficial effect on tooth enamel, resisting dental caries.
Major source is fluoridated drinking water and tea leaves.

k. Chromium
RDA—(50–200 μg/day). In self-selected diet of 2300 kcal, average intake is 33 μg/day.
Chromium potentiates insulin action and, therefore, influences carbohydrate, lipid, and protein metabolism. In 1977, patients receiving total parenteral nutrition (TPN) exhibited abnormalities of glucose metabolism reversed by chromium supplementation. Proposed role as "glucose tolerance factor" is controversial.
Dietary sources: Difficult to assess because biologically available and inorganic chromium cannot be distinguished from each other. Brewer's yeast, oysters, liver, and potatoes have high concentrations.
Absorption: Organic and inorganic forms are absorbed differently. Organic is easily absorbed but quickly passes out of the body. Less than 2% of trivalent chromium consumed is absorbed. There appears to be a commonality with iron absorption pathways. Is carried by transferrin.
Strenuous exercise increases excretion of chromium.
Deficiency: Mertz (1993) (2) concluded the following:

1. Chromium deficiency results in insulin resistance.
2. Insulin resistance caused by chromium deficiency can be ameliorated by chromium supplementation.
3. Chromium deficiency does occur in populations in the United States and may be an important cause of insulin resistance. In animals, deficiency signs include impaired growth, elevated serum cholesterol and triglyceride concentrations, increased aortic plaques, corneal lesions, and decreased fertility and sperm count.
4. Chromium for weight loss: In a study by Grant et al. (1) using 43 obese women, the women on 400 μg of chromium picolinate gained weight, whereas those on chromium nicotinate lost weight if they were engaged in exercise as well. Recent meta-analyses of studies of chromium suggest only minimal effects on weight loss. It has been shown to be toxic in bacterial cultures.

l. Molybdenum
Required in enzymes which catalyze oxidation–reduction reactions.
Distributed widely in commonly used foods, such as legumes, whole grain cereals, milk, and milk products.

VEGETARIANISM

(a) *Lacto-ovo vegetarian*—Eats no meat, fish, or poultry. Does include milk, cheese, dairy products, and eggs.
(b) *Lactovegetarian*—Eats no meat, fish, poultry, or eggs. Does include milk, cheese, and other dairy products.
(c) *Vegan*—Eats no food of animal origin.

The only variety of vegetarianism which incorporates any real risk of inadequate nutrition. This can be avoided with careful planning.

1. *Iron*—Assimilation of nonheme iron in fruits, vegetables, and unrefined cereals aided with ascorbic acid.
2. *Calcium*—Without dairy products, calcium and vitamin D intake may be low.
3. B_{12}—Megaloblastic anemia may develop in long-standing vegans. B_{12} occurs only in foods of animal origin. High levels of folate may mask the neurological damage of this deficiency. Vegans need a reliable source, such as fortified cereals, soy beverages, or supplements.

4. *Protein*—Lower content than most omnivores. Usually results in lower intake of dietary fat. Sources should be varied (cereals + legumes) to ensure complimentary proteins.

BARIATRIC SURGERY-RELATED NUTRITIONAL PROBLEMS

Highly dependent on the type of surgery done. In the Roux-en-Y procedure the duodenum and part of the jejunum are eliminated. The absorption of Ca, iron, and B_{12} is depressed. This can result in anemia from lack of iron and B_{12} and osteoporosis from lack of Ca.

Dumping syndrome results from rapid passage of food into the small intestine, which shifts fluid too quickly into the intestine. The result is often diarrhea and dehydration. Cramping, sweating, flushed appearance, dizziness, weakness, and headaches characterize dumping syndrome. This results in electrolyte imbalance and reduced fat-soluble vitamin absorption.

REFERENCES

1. Grant KE, Chandler RM, Castle AL, et al. Chromium and exercise training: effect on obese women. Med Sci Sports Exerc 1997; 29(8):992–998.
2. Mertz W. Chromium in Human Nutrition: A review. J Nut 1993; 123(4):626–636.

BIBLIOGRAPHY

Barrett S, Herbert V. The Vitamin Pushers. Amherst, NY: Prometheus Books, 1994.

(Written by two physicians respected for their work in exposing quackery in medicine. Reviews many of the common myths regarding vitamins and supplementation. Old but still of interest.)

Charles VanWay III, Carol Ireton-Jones. Nutrition Secrets. Hanley and Belfus, 2003.

Food and Nutrition Board—National Research Council. Recommended Dietary Allowances. 10th ed. Washington, DC: National Academy Press, 1989.

(Published by the National Research Council, the basics on RDAs. Now out of print, will be replaced by the various reports of DRIs released in a serial fashion.)

Mahan L, Escott-Stump S. Krause's Food, Nutrition, & Diet Therapy. 12th ed. Philadelphia, PA: WB. Saunders Co, 2005.

(An up-to-date comprehensive text for nutrition professionals. An in-depth look at nutrition in health and disease. Despite its size, very readable.)

Mahan LK, Sylvia E-S. Nutritional Concepts and Controversies. 11th ed. Philadelphia, PA: Saunders, 2008.

Rinzler CA. Nutrition for Dummies. 2nd ed. New York, NY: Hungry Minds, 1999. (Fun, easy book on basic nutrition.)

Appendix B
Behavioral modification forms

Erin Chamberlin-Snyder

Patient Medical History Form

Name: ______________________________________ Age:________ Sex: M F

Present Status:

1. Are you in good health at the present time to the best of your knowledge? Yes No
   Explain a "no" answer:

2. Are you under a doctor's care at the present time? Yes No
   If yes, for what?

3. Are you taking any medications at the present time? Yes No

   Prescription Drugs: List all
   Drug: Dosage:

   Over-the-Counter medications, vitamins, supplements: List all Yes No
   Product Dosage

4. Any allergies to any medications? Yes No
   Please list:

5. History of High Blood Pressure? Yes No

6. History of Diabetes? Yes No
   At what age: ____________

7. History of Heart Attack or Chest Pain or other heart condition? Yes No

8. History of Swelling Feet Yes No

9. History of Frequent Headaches? Yes No
   Migraines? Yes No Medications for Headaches: ___________________________

10. History of Constipation (difficulty in bowel movements)? Yes No

11. History of Glaucoma? Yes No

12. History of Sleep Apnea? Yes No

13. Gynecologic History:
    Pregnancies: Number: ________________ Dates: ________________________
    Natural Delivery or C-Section (specify): ________________________________
    Menstrual: Onset: ________________
    Duration: ________________
    Are they regular: Yes No
    Pain associated: Yes No
    Last menstrual period: ________________________________
    Hormone Replacement Therapy: Yes No
    What: ____
    Birth Control Pills: Yes No
    Type: ____
    Last Check Up: ____

14. Serious Injuries: Yes No
    Specify (list all) Date

15. Any Surgery: Yes No
    Specify: (List all) Date

16. Family History:

	Age	Health	Disease	Cause of Death	Overweight?
Father:					
Mother:					
Brothers:					
Sisters:					

Has any blood relative ever had any of the following:

Glaucoma:	Yes	No	Who: ________________
Asthma:	Yes	No	Who: ________________
Epilepsy:	Yes	No	Who: ________________
High Blood Pressure	Yes	No	Who: ________________
Kidney Disease:	Yes	No	Who: ________________
Diabetes:	Yes	No	Who: ________________
Psychiatric Disorder	Yes	No	Who: ________________
Heart Disease/Stroke	Yes	No	Who: ________________

Past Medical History: (check all that apply)

_______ Polio	_______ Measles	_______ Tonsillitis
_______ Jaundice	_______ Mumps	_______ Pleurisy
_______ Kidneys	_______ Scarlet Fever	_______ Liver Disease
_______ Lung Disease	_______ Whooping Cough	_______ Chicken Pox
_______ Rheumatic Fever	_______ Bleeding Disorder	_______ Nervous Breakdown
_______ Ulcers	_______ Gout	_______ Thyroid Disease
_______ Anemia	_______ Heart Valve Disorder	_______ Heart Disease
_______ Tuberculosis	_______ Gallbladder Disorder	_______ Psychiatric Illness
_______ Drug Abuse	_______ Eating Disorder	_______ Alcohol Abuse
_______ Pneumonia	_______ Malaria	_______ Typhoid Fever
_______ Cholera	_______ Cancer	_______ Blood Transfusion
_______ Arthritis	_______ Osteoporosis	_______ Other: _________

Nutrition Evaluation:

1. Present Weight: __________ Height (no shoes): ___________ Desired Weight: _____________

2. In what time frame would you like to be at your desired weight? ________________________________

3. Birth Weight: _____ Weight at 20 years of age: ___________ Weight one year ago: _______________

4. What is the main reason for your decision to lose weight? ____________________________________

5. When did you begin gaining excess weight? (Give reasons, if known): ________________________

   ____

6. What has been your maximum lifetime weight (nonpregnant) and when?_________________________

7. Previous diets you have followed: Give dates and results of your weight loss:

8. Is your spouse, fiancee, or partner overweight? Yes No

9. By how much is he or she overweight? ____

10. How often do you eat out? ____

11. What restaurants do you frequent?____

12. How often do you eat "fast foods?"____

13. Who plans meals? _________________________ Cooks? ____________________ Shops?_________

14. Do you use a shopping list? Yes No

15. What time of day and on what day do you usually shop for groceries? ________________________

16. Food allergies: ____

17. Food dislikes: ____________________

18. Food(s) you crave: ____________________

19. Any specific time of the day or month do you crave food? ____________________

20. Do you drink coffee or tea? Yes No How much daily? ____________________

21. Do you drink cola drinks? Yes No How much daily? ____________________

22. Do you drink alcohol? Yes No

    What? ____________ How much daily? ________ Weekly? ________

23. Do you use a sugar substitute? ______ Butter? ________ Margarine? ________

24. Do you awaken hungry during the night? Yes No

    What do you do? ____________________

25. What are your worst food habits? ____________________

26. Snack Habits:

    What? ____________ How much? ____________ When? ________

    ____________ ____________ ________

27. When you are under a stressful situation at work or family related, do you tend to eat more? Explain:

    ____

    ____

28. Do you thing you are currently undergoing a stressful situation or an emotional upset? Explain:

    ____

    ____

29. Smoking Habits: **(answer only one)**

    ___ You have never smoked cigarettes, cigars, or a pipe.
    ___ You quit smoking ____ years ago and have not smoked since.
    ___ You have quit smoking cigarettes at least one year ago and now smoke cigars or a pipe without inhaling smoke.
    ___ You smoke 20 cigarettes per day (1 pack).
    ___ You smoke 30 cigarettes per day (1-1/2 packs).
    ___ You smoke 40 cigarettes per day (2 packs).

30. Typical Breakfast

Typical Breakfast	Typical Lunch	Typical Dinner
________________	________________	________________
________________	________________	________________
________________	________________	________________
________________	________________	________________
Time eaten: ________	Time eaten: ________	Time eaten: ________
Where: ________	Where: ________	Where: ________
With whom: ________	With whom: ________	With whom: ________

31. Describe your usual energy level: ____

32. Activity Level: **(answer only one)**
    ___ Inactive—no regular physical activity with a sit-down job.
    ___ Light activity—no organized physical activity during leisure time.
    ___ Moderate activity—occasionally involved in activities such as weekend golf, tennis, jogging, swimming, or cycling.
    ___Heavy activity—consistent lifting, stair climbing, heavy construction, etc., or regular participation in jogging, swimming, cycling, or active sports at least three times per week.
    ___Vigorous activity—participation in extensive physical exercise for at least 60 minutes per session four times per week.

33. Behavior style: **(answer only one)**
    ___ You are always calm and easygoing.
    ___ You are usually calm and easygoing.
    ___ You are sometimes calm with frequent impatience.
    ___ You are seldom calm and persistently driving for advancement.
    ___ You are never calm and have overwhelming ambition.
    ___ You are hard-driving and can never relax.

34. Please describe your general health goals and improvements you wish to make: ____________

    ____

    ____

    ____

This information will assist us in assessing your particular problem areas and establishing your medical management. Thank you for your time and patience in completing this form.

American Medical Association
Physicians dedicated to the health of America

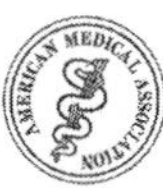

Weight Loss Questionnaire

Name ______________________ Date __________

Please complete this questionnaire, which will help you and your physician develop the best management plan for you.

1. Is there a reason you are seeking treatment at this time? ______________________
2. What are your goals about weight control and management? ______________________
3. Your level of interest in losing weight is:

Not interested	1	2	3	4	5	Very interested

4. Are you ready for lifestyle changes to be a part of your weight control program?

Not ready	1	2	3	4	5	Very ready

5. How much support can your family provide?

No support	1	2	3	4	5	Much support

6. How much support can your friends provide?

No support	1	2	3	4	5	Much support

7. What is the hardest part about managing your weight? ______________________
8. What do you believe will be of most help to assist you in losing weight? ______________________
9. How confident are you that you can lose weight at this time?

Not interested	1	2	3	4	5	Very interested

Weight history

10. As best as you can recall, what was your body weight at each of the following time points (if they apply)?
Grade school _______ High school _______ College _______ Ages 20-29 _______ 30-39 _______ 40-49_______ 50-59 _______
11. What has been your lowest body weight as an adult?_______ What has been your heaviest body weight as an adult? _______
12. At what age did you start trying to lose weight?___________
13. Please check all previous programs you have tried in order to lose weight. Include dates and your length of participation.

Program	Date	Weight (lost or gained)	Length of participation
• TOPS			
• Weight Watchers			
• Overeaters Anonymous			
• Liquid diets (eg, Optifast)			
• Diet pills: Meridia, Xenical			
• Diet pills: phen-fen, Redux,			
• NutriSystem / Jenny Craig			
• OTC diet pills			
• Obesity Surgery			
• Registered Dietitian			
• Other			

14. Have you maintained any weight loss for up to 1 year on any of these programs? Yes ☐ No ☐
15. What did you learn from these programs regarding your weight? ______________________
16. What did not work about these programs? ______________________
17. Have you been involved in physical activity programs to help with weight loss? Yes ☐ No ☐
Which ones or in what way? ______________________

Adapted with permission from the Wellness Institute, Northwestern Memorial Hospital. Source: American Medical Association.

This project was funded by the American Medical Association and The Robert Wood Johnson Foundation. • November 2003 SEE:03-0107:4M:11/03

American Medical Association
Physicians dedicated to the health of America

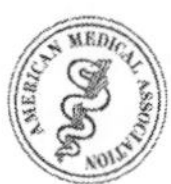

Roadmaps for Clinical Practice
Case Studies in Disease Prevention and Health Promotion
Assessment and Management of Adult Obesity: A Primer for Physicians

Assessment of patient readiness

Patient Readiness Checklist

Motivation/support
- ☐ How important is it that you lose weight at this time?
- ☐ Have you tried to lose weight before? What factors have led to your success and what has made weight loss difficult? (For example, cost, peer pressure, family, etc.)
- ☐ Is your decision to lose weight your own, or for someone else?
- ☐ Is your family supportive?
- ☐ Who, if anyone, is supportive of your decision to begin a weight loss program?
- ☐ What do you consider the benefits of weight loss?
- ☐ What would you have to sacrifice? What are the down sides?

Stressful life events
- ☐ Are there events in your life right now that might make losing weight especially difficult? (For example, work responsibilities, family commitments)
- ☐ If now is not a convenient time for weight loss, what would it take for you to be ready to lose weight? When do you think you might be ready to begin losing weight?

Psychiatric issues
- ☐ What is your mood like most of the time? Do you feel you have the needed energy to lose weight? (may need to assess for depression)
- ☐ Do you feel that you eat what most people would consider a large amount of food in a short period of time? Do you feel out of control during this time? (may need to assess for binge eating disorders)
- ☐ Do you ever forcibly vomit, use laxatives, or engage in excessive physical activity as a means of controlling weight? (may need to assess for bulimia nervosa)

Time availability/constraints
- ☐ How much time are you able to devote to physical activity on a weekly basis?
- ☐ Do you believe that you can make time to record your caloric intake?
- ☐ Can you take time out of your schedule to relax and engage in personal activities?

Weight-loss goals/expectations
- ☐ How much weight do you expect to lose?
- ☐ How fast do you expect to lose weight?
- ☐ What other benefits do you expect to experience as a result of weight loss?

Adapted with permission from the Wellness Institute, Northwestern Memorial Hospital.

This project was funded by the American Medical Association and The Robert Wood Johnson Foundation. • November 2003. Source: American Medical Association. SEE:03-0107:2M:11/03

American Medical Association
Physicians dedicated to the health of America

Food and Activity Diary

As part of your dietary management plan, you may want to utilize a Food and Activity Diary. This sample log is a good tool to help you keep track of what you are eating and doing and when. Be sure to record the following information each day and review it with you health care provider at your next visit.

1. Date, time, and place of your meals, snacks, or nibbles.
2. Describe the foods eaten and estimate the portion size.
   - Meat, poultry, fish, and cheese are best described in ounces (3 oz. is approximately equal to the size of a deck of cards)
   - Vegetables and cut fruit are best described in relation to cups (1 cup is approximately the size of a woman's fist)
   - Beverages are best described in terms of fluid ounces (1 cup = 8 fluid ounces)
3. Rate your hunger before eating:
   0 = Not hungry and uninterested in eating
   1 = Not hungry but could still be interested
   2 = Neutral
   3 = Mild to moderately hungry
   4 = Moderately to extremely hungry
4. List, describe, and estimate the time spent on any physical activity performed throughout the day. Be specific.
5. Remember to also record the following:
   - All condiments (1 t. butter, 1 T. mayonnaise, 3 T. sour cream, etc.)
   - Combination foods by breaking them down (eg, 2 c. noodles, 1/2 c. marinara sauce)
   - How food is prepared (home, restaurant, fast food — baked, broiled, fried, etc.)

Time	Amount	Food selection	Hunger rating
12:30	1 large	onion pita	3
	3 oz.	turkey, white	
	2 oz.	American cheese	
	1 c.	lettuce	
	1 slice	tomato	
	8 oz.	yogurt, custard style	
	1 large	banana	
	16 oz.	root beer	

Type of activity (10 minutes per circle)
Laundry, cleaning house ●●○

Adapted with permission from the Wellness Institute, Northwestern Memorial Hospital

___/___/___ **Sunday**

Time	Amount	Food selection	Hunger rating

Type of activity (10 minutes per circle)

Water (8 fluid oz per circle)

___/___/___ **Monday**

Time	Amount	Food selection	Hunger rating

Type of activity (10 minutes per circle)

Water (8 fluid oz per circle)

___/___/___ **Tuesday**

Time	Amount	Food selection	Hunger rating

Type of activity (10 minutes per circle)

Water (8 fluid oz per circle)

This project was funded by the American Medical Association and The Robert Wood Johnson Foundation. © November 2003

SEE:03-0107:4M:11/03

Food and Activity Log (front)

Enlarge the activity log 127% from letter (8 1/2" x 11") to legal size (8 1/2" x 14") on a copy machine. You may make copies of this sheet to record information weekly.
Source: American Medical Association.

__/__/__ Wednesday

Time	Amount	Food selection	Hunger rating

Type of activity (10 minutes per circle)

Water (8 fluid oz per circle)

__/__/__ Thursday

Time	Amount	Food selection	Hunger rating

Type of activity (10 minutes per circle)

Water (8 fluid oz per circle)

__/__/__ Friday

Time	Amount	Food selection	Hunger rating

Type of activity (10 minutes per circle)

Water (8 fluid oz per circle)

__/__/__ Saturday

Time	Amount	Food selection	Hunger rating

Type of activity (10 minutes per circle)

Water (8 fluid oz per circle)

Record your weight

Food and Activity Log (back)

Enlarge the activity log 127% from letter (8 1/2" x 11") to legal size (8 1/2" x 14") on a copy machine. You may make copies of this sheet to record information weekly. Source: American Medical Association.

Nutrition: Keeping a Food Diary

Instructions: The information you record in your food diary will help you and your family doctor design an eating program to meet your needs. These instructions will help you get the most out of your food diary. Generally, food diaries are meant to be used for a whole week, but studies have shown that keeping track of what you eat for even 1 day can help you make changes to your diet.

How much:
In this space indicate the amount of the particular food item you ate. Estimate the size (2″ × 1″ × 1″), the volume (1/2 cup), the weight (2 ounces) and/or the number of items (12) of that type of food.

What kind:
In this column, write down the type of food you ate. Be as specific as you can. Include sauces and gravies. Don't forget to write down "extras," such as soda, salad dressing, mayonnaise, butter, sour cream, sugar, and ketchup.

Time:
Write the time of day you ate the food.

Where:
Write what room or part of the house you were in when you ate. If you ate in a restaurant, fast-food chain, or your car, write that location down.

Alone or With Someone:
If you ate alone, write "alone." If you were with friends or family members, list them.

Activity:
In this column, list any activities you were doing while you were eating (for example, working, watching TV, or ironing).

Mood:
How were you feeling when you were eating (for example, sad, happy, or depressed)?

Some basic rules to remember:

Write everything down:
Keep your form with you all day and write down everything you eat or drink. A piece of candy, a handful of pretzels, a can of soda pop, or a small donut may not seem like much at the time, but over a week these calories add up!

Do it now:
Don't depend on your memory at the end of the day. Record your eating as you go.

Be specific:
Make sure you include "extras," such as gravy on your meat or cheese on your vegetables. Do not generalize. For example, record french fries as french fries, not potatoes.

Estimate amounts:
If you had a piece of cake, estimate the size (2″ × 1″ × 2″) or the weight (3 ounces). If you had a vegetable, record how much you ate (1/4 cup). When eating meat, remember that a 3-ounce cooked portion is about the size of a deck of cards.

American Weight Loss Center
Food/Activity and Behavior Diary

TIME		Amounts	Carbs	Protein	Fat	Calorie	Location	Why Trigged	Mood	W/Whom	How Long	Meds	Symptoms BP/BS, etc	Solution
	Wake-Up													
	Breakfast													
	Liquid													
	Snack													
	Exercise													
	Liquid													
	Lunch													
	Liquid													
	Snack													
	Exercise													
	Liquid													
	Dinner													
	Exercise													
	TV, other													
	Bed													

Record all items placed in mouth, including fluids, condiments, vitamins/meds. Type and how many minutes spent on physical activity

Record why you ate, i.e., hunger, tired, bored, anxious, persuasion, someone told you to eat, the item was around trigger, item was present, sugar or comfort craving, planned for it

Record any physical symptoms and the time, i.e., light-headed, nausea, tired, headache, depressed, and blood pressure/sugars

Record possible solutions; ways to avoid the trigger event that led to a less healthy food choice or avoid getting too hungry, tired, bored, etc.

Quality of Life Self-Assessment

Please use the following scale to rate how satisfied you feel now about different aspect of your daily life. Choose any number from this list (1 to 9) and indicate your choice on the questions below.

1 = Extremely Dissatisfied	6 = Somewhat satisfied
2 = Very Dissatisfied	7 = Moderately Satisfied
3 = Moderately Dissatisfied	8 = Very Satisfied
4 = Somewhat Dissatisfied	9 = Extremely Satisfied
5 = Neutral	

---

1. ____ Mood (feelings of sadness, worry, happiness, etc.)
2. ____ Self-esteem
3. ____ Confidence, self-assurance, and comfort in social situations
4. ____ Energy and feeling healthy
5. ____ Health problems (diabetes, high blood pressure, etc.)
6. ____ General appearance
7. ____ Social life
8. ____ Leisure and recreational activities
9. ____ Physical mobility and physical activity
10. ____ Eating habits
11. ____ Body image
12. ____ Overall quality of life

DIET READINESS TEST QUESTIONNAIRE

For each question, circle the answer that best describes how you feel.

Section 1: Goals and Attitudes

1. Compared to previous attempts, how motivated to lose weight are you this time?

1	2	3	4	5
Not At All Motivated	Slightly Motivated	Somewhat Motivated	Quite Motivated	Extremely Motivated

2. How certain are you that you will stay committed to a weight loss program for the time it will take to reach your goal?

1	2	3	4	5
Not At All Certain	Slightly Certain	Somewhat Certain	Quite Certain	Extremely Certain

3. Consider all outside factors at this time in your life (the stress you are feeling at work, your family obligations, etc.). To what extent can you tolerate the effort required to stick to a diet?

1	2	3	4	5
Cannot Tolerate	Can Tolerate Somewhat	Uncertain	Can Tolerate Well	Can Tolerate Easily

4. Think honestly about how much weight you hope to lose and how quickly you hope to lose it. Figuring a weight loss of 1 to 2 pounds per week, how realistic is your expectation?

1	2	3	4	5
Very Unrealistic	Somewhat Unrealistic	Moderately Unrealistic	Somewhat Realistic	Very Realistic

5. While dieting, do you fantasize about eating a lot of your favorite foods?

1	2	3	4	5
Always	Frequently	Occasionally	Rarely	Never

6. While dieting, do you feel deprived, angry, and/or upset?

1	2	3	4	5
Always	Frequently	Occasionally	Rarely	Never

Section 1—TOTAL Score ______

6--16
17--23
24--30

Section 2: Hunger and Eating Cues

7. When food comes up in conversation or in something you read, do you want to eat even if you are not hungry?

1	2	3	4	5
Never	Rarely	Occasionally	Frequently	Always

8. How often do you eat because of **physical hunger**?

1	2	3	4	5
Always	Frequently	Occasionally	Rarely	Never

9. Do you have trouble controlling your eating when your favorite foods are around the house?

1	2	3	4	5
Never	Rarely	Occasionally	Frequently	Always

Section 2—TOTAL Score ______

3–6

7–9
10–15

Section 3: Control Over Eating

If the following situations occurred while you were on a diet, would you be likely to eat **more** or **less** immediately afterward and for the rest of the day?

10. Although you planned on skipping lunch, a friend talks you into going out for a midday meal.

1	2	3	4	5
Would Eat Much Less	Would Eat Somewhat Less	Would Make No Difference	Would Eat Somewhat More	Would Eat Much More

11. You "break" your diet by eating a fattening, "forbidden" food.

1	2	3	4	5
Would Eat Much Less	Would Eat Somewhat Less	Would Make No Difference	Would Eat Somewhat More	Would Eat Much More

12. You have been following your diet faithfully and decide to test yourself by eating something you consider a treat.

1	2	3	4	5
Would Eat Much Less	Would Eat Somewhat Less	Would Make No Difference	Would Eat Somewhat More	Would Eat Much More

Section 3—TOTAL Score ______

3–7

8–11

12–15

Section 4: Binge Eating and Purging

13. Aside from holiday feasts, have you ever eaten a large amount of food rapidly and felt afterward that this eating incident was excessive and out of control?

2	0
Yes	No

14. If you answered yes to #13 above, how often have you engaged in this behavior during the last year?

1	2	3	4	5	6
Less Than Once A Month	About Once A Month	A Few Times A Month	About Once A Week	About Three Times A Week	Daily

15. Have you ever purged (used laxatives, diuretics, or induced vomiting) to control your weight?

5	0
Yes	No

16. If you answered yes to #15 above, how often have you engaged in this behavior during the last year?

1	2	3	4	5	6
Less Than Once A Month	About Once A Month	A Few Times A Month	About Once A Week	About Three Times A Week	Daily

Section 4—TOTAL Score ______

0–1
2–11
12–19

Section 5: Emotional Eating

17. Do you eat more than you would like to when you have negative feelings such as anxiety, depression, anger, or loneliness?

1	2	3	4	5
Never	Rarely	Occasionally	Frequently	Always

18. Do you have trouble controlling your eating when you have positive feelings---do you celebrate feeling good by eating?

1	2	3	4	5
Never	Rarely	Occasionally	Frequently	Always

19. When you have unpleasant interactions with others in your life, or after a difficult day at work, do you eat more than you would like?

1	2	3	4	5
Never	Rarely	Occasionally	Frequently	Always

Section 5—TOTAL Score ______

3–8
9–11
12–15

Section 6: Exercise Patterns and Attitudes

20. How often do you exercise?

1	2	3	4	5
Never	Rarely	Occasionally	Somewhat	Frequently

21. How confident are you that you can exercise regularly?

1	2	3	4	5
Not At All Confident	Slightly Confident	Somewhat Confident	Highly Confident	Completely Confident

22. When you think about exercise, do you develop a positive or negative picture in your mind?

1	2	3	4	5
Completely Negative	Somewhat Negative	Neutral	Somewhat Positive	Completely Positive

23. How certain are you that you can work regular exercise into your daily schedule?

1	2	3	4	5
Not At All Certain	Slightly Certain	Somewhat Certain	Quite Certain	Extremely Certain

Section 6---TOTAL Score ______

4–10
11–16
17–20

THE DIET READINESS TEST
SCORING GUIDE
(For use with the Diet Readiness Test)

After the patient completes each of the six sections, add the numbers of answers and compare them with the scoring guide below:

Section 1: Goals and Attitudes

TOTAL Score _____

If you scored:

6 to 16: This may not be a good time for you to start a weight loss program. Inadequate motivation and commitment together with unrealistic goals could block your progress. Think about those things that contribute to this and consider changing them before undertaking a diet program.

17 to 23: You may be close to being ready to begin a program but should think about ways to boost your preparedness before you begin.

24 to 30: The path is clear with respect to goals and attitudes.

Section 2: Hunger and Eating Cues

TOTAL Score _____

If you scored:

3 to 6: You might occasionally eat more than you would like, but it does not appear to be a result of high responsiveness to environmental cues. Controlling the attitudes that make you eat may be especially helpful.

7 to 9: You may have a moderate tendency to eat just because food is available. Dieting may be easier for you if you try to resist external cues and eat only when you are physically hungry.

10 to 15: Some or most of your eating may be in response to thinking about food or exposing yourself to temptations to eat. Think of ways to minimize your exposure to temptations, so that you eat only in response to physical hunger.

Section 3: Control Over Eating

TOTAL Score _____

If you scored:

3 to 7: You recover rapidly from mistakes. However, if you frequently alternate between eating out of control and dieting strictly, you may have a serious eating problem and should get professional help.

8 to 11: You do not seem to let unplanned eating disrupt your program. This is a flexible, balanced approach.

12 to 15: You may be prone to overeat after an event breaks your control or throws you off track. Your reaction to these problem-causing eating events can be improved.

Section 4: Binge Eating and Purging

TOTAL Score _____

If you scored:

0 to 1: It appears that binge eating and purging is not a problem for you.

2 to 11: Pay attention to these eating patterns. Should they arise more frequently, get professional help.

12 to 19: You show signs of having a potentially serious eating problem. See a counselor experienced in evaluating eating disorders right away.

Section 5: Emotional Eating

TOTAL Score _____

If you scored:

3 to 8: You do not appear to let your emotions affect your eating.

9 to 11: You sometimes eat in response to emotional highs and lows. Monitor this behavior to learn when and why it occurs and be prepared to find alternative activities.

12 to 15: Emotional ups and downs can stimulate your eating. Try to deal with feelings that trigger the eating and find other ways to express them.

Section 6: Exercise Patterns and Attitudes

TOTAL Score _____

If you scored:

4 to 10: You are probably not exercising as regularly as you should. Determine whether your attitudes about exercise are blocking your way, then change what you must and put on those walking shoes.

11 to 16: You need to feel more positive about exercise so that you can do it more often. Think of ways to be more active that are fun and fit your lifestyle.

17 to 20: It looks like the path is clear for you to be active. Now think of ways to get motivated.

Food Addiction Questionnaire
Do you see yourself in some of these questions?

1. Has anyone expressed concern about your thoughts and/or behavior around your eating, body, or weight?

2. Do you think or obsess about food, your eating, your body, and/or your weight much of the time?

3. Do you binge on a regular basis, eating a relatively large quantity of food at one sitting?

4. Do you eat to relieve unpleasant emotions?

5. Do you eat when you are not hungry?

6. Do you hide food for yourself or eat in secret?

7. Can you stop eating without difficulty after one or two bites of a snack food or sweets?

8. Do you often eat more than you originally planned to eat?

9. Do you have feelings of guilt, shame, or embarrassment when you eat---or afterward?

10. Do you spend a lot of time calculating the calories you ate and the calories you burned?

11. Do you feel anxious about your weight, body, or eating?

12. Are you fearful of gaining weight?

13. Do you tell yourself you'll be happy when you achieve a certain weight?

14. Do you feel like your whole life is a struggle with food and your weight?

15. Do you feel hopeless about your behavior with food, and/or your obsession with your body and weight?

16. Do you entertain yourself with thoughts of food and what you are going to eat next?

17. Do you weigh yourself once, twice, or more daily?

18. Do you exercise excessively to control your weight?

19. Do you avoid eating or severely limit the amount of food you will eat?

20. Being totally honest with yourself, do you think you have a problem with food?

Index